P9-DHD-048

▲ ▲

Patient Care Guidelines for Nurse Practitioners

FOURTH EDITION

▼

Patient Care Guidelines for Nurse Practitioners

FOURTH EDITION

Axalla J. Hoole, M.D.

*Professor of Medicine, University of North Carolina at Chapel Hill School of Medicine;
Attending Physician, Department of Medicine, North Carolina Memorial Hospital,
Chapel Hill, North Carolina*

C. Glenn Pickard, Jr., M.D.

*Professor of Medicine, University of North Carolina at Chapel Hill School of Medicine;
Attending Physician, Department of Medicine, North Carolina Memorial Hospital,
Chapel Hill, North Carolina*

Ruth M. Ouimette, R.N., M.S.N., A.N.P

*Clinical Assistant Professor, Duke University School of Nursing,
Duke University Medical Center, Durham, North Carolina*

Jacob A. Lohr, M.D.

*Professor of Pediatrics, Chief of Community Pediatrics,
Associate Chair for Ambulatory Services,
University of North Carolina at Chapel Hill School of Medicine*

Robert A. Greenberg, M.D.

*Professor of Pediatrics, Department of Pediatrics, School of Medicine,
Tulane University, New Orleans, Louisiana*

J.B. Lippincott Company
PHILADELPHIA

Sponsoring Editor: Jennifer E. Brogan
Coordinating Editorial Assistant: Danielle J. Di Palma
Production Editor: Mary Kinsella
Indexer: Maria Coughlin
Cover Designer: Tom Jackson
Production Manager: Janet Greenwood
Production Service: Berliner, Inc.
Printer/Binder: RR Donnelley & Sons, Crawfordsville
Cover Printer: New England Book Components

Fourth Edition

Copyright © 1995, by J. B. Lippincott Company. Copyright © 1976, 1982, 1988, by Axalla J. Hoole, Robert A. Greenberg, and C. Glenn Pickard, Jr. All rights reserved. No part of this book may be used or reproduced in any manner whatsoever without written permission except for brief quotations embodied in critical articles and reviews. Printed in the United States of America. For information write J.B. Lippincott Company, 227 East Washington Square, Philadelphia, Pennsylvania 19106.

6 5 4 3 2 1

Library of Congress Cataloging in Publications Data
Patient care guidelines for nurse practitioners / edited by Axalla J.
    Hoole ...[et al.]. — 4th ed.
        p.   cm.
    Includes index.
    ISBN 0-397-55060-X
    1. Nurse practitioners.   2. Medical protocols.   I. Hoole, Axalla
J., 1938–   .
    [DNLM: 1. Nursing Care—handbooks.   2. Nurse Practitioners—
handbooks.   3. Nursing—handbooks.   WY 39 P298 1995]
RT82.8.P37   1995
610.73—dc20
DNLM/DLC
for Library of Congress   94-13710
                                                                CIP

Any procedure or practice described in this book should be applied by the health-care practitioner under appropriate supervision in accordance with professional standards of care used with regard to the unique circumstances that apply in each practice situation. Care has been taken to confirm the accuracy of information presented and to describe generally accepted practices. However, the authors, editors, and publisher cannot accept any responsibility for errors and omissions or for any consequences from application of the information in this book and make no warranty, express or implied, with respect to the contents of the book.

Every effort has been made to ensure that drug selections and dosages are in accordance with current recommendations and practice. Because of ongoing research, changes in government regulations and the constant flow of information on drug therapy reactions and interactions, the reader is cautioned to check the package insert for each drug for indications, dosages, warnings, and precautions, particularly if the drug is new or infrequently used.

▲ Contributors

ELLEN DE FLORA, Fellow, Department of Pediatrics, University of North Carolina at Chapel Hill School of Medicine, Chapel Hill, North Carolina.

LAMAR E. EKBLADH, M.D. Professor, Milton S. Hershey Medical Center, Department of Obstetrics and Gynecology, Hershey, Pennsylvania.

CYNTHIA M. FREUND, B.S.N., M.S.N., PH.D. Professor of Nursing, Dean of School of Nursing, University of North Carolina at Chapel Hill, Chapel Hill, North Carolina.

ROBERT A. GREENBERG, M.D. Professor of Pediatrics, Department of Pediatrics, School of Medicine, Tulane University, New Orleans, Louisiana.

HARVEY J. HAMRICK, M.D. Professor of Pediatrics, University of North Carolina at Chapel Hill School of Medicine; Attending Physician and Director of the Pediatric Residency Training Program, Department of Pediatrics, North Carolina Memorial Hospital, Chapel Hill, North Carolina.

AXALLA J. HOOLE, M.D. Professor of Medicine, University of North Carolina at Chapel Hill School of Medicine; Attending Physician, Department of Medicine, North Carolina Memorial Hospital, Chapel Hill, North Carolina.

GREGOR S. LIPTAK, M.D., M.P.H. George Washington Goler Associate Professor of Pediatrics, University of Rochester School of Medicine and Dentistry; Director of Birth Defects Center, Department of Pediatrics, Strong Memorial Hospital, Rochester, New York.

FRANK A. LODA, M.D. Professor of Pediatrics and Adjunct Professor of Maternal and Child Health, University of North Carolina at Chapel Hill School of Medicine; Director of Center for Early Adolescent, Department of Pediatrics, School of Medicine, North Carolina Memorial Hospital, Chapel Hill, North Carolina.

JACOB A. LOHR, M.D. Professor of Pediatrics, Chief of Community Pediatrics, Associate Chair for Ambulatory Services, University of North Carolina at Chapel Hill School of Medicine

RUTH M. OUIMETTE, R.N., M.S.N., A.N.P. Clinical Assistant Professor, Duke University School of Nursing; Duke University Medical Center, Durham, North Carolina.

PEDEN, DAVID B., M.D., Associate Professor of Pediatrics, University of North Carolina at Chapel Hill School of Medicine; Associate Attending Physician, Department of Pediatrics, North Carolina Memorial Hospital, Chapel Hill, North Carolina.

C. GLENN PICKARD, JR., M.D. Professor of Medicine, University of North Carolina at Chapel Hill School of Medicine; Attending Physician, Department of Medicine, North Carolina Memorial Hospital, Chapel Hill, North Carolina.

JAMES E. SCHWANKL, M.D., M.P.H. Clinical Assistant Professor of Pediatrics, University of North Carolina at Chapel Hill School of Medicine; Attending Physician, Chatham Hospital, Siler City, North Carolina.

NELSON A. WARNER, M.D. Attending Dermatologist, Winter Haven Hospital, Winter Haven, Florida.

MARGARET J. WILKMAN, R.N., F.N.P., C.D.E., M.P.H. Clinical Nurse Specialist, Department of Nursing, Clinical Associate in School of Nursing, Duke University Medical Center, Durham, North Carolina.

▲ FOREWORD

In the mid-sixties, the United States faced a "primary care crisis." Due to the shortage and maldistribution of physicians and other health professionals, the crisis was particularly severe in rural and inner city areas. Health professionals, government officials and policy-makers, business and labor leaders, and others all searched for solutions. One solution proposed was the creation of a new breed of nursing professional—the nurse practitioner. The Schools of Nursing, Medicine and Public Health at the University of North Carolina at Chapel Hill were advocates of the approach, and in the late sixties, they developed one of the first three Family Nurse Practitioner Programs in the country.

During the late sixties and throughout the seventies, nurse practitioners were deployed in rural and inner city areas to alleviate the shortage of doctors and meet the burgeoning need for primary care. During this period, nurse practitioners were found to be cost-effective primary care providers; they located in underserved areas (rural communities and inner cities) at a greater rate than did physicians. It had been well documented that nurse practitioners provide high quality care that is comparable to that of physicians. In other words, after almost two decades of demonstration and study, it was clear: nurse practitioners were well qualified, cost-effective providers of primary care services.

As we came into the eighties, the country faced skyrocketing health care costs. The national health agenda turned to cost containment. By necessity, attention was focused on hospital costs and how to contain the acceleration of these costs. Despite the lack of attention to primary care, nurse practitioners continued to provide primary care services in underserved areas.

Today, with health care reform an emerging reality, primary care and clinical preventive services are being given renewed emphasis. Because the majority of physicians have chosen specialty practice and because the number of providers in underserved areas continues to be inadequate, the country faces its second-generation primary care crisis. Nurse practitioners and other advanced practice nurses are being viewed again as a ready and well qualified group of providers that can help meet the increased demand for primary care and clinical preventive services.

Since the mid-sixties, despite the ebb and flow of attention to primary care, the University of North Carolina at Chapel Hill has maintained its commitment to primary care and to the preparation of Family Nurse Practitioners. We will continue to do so because of our belief that nurse practitioners make a significant contribution to the health of the public by providing primary care and preventive services.

Recognizing that nurse practitioners are engaging in what has previously been called "medical practice," these guidelines represent a statement of the collaboration between doctors and nurse practitioners in agreeing to standards of care for medical problems. The guidelines were developed by physicians and nurses who, from the beginning to the present day, have given their support to the concept of nurse practitioners and to the education and practice of nurse practitioners.

Cynthia M. Freund, BSN, MSM, PhD
Dean, School of Nursing
University of North Carolina at Chapel Hill
Chapel Hill, North Carolina

▲ PREFACE

In the decade from 1965 to 1975, the United States was confronted with a medical care "crisis" involving the quality, quantity, and accessibility of primary health care services that particularly affected the rural areas and the inner cities. The disappearance of the general practitioner from small towns and villages in rural areas and the flight of physicians from the inner cities to the suburbs created major problems in medical care delivery that stimulated a wide variety of programs designed to alleviate the crisis.

As one response to this crisis, the Schools of Nursing, Public Health, and Medicine at the University of North Carolina at Chapel Hill developed a training program for Family Nurse Practitioners (FNPs). In conjunction with the training program, faculty members of the schools participated in an innovative primary health care delivery program in which FNPs staffed satellite rural clinics, while physicians from the medical center provided consultation and supervision for the medical practice of the FNPs.

The patient care guidelines presented in this manual were initially developed in the training program and the demonstration practice. Subsequently, they have been modified and changed repeatedly based on our own experience and the experience of others across the nation who are engaged in similar practices. They still represent our approach to management. Accordingly, this book is not intended as an exhaustive treatise on the conditions covered nor as an exposition of all the ways in which each condition can be managed. Rather, it is intended as a codification of acceptable criteria for diagnosing an illness or condition and of acceptable plans for management.

Although many individuals are predicting that as more physicians are trained and enter practice, the importance of the nurse practitioner will decline, we have found, rather, a shift in locations. Many nurse practitioners are still in practice in rural satellite clinics, but in recent years an increasing number have gone to large urban clinics—particularly to HMOs; to highly specialized areas of practice, such as oncology clinics; and to rest and retirement homes, where nurse practitioners often assume the role of the primary coordinator of care. We still feel that the nurse practitioner–physician team approach to primary care practice capitalizes maximally on the skills of the nurse and physician and can bring to patient care a rational system of high quality not easily obtainable in traditional practice patterns.

We would like to acknowledge the many helpful comments and criticisms we have received from practitioners throughout the country. Their willingness to take the time to offer criticism of our work is greatly appreciated. Their suggestions have been quite helpful in our efforts to improve this work. We encourage all who use these guidelines to let us know about errors, points of disagreement, or significant alterations to our guidelines.

A. J. H.
R. A. G.
C. G. P.
R. M. O.
J. A. L.

▲ INTRODUCTION

USE OF PATIENT CARE GUIDELINES

Several fundamental concepts underlie these patient care guidelines and need to be made clear at the outset:

1. A nurse practitioner cannot legally carry out medical-practice acts without having a working relationship with a physician who agrees to be ultimately responsible for the medical practice acts of the nurse and to be always available for consultation or referral or both. Normal procedures of nursing practice, carried out by the nurse practitioner, are not under the supervision of the physician.
2. The guidelines must be thoroughly reviewed, changed if necessary, and mutually agreed to by the nurse practitioner and physician before they are implemented.
3. The patient care guidelines define the boundaries of the medical practice acts available to the nurse practitioner. If there is no guideline defining a medical condition and its management, the nurse practitioner must not diagnose or treat the condition without the direct involvement of the physician.
4. The nurse practitioner and responsible physician must assure one another through supervised practice that the nurse practitioner has the knowledge and skills to make the diagnosis contained in the guidelines and to render treatment as outlined. The guidelines are *not* intended to serve as a "cookbook" reference work to assist in making diagnoses. Rather, they are an attempt to codify the knowledge and practices of the nurse and physician.

In settings in which we have had experience, the guidelines cover about 75% of the presenting problems of patients seeking primary health care. Obviously, in certain settings other conditions may occur more frequently, and the need to develop additional guidelines may arise. Thus, the need to review one's practice and to develop or revise guidelines is constant.

In practice, the guidelines have been used to enable the nurse practitioner legally and ethically to engage in medical practice acts without the physician's personally seeing each patient. In certain settings, the nurse and physician may be geographically separated, as when the nurse practitioner operates a satellite clinic. In this context, the guidelines are often referred to as *standing orders*. The clinical note should contain adequate information to assure anyone reading it that the patient's condition fits the guideline being followed. In practice, the nurse practitioner needs to refer to the guidelines for common conditions only as a check; the condition being managed and the correct procedures for treating it usually are known before the guidelines are checked.

An additional use for the guidelines is a standard of care in medical audit procedures. Effective use of the guidelines in this manner, however, demands that the practitioners being audited have an opportunity to review, discuss, and modify the guidelines *before* any audit begins to ensure that they are appropriate standards for the geographic area and the specific practice.

We do not presume to assert that the guidelines we have developed apply immediately everywhere as standards of care. They should simply serve as a point of departure from which to develop guidelines that suit local norms and conditions.

A final word about the format. Originally we experimented with clinical algorithms, or branching logic trees. Although we found these useful in attempting to analyze the clinician's approach to clinical problem solving, we found them unworkable as guides to practice. Experienced, well-trained practitioners simply do not follow the same branching logic in dealing with every patient. The same key observations are made, but not necessarily in that order. We therefore abandoned that format.

We again wish to emphasize that this is, and should remain, an unfinished work. In this regard, we welcome the comments and suggestions of others. We sincerely hope that this book will contribute to the continuing effort to provide improved patient care.

▲ Contents

1

HEALTH MAINTENANCE

▲ USE OF THE HEALTH MAINTENANCE FLOW SHEET: AGE TWO WEEKS TO SEVENTEEN YEARS

I. Purpose of the Health Maintenance Flow Sheet (Figure 1-1)

A. To guide the health care provider in recommended health maintenance procedures.

B. To serve as a data sheet for recording the results of procedures.

C. To individualize a patient's health maintenance program appropriately.

D. To summarize a patient's health maintenance status.

II. General Instructions

A. At the patient's first health maintenance visit after registration, the recommended procedures that are appropriate for the patient's age are done; see Age-Specific Health Maintenance Guidelines: Pediatric.

B. The date (month and year) are recorded beside each completed procedure in the first blank column.

Patient Care Guidelines for Nurse Practitioners, 4th ed. by Axalla J. Hoole, C. Glenn Pickard, Jr., Ruth M. Ouimette, Jacob A. Lohr, and Robert A. Greenberg. Copyright © 1995 by J. B. Lippincott Company.

FIGURE 1-1

HEALTH MAINTENANCE FLOW SHEET: 12 WEEKS TO 17 YEARS

PROCEDURES AND AGES										
Assessments: 2 wk;	Date scheduled									
2, 4, 6, 9, 12, 15, 18 mo;	Date seen									
2, 3, 5, 8, 11, 13, 15, 17 yr	Age									
	Provider									
Complete history	Date									
Complete examination	Date									
Immunizations (record dates below)										
DPT										
OPV										
MMR										
Hib										
Td										
Tuberculin test if at risk 1, 3, 5, 11, 15 yr	Pos/Neg									
Hematocrit 1, 5, 13 yr	Result									
Urine culture (female) optional 5, 8 yr	Nl/Abn/									
Blood pressure 3 yr and each subsequent visit	Result									
Development each visit	Nl/Abn/?									
Hearing 6 mo; 1, 3 yr; and each subsequent visit	P/F									
Vision 4 mo; 1, 3 yr; and each subsequent visit	P/F									
Language 2, 3, 5 yr	P/F									
Dental care each visit										
Counseling: each visit										
Nutrition										
Physical care										
Behavior/psychosocial										
Sex education										
Stimulation										
Safety										
Family planning										
Other										

C. The date of the next scheduled assessment is written in the top box of the second blank column (opposite the heading "Date scheduled").

D. Moving down the second column, the boxes of the procedures to be done at the next assessment should be outlined by the provider with a red pencil. No other columns are marked in advance, because the purpose of outlining the procedure boxes in each column is to indicate which procedures should be done at or before the next assessment. This can be determined only by what was actually done by the end of the previous assessment.

E. If procedures are done before the next scheduled assessment, the date they are done and the results are recorded in the red-outlined box.

F. This sequence is repeated at each scheduled assessment. If a patient develops a problem that requires more frequent visits, the regular medical record—not the health maintenance flow sheet—is used for such extra visits.

G. If an indicated procedure is not done or needs to be repeated, the appropriate box of the next assessment is outlined at each visit until the procedure is done. At that time, a check mark is placed in the box or a result is recorded.

H. The information recorded on the health maintenance flow sheet does not have to be recorded in the regular medical record entry. The regular medical record entry should contain the interval medical history, whatever physical examination is done, any medication prescribed, and any details that the provider feels will be helpful for future visits (e.g., certain counseling subjects that will need particular emphasis at future visits).

Note: Unlike most health maintenance flow sheets, this one is based on the procedures this particular patient has actually had and on those needed by the specific date of the next scheduled assessment. By merely looking down the column after the date of a scheduled assessment has passed, one can tell what procedures a patient still needs. Thus, audit of health maintenance status is simplified.

III. **Specific Procedures**

A. **Assessments.** Record the date the patient was seen, the patient's age, and the health care provider's initials. The 2-week assessment ideally is carried out in the home, subsequent ones in the clinic. Enter the date of the next scheduled assessment in the next column. Note that the assessment intervals given represent the minimum number of assessments that all patients should have. If problems are discovered, more frequent assessments may be needed. These additional assessments are recorded not on this flow sheet but in the medical record. A flow sheet for a specific problem (e.g., urinary tract infection) may be indicated.

B. **Complete history.** The complete health history should include past medical history, family history, social history, and review of systems. An age-specific health questionnaire, which is reviewed with the parent or patient, or both, and commented on in the medical record, is recommended. The history should be taken as soon as possible after registration. The date that it is completed is entered in the space provided. At each assessment, an appropriate interval medical history is taken, but it need not be noted on the health maintenance flow sheet.

C. **Complete examination.** A complete physical examination should be performed as soon as possible after registration. Enter the date it is completed in the space provided. The extent of subsequent physical examinations, which need not be recorded on the flow sheet, is determined by the age-specific health maintenance guidelines (discussed later in this chapter) and by clinical judgment based on the interval medical history and the patient's age and problem list.

D. **Immunizations.** See Age-Specific Health Maintenance Guidelines: Pediatric for recommended program. Contraindications should be carefully reviewed before giving any vaccine. Contraindications for administering specific vaccines are indicated in the manufacturer's package insert and in chapters on vaccine-preventable diseases in the *Report of the Committee on Infectious Diseases* (the "Red Book") of the American Academy of Pediatrics.* Minor illness is not a contraindication to using a vaccine; deferring the administration of a vaccine in such circumstances frequently results in unimmunized children vulnerable to vaccine-preventable diseases. Fever per se is not a contraindication to immunizations, unless associated with other signs of a more serious illness. General contraindications for all live virus vaccines include (1) immunosuppressive therapy (radiation therapy, corticosteroids, antimetabolites, alkylating agents, and cytotoxic drugs); (2) immunodeficiency disorders, including AIDS; (3) leukemia, lymphoma, or generalized malignancy; (4) pregnancy; and (5) recent (within 8 weeks) immune globulin, plasma, or blood transfusions. Refer to the "Red Book" for further details. If a patient will need an immunization by the next scheduled assessment, outline the box in the next scheduled assessment column and write in the immunization that will be needed. Place a check mark in the most recently outlined box when immunizations are up to date. A record of the date that each specific immunization is given is entered in the appropriate box in the Procedures column and also on the immunization record card that is given to patients.

---

*This report is revised and published every few years by the American Academy of Pediatrics, PO Box 1034, Evanstown, Illinois 60204.

Informed consent: The patient, parent, and/or legal guardian should be educated about the major benefits to be derived from vaccines in preventing disease in individuals and in the community, and about the risks of those vaccines. Benefit and risk statements should be presented in lay terminology. The National Childhood Vaccine Injury Act of 1986 includes requirements for detailed notification of patients and parents about vaccine benefits and risks in both the private and public sectors. This legislation requires the use of standardized benefit and risk statements (available since October 1990) when administering vaccines for which vaccine injury compensation is available. (See Federal Vaccine Injury Compensation Table, the "Red Book.")

E. **Tuberculin test.** The decision to administer this test can depend on the prevalence of tuberculosis in the population. Record the date the test is given and the result as positive (pos) or negative (neg).

F. **Hematocrit.** Record the date the test is done and the hematocrit value (see Table 1-1).

G. **Urine culture.** Record the date the specimen is collected and the result as normal (Nl) or abnormal (Abn). Normal is less than 10,000 organisms per milliliter on a clean midstream specimen. Consult Chapter 9, Urinary Tract Infection: Pediatric, **IV**, p. 232, if the culture has more than 10,000 organisms per milliliter.

H. **Blood pressure.** Record the date and the blood pressure. Be sure to use a cuff that covers two thirds of the arm, with the inflatable portion completely encircling the arm. Table 1-2 shows normal blood pressure values.

I. **Development.** The Denver Prescreening Developmental Questionnaire* or a similar, established instrument should be used. Record the date when the test is done. Results are recorded as normal (Nl), abnormal (Abn), or questionable (?).

TABLE 1-1
MINIMUM NORMAL HEMATOCRIT VALUES AT DIFFERENT AGES

AGE	HEMATOCRIT
6 months to 6 years	33
6–14 years	35
Over 14	
Female	36
Male	40

---

*Ladoca Project and Publishing Foundation Inc., East 51st Ave and Lincoln Street, Denver, CO 80216.

TABLE 1-2

MAXIMUM NORMAL VALUES OF BLOOD PRESSURE RECORDED IN THE SUPINE POSITION

AGE (YEARS)	SYSTOLIC/DIASTOLIC (MMHG)
0–3	110/65
3–7	120/70
7–10	130/75
10–13	140/80
13–15	
Male	140/80
Female	140/85
Over 15	140/90

J. Hearing. Record the date and the result as pass (P) or fail (F). The following screening tests should be used:

1. **Six to twenty-four months**

   a. Parent gives a history of infant's vocalization and response to sound; see Age-Specific Health Maintenance Guidelines: Pediatric.

   b. Infant ceases activity on hearing a conversational voice or orients himself toward the voice, or both.

   c. With the infant held, his attention should be fixed on a visual stimulus. The source of sound should be held 4 feet to one side of the infant's head, out of peripheral vision. The infant should respond to low-pitched (clacker or block and hammer), medium-pitched (squeaky toy), and high-pitched (bell) sounds.

2. **Three to seventeen years.** Pure-tone audiometry.*

K. Vision. Record the date and the result as pass (P) or fail (F). In addition, record actual visual acuity in the medical record when the Snellen E test is used. The following screening tests should be performed:

1. **Under four years**

   a. Pupil size, shape, and reaction to light.

   b. Ability to follow light.

---

*For procedure, see *Pediatric Outpatient Procedures.* Philadelphia: J. B. Lippincott, 1991.

    c. Ability to pick up small, raisin-sized object (over 9 months of age).

    d. Evidence of strabismus by history, position of light reflection on cornea, and extraocular movements.

    e. Evidence of latent strabismus by cover–uncover test.

  2. Four years and over

    a. Pupil size, shape, and reaction to light.

    b. Evidence of strabismus by history, position of light reflection on cornea, and extraocular movements.

    c. Evidence of latent strabismus by cover–uncover test.

    d. Snellen E test

      (1) Place the child 20 feet from the well-illuminated chart. Each child is tested on the 20/50, 20/40, 20/30, and 20/20 lines of the chart, using both eyes and each alone, until the criteria for failure are met. A child who wears glasses should be tested with and without the glasses. The examiner should watch for signs of visual problems, such as excessive blinking, squinting, crossed eyes, or tearing.

      (2) Visual acuity is recorded as the lowest line on the chart that is passed. The first number is the distance from the testing chart; the second number is the distance at which the particular line of the chart is readable by the normal person. Criteria for failure are as follows:

        (a) Failure to read more than half the letters of the 20/30 line successfully.

        (b) Difference in acuity between eyes of more than one line—if an entire line is exposed for testing at a time; *or,* difference in acuity between eyes of one line—if only one E is exposed for testing at a time.

        (c) Observation of visual problems by the examiner.

 L. Language. For procedures, see Age-Specific Health Maintenance Guidelines: Pediatric. Record the date and the result as pass (P) or fail (F).

M. Dental care. Record date. Teeth and gums should be examined and parents and patients counseled on dental care. See Age-Specific Health Maintenance Guidelines: Pediatric for details. Patients are referred to a dental service for screening and health education at 3 years of age, or at the time of registration if they are older.

N. Counseling. See Age-Specific Health Maintenance Guidelines: Pediatric for counseling under each category. Place a check mark in the appropriate box when counseling has been done.

O. **Other.** At the bottom of the flow sheet are empty spaces for other procedures that the provider would like to have as part of an individual's health maintenance program.

▲ AGE-SPECIFIC HEALTH MAINTENANCE GUIDELINES: PEDIATRIC

TWO-WEEK VISIT

I. Provider
Nurse practitioner (optimally conducts visit in the patient's home).

II. History
A. Review obstetric and newborn hospital record.

B. Take interval medical history.

III. Examination
Inspection of baby completely undressed.

IV. Procedures
None.

V. Dental Care
A. Content of fluoride in drinking water should be 0.7–2.3 ppm.

B. If concentration of fluoride in drinking water or water intake is inadequate, supplemental fluoride should be given in the form of sodium fluoride (Luride) drops, containing 0.125 mg of fluoride per drop. If water supply has less than 0.3 ppm or baby is breast-fed, give 2 drops per day.

VI. Counseling
A. **Nutrition**

  1. Discuss breast-feeding:

    a. Breast and nipple care.

    b. Normal balanced diet and good fluid intake for mother.

    c. Feeding technique and schedule.

    d. Misconceptions.

    e. Supplemental vitamin D.

    f. Encouragement.

    g. Scheduling for future counseling if needed.

  2. Discuss bottle feeding:

    a. Milk formula selection.

    b. Preparation and storage techniques.

    c. Supplemental vitamins if not in formula.

       d. Feeding technique and schedule.

B. Physical care

  1. Assess adequacy of physical environment for newborn with appropriate counseling or agency referral, or both, as needed.

  2. Discuss fever management. Note that fever in infants less than two months of age has high association with significant illness.

  3. Discuss skin care for baby.

    a. Minor and periodic variations in normal skin.

    b. Bathing techniques.

    c. Care of diaper area.

    d. Care of umbilical cord stump.

    e. Clothing (avoid overheating).

  4. Discuss parents' questions.

C. Behavior and psychosocial environment

  1. Assess adequacy of emotional environment:

    a. Postpartum depression. Evaluate available supports, such as father, grandparents, public health nurse, caretaker, day nursery, social worker.

    b. Mother–infant interaction. Was baby wanted? Is it of the desired sex? What are the mother's expectations of baby?

    c. Role of father. Evaluate degree of support he can provide and his expectations of baby.

    d. Adjustment of siblings to baby.

  2. Discuss infant behavior and normal variations.

    a. Crying.

    b. Sleeping and breathing patterns.

    c. Bowel movements.

  3. Assess appropriateness of concepts of discipline and punishment.

  4. Discuss parents' questions.

D. Stimulation. See Infant and Child Stimulation Guidelines.

E. Safety and environment. Advise patients on the following safety and environmental practices:

  1. Eliminate tobacco smoking in the baby's home and care environments and, if possible, elsewhere. (See Smoking Assistance Counseling.)

  2. Be certain smoke detectors are properly placed in the home and are in working order.

  3. Use special infant car seat for automobile travel. Parent's lap is *not* safe.

    4. Be certain crib meets safety standards of the Consumer Product Safety Commission.

    5. Never leave infant without protection to prevent falling from a surface.

    6. Never leave infant alone in the bath water.

    7. Temperature of hot water from faucet should be below 130 °F to prevent accidental burns.

    8. Protect from young siblings and pets.

  F. Family planning.

  G. Other topics, based on the parents' concerns.

VII. Follow-Up

  A. Explain the purpose of health maintenance visits. Review flow sheet with parents.

  B. Give clinic telephone number.

  C. Schedule first appointment.

  D. Leave medical questionnaire with parent to be completed just before first clinic visit and brought to clinic.

  E. Emphasize availability of health care and counseling before scheduled clinic visit, if needed.

TWO-MONTH CLINIC VISIT

I. Provider

Physician.

II. History

  A. Review neonatal hospital summary.

  B. Review record of 2-week visit.

  C. Take dietary history.

  D. Take developmental history.

  E. Take family medical history.

  F. Take social history.

  G. Review systems.

III. Examination

  A. Measurements (record on growth chart):

    1. Weight.

    2. Length.

    3. Head circumference.

  B. Complete physical examination.

IV. Procedures*

    A. Immunizations, after reviewing contraindications and discussing side effects:

        1. Diphtheria–pertussis–tetanus vaccine #1.

        2. Oral polio vaccine (trivalent) #1.

        3. Hemophilus influenza vaccine #1.

        4. Hepatitis B vaccine #2 (#1 should have been administered in the newborn nursery.

    B. Developmental appraisal.

V. Dental Care

Give supplemental fluoride, if necessary (see Two-Week Visit, **V**, p. 8).

VI. Counseling

    A. Nutrition

        1. Review milk formula or breast-feeding or both.

        2. Review preparation and storage techniques.

        3. Discuss the adequacy of milk alone as the source of nutrition until at least 4 months of age.

        4. Give supplemental vitamins if not in formula or vitamin D if the mother is breast-feeding.

        5. Discuss iron requirements:

            a. Breast milk will supply sufficient iron for full-term babies.

            b. Iron-fortified formula

              or

            c. Ferrous sulfate (Fer-In-Sol) drops (15 mg elemental iron per 0.6 mL). For infants weighing 4–7 kg (8–14 lb), give 0.3 mL once a day in water or fruit juice. For infants weighing more than 7 kg (more than 14 lb) and for all premature babies, give 0.6 mL once a day.

        6. Discuss parents' questions.

    B. Physical care

        1. Discuss baby's response to common respiratory and gastrointestinal illnesses, home management, and indications for seeking medical care.

        2. Discuss parents' questions.

    C. Behavioral and psychosocial environment

        1. Assess adequacy of emotional environment, with counseling when appropriate:

---

*See Use of the Health Maintenance Flow Sheet, pp. 1–5, for details.

      a. Mother–infant interaction. Observe for overprotectiveness, lack of warmth toward baby, signs of maternal depression.

      b. Role of father.

      c. Role of siblings—management of sibling rivalry.

      d. Role of extended family and support systems (grandparents, friends).

    2. Discuss behavior changes expected before next visit.

    3. Discuss parents' questions.

  D. Stimulation. See Infant and Child Stimulation Guidelines, pp. 39–45.

  E. Safety and environment. Advise parents on the following safety and environmental practices:

    1. Use special infant car seat for automobile travel. Parent's lap is *not* safe.

    2. Be certain smoke detectors are properly installed in the house and are in working order.

    3. Eliminate tobacco smoking in the baby's home and care environments and, if possible, elsewhere (see Smoking Cessation Counseling).

    4. Be certain crib meets safety standards of the Consumer Product Safety Commission.

    5. Never leave infant without protection to prevent falling from a surface.

    6. Never leave infant alone in the bath water.

    7. Temperature of hot water from the faucet should be below 130° F to prevent accidental burns.

    8. Keep objects or toys that are sharp, breakable, ingestible, or that have cords away from baby.

    9. Protect from young siblings and pets.

    10. Avoid more than minimal direct exposure of baby's skin to sun rays.

  F. Family planning.

  G. Other topics, based on the parents' concerns.

VII. Follow-Up

In 2 months or sooner, if necessary.

FOUR-MONTH CLINIC VISIT

I. Provider

Nurse practitioner.

II. History

Interval medical history.

III. Examination

   A. Measurements (record on growth chart):

      1. Weight.

      2. Length.

      3. Head circumference.

   B. Inspection of baby completely undressed.

   C. Extent of further examination is based on interval medical history and patient's problem list.

IV. Procedures*

   A. Immunizations, after reviewing contraindications and discussing side effects:

      1. Diphtheria-pertussis-tetanus vaccine #2.

      2. Oral polio vaccine (trivalent) #2.

      3. Hemophilus influenza vaccine #2.

   B. Developmental appraisal.

V. Dental Care

   A. Give supplemental fluoride, if necessary (see Two-Week Visit, V, p. 8).

   B. Discuss teething and the use of teething toys and hard crackers.

VI. Counseling

   A. Nutrition

      1. Continue milk formula or breast-feeding, or both.

      2. Discuss gradual introduction of solid foods.

      3. Give supplemental vitamins if not in formula or if the mother is breast-feeding.

      4. Discuss iron requirements:

         a. Breast-feeding plus iron-fortified cereal by 6 months of age.

         b. Iron-fortified formula

          or

         c. Ferrous sulfate (Fer-In-Sol) drops (15 mg elemental iron per 0.6 mL). For infants weighing 7 kg or less (14 lb or less), give 0.3 mL once a day in water or fruit juice. For infants weighing over 7 kg (over 14 lb) and all premature babies, give 0.6 mL once a day.

      5. Discuss parents' questions.

   B. Physical care

      1. Review baby's response to common respiratory and gastrointestinal illnesses, home management, and indications for seeking medical care.

---

*See Use of the Health Maintenance Flow Sheet, pp. 1–5, for details.

2. Discuss parents' questions.

C. **Behavioral and psychosocial environment**

1. Assess mother–infant interaction and role of father.

2. Discuss alternative caretakers to allow mother time free from baby. Discuss attitude toward mother's returning to work and using day care.

3. Discuss behavior changes expected before next visit.

4. Discuss parents' questions.

D. **Stimulation.** See Infant and Child Stimulation Guidelines, p. 39.

E. **Safety and environment.** Advise parents on the following safety and environmental practices:

1. Use special infant car seat for automobile travel. Parent's lap is *not* safe.

2. Be certain smoke detectors are properly installed in the house and are in working order.

3. Eliminate tobacco smoking in the baby's home and care environments and, if possible, elsewhere (see Smoking Cessation Counseling).

4. Be certain crib meets safety standards of the Consumer Product Safety Commission.

5. Discuss infant's increasing mobility and risk of rolling off surfaces. Keep crib sides up.

6. Never leave infant alone in the bath water.

7. Temperature of hot water from the faucet should be below 130 °F to prevent accidental burns.

8. Keep objects or toys that are sharp, breakable, ingestible, or that have cords away from baby.

9. Protect from young siblings and pets.

10. Avoid more than minimal direct exposure of baby's skin to sun rays.

F. **Other topics,** based on the parents' concerns.

VII. **Follow-Up**

In 2 months or sooner, if necessary.

SIX-MONTH CLINIC VISIT

I. **Provider**

Nurse practitioner.

II. **History**

Interval medical history.

III. **Examination**

A. Measurements (record on growth chart):
   1. Weight.
   2. Length.
   3. Head circumference.
B. Complete physical examination.

IV. Procedures*

A. **Immunizations.** After reviewing contraindications and discussing side effects:
   1. Diphtheria–pertussis–tetanus vaccine #3.
   2. Oral polio vaccine (trivalent) #3 (optional).
   3. Hemophilus influenza vaccine #3.
   4. Hepatitis B vaccine #3.
B. **Developmental appraisal.**
C. **Hearing screening.** Ask parents these questions:
   1. Does your baby stir or awaken when sleeping quietly and someone talks or makes a loud noise nearby? (The baby does not have to do this all the time, but should occasionally.)
   2. Does your baby sometimes start or jump when there is a very loud noise, such as a cough, dog bark, or object dropped?

V. Dental Care

A. **Give supplemental fluoride.** If necessary (see Two-Week Visit, **V**, p. 8).
B. **Discuss teething** and the use of teething toys and hard crackers.
C. **Caries Prevention.** Tell parents not to leave a nursing bottle in the crib with the baby after teeth have erupted.

VI. Counseling

A. **Nutrition**
   1. Continue milk formula or breast-feeding, or both.
   2. Watch for excessive weight gain.
   3. Discuss importance of basic food groups and of avoiding non-nutritious sugared commercial foods.
   4. Discuss need for supplemental vitamins if not in formula or vitamin D if breast-feeding.
   5. Discuss iron requirements:
      a. Iron-fortified formula
         or
      b. Ferrous sulfate (Fer-In-Sol) drops (15 mg elemental iron per

---

*See Use of the Health Maintenance Flow Sheet, pp. 1–5, for details.

0.6 mL) 0.6 mL once a day in water or fruit juice
and,

c. for breast- and bottle-fed infants,
Iron-fortified cereals and iron containing foods.

6. Discuss parents' questions.

B. Physical care

1. Review parental management of illnesses occurring since previous visit.

2. Discuss parents' questions.

C. Behavioral and psychosocial environment

1. Assess maternal–infant interaction and role of father.

2. Discuss parents' attitude toward discipline. Emphasize that the baby is too young to "behave."

3. Discuss adjustment of siblings to baby.

4. Discuss stranger anxiety—baby sitter should be familiar to the baby before parents leave.

5. Discuss parents' questions.

D. Stimulation. See Infant and Child Stimulation Guidelines, pp. 39–45.

E. Safety and environment. Advise parents on the following safety and environmental practices:

1. Use special infant car seat for automobile travel. Parent's lap is *not* safe.

2. Be certain smoke detectors are properly installed in the house and are in working order.

3. Eliminate tobacco smoking in the baby's home and care environments and, if possible, elsewhere (see Smoking Cessation Counseling).

4. Be certain crib meets safety standards of the Consumer Product Safety Commission.

5. Never leave infant alone in the bath water or near a pool.

6. Temperature of hot water from the faucet should be below 130 °F to prevent accidental burns.

7. Prepare house for infant's increasing mobility:

   a. Cover electric outlets with plug guards.

   b. Disconnect all cords to appliances when not in use.

   c. Keep sharp, breakable, or ingestible objects out of reach, off floor and low tables.

   d. Avoid small, hard foods that could be aspirated into airway (e.g., peanuts).

   e. Lock medicines, cleaning materials, and poisons away and

out of reach (review the use of syrup of ipecac as described in Chapter 2, Ingestions and Poisonings: Pediatric, **VI.E**, p. 80).

    f. Keep handles of pots turned away from reach.

    g. Keep hot food containers out of reach on tables, and do not use table cloths that can be pulled down.

    h. Put gate across top of stairs.

    i. Place screens or guards in front of space heaters, heating stoves, and radiators.

    j. Keep screens in open windows.

    k. Keep child in enclosed space when outdoors and not in the company of an adult.

  8. Avoid more than minimal direct exposure of baby's skin to sun rays.

  9. Avoid use of infant walkers.

F. Other topics, based on parents' concerns.

VII. Follow-Up

In 3 months, or sooner if necessary.

NINE-MONTH CLINIC VISIT

I. Provider

Nurse practitioner.

II. History

Interval medical history.

III. Examination

  A. Measurements (record on growth chart):

    1. Weight.

    2. Length.

    3. Head circumference.

  B. Inspection of baby completely undressed.

  C. Extent of further examination is based on interval history and patient's problem list.

IV. Procedures*

  A. Review flow sheet to be certain that procedures indicated at previous visits have been completed.

  B. Developmental appraisal.

V. Dental Care

  A. Examine teeth.

---

*See Use of the Health Maintenance Flow Sheet, pp. 1–5, for details.

    B. Give supplemental fluoride, if necessary (see Two-Week Visit, V, p. 8).

    C. To prevent caries, tell parents not to leave a nursing bottle in the crib with the baby.

    D. Tell parents to clean teeth with gauze pad once a day.

VI. Counseling

    A. Nutrition

        1. Continue milk formula or breast-feeding, or both.

        2. Review diet. Counsel on importance of basic food groups and of avoiding nonnutritious sugared commercial foods. Consider family preferences and economic factors.

        3. Give supplemental vitamins if not in formula or vitamin D if breast-feeding.

        4. Discuss iron requirements:

            a. Iron-fortified formula

            or

            b. Ferrous sulfate (Fer-In-Sol) drops (15 mg elemental iron per 0.6 mL) 0.6 mL once a day in water or fruit juice.

            c. Iron-fortified cereals and iron-containing foods.

        5. Discuss management of food preferences and possible decrease in appetite.

    B. Physical care

        1. Review parental management of illnesses occurring since previous visit.

        2. Discuss parents' questions.

    C. Behavioral and psychosocial environment

        1. Assess family's response to annoying behavior. Help parents to realize that baby is not yet able to be disciplined.

        2. Discuss stranger and separation anxiety.

        3. Discuss child's desire to use spoon and cup for feeding and expected messiness.

        4. Discuss parents' questions and expectations of baby.

    D. Stimulation. See Infant and Child Stimulation Guidelines, pp. 39–45.

    E. Safety and environment. Advise parents on the following safety and environmental practices:

        1. Use special infant car seat for automobile travel. Parent's lap is *not* safe.

        2. Be certain smoke detectors are properly installed in the house and are in working order.

        3. Eliminate tobacco smoking in the baby's home and care environments and, if possible, elsewhere (see Smoking Cessation Counseling).

4. Be certain crib meets safety standards of the Consumer Product Safety Commission.

5. Never leave infant alone in the bath water or near a pool.

6. Temperature of hot water from the faucet should be below 120 °F to prevent accidental burns.

7. Prepare house for infant's increasing mobility:

   a. Cover electric outlets with plug guards.

   b. Disconnect all cords to appliances when not in use.

   c. Keep sharp, breakable, or ingestible objects out of reach, off floor and low tables.

   d. Avoid small, hard foods that could be aspirated into airway (e.g., peanuts). Avoid eating/chewing certain foods (popcorn, gum) during play (running).

   e. Lock medicines, cleaning materials, and poisons away and out of reach (review the use of syrup of ipecac as described in Chapter 2, Ingestions and Poisonings: Pediatric, **VI.E**, p. 80).

   f. Keep handles of pots turned away from reach.

   g. Keep hot food containers out of reach on tables, and do not use table cloths that can be pulled down.

   h. Put gate across top of stairs.

   i. Place guards in front of space heaters, heating stoves, and radiators.

   j. Keep screens or guards in open windows.

   k. Keep child in enclosed space when outdoors and not in the company of an adult.

F. **Other topics**, based on parents' concerns.

VII. Follow-Up

In 3 months, or sooner if necessary.

TWELVE-MONTH CLINIC VISIT

I. Provider

Physician.

II. History

Interval medical history.

III. Examination

A. Measurements (record on growth chart):

   1. Weight.

   2. Length.

   3. Head circumference.

B. Complete physical examination.

IV. Procedures*

A. **Hematocrit determination** (normal is greater than 32%).

B. **Developmental appraisal.**

C. **Hearing screening.** Ask parents these questions:

   1. Does your baby turn his head in any direction to find an interesting sound or the person speaking?

   2. Does your baby stir or waken when sleeping quietly and someone talks or makes a loud sound nearby?

D. **Vision screening.**

E. **Tuberculin skin test**, depending on the prevalence of tuberculosis in the population.

V. Dental Care

A. Examine teeth.

B. Give supplemental fluoride, if necessary (see Two-Week Visit, **V**, p. 8).

C. To prevent caries, tell parents not to leave a nursing bottle in the crib with the baby.

D. Describe rationale for avoiding frequent snacks or sugar-containing foods.

E. Remind parents to clean teeth with soft toothbrush or gauze pad once a day.

VI. Counseling

A. **Nutrition**

   1. Try to keep milk intake under 20 ounces if a balanced diet is available.

   2. Review diet. Counsel again, if necessary, on importance of basic food groups and of avoiding nonnutritious sugared commercial foods. Consider family preferences and economic factors.

   3. Continue iron-fortified formula or ferrous sulfate (Fer-In-Sol) drops (15 mg elemental iron per 0.6 mL) 0.6 mL once a day in water or fruit juice. Give supplemental vitamins if not in formula or vitamin D if breast-feeding.

   4. If necessary, discuss management of food preferences and possible decrease in appetite.

B. **Physical care**

   1. Review baby's response to common respiratory and gastrointestinal illnesses, home management, and indications for seeking medical care.

   2. Discuss parents' questions.

---

*See Use of the Health Maintenance Flow Sheet, pp. 1–5, for details.

C. **Behavioral and psychosocial environment**

1. Discuss parents' concept of acceptable behavior and discipline and their expectations.

2. Discuss adjustment of family to curiosity, mobility, and negativity of baby and their tolerance of noise from baby and siblings.

3. Discuss management of separations.

4. Explore parents' concept of toilet training.

5. Discuss child's progress toward drinking mainly from cup.

6. Discuss parents' questions.

D. **Stimulation.** See Infant and Child Stimulation Guidelines, pp. 39–45.

E. **Safety and Environment.** See Nine-Month Clinic Visit, **VI.E**, p. 18.

F. **Other topics,** based on the parents' concerns.

VII. **Follow-Up**

Measles–mumps–rubella and *Haemophilus influenzae* b vaccine to be given at age 15 months. Routine health maintenance visit in 6 months, or sooner if necessary.

Eighteen-Month Clinic Visit

I. **Provider**

Nurse practitioner.

II. **History**

A. Interval medical history.

B. Review and revision of family and social history.

III. **Examination**

A. Measurements (record on growth chart):

1. Weight.

2. Length.

3. Head circumference.

B. Inspection of baby completely undressed.

C. Extent of further examination is based on interval history and patient's problem list.

IV. **Procedures***

A. **Immunizations,** after reviewing contraindications and discussing side effects:

1. Diphtheria–pertussis–tetanus vaccine.

2. Oral polio vaccine (trivalent).

---

*See Use of Health Maintenance Flow Sheet, pp. 1–5, for details.

B. Developmental appraisal.

V. Dental Care

A. Examine teeth.

B. Give supplemental fluoride, if necessary (see Two-Week Visit, **V**, p. 8).

C. Discuss rationale for avoiding frequent snacks or sugar-containing foods.

D. Remind parents to clean teeth with soft toothbrush or gauze pad twice a day.

VI. Counseling

A. Nutrition

1. Review diet. Counsel again, if necessary, on importance of basic food groups and of avoiding nonnutritious sugared commercial foods. Consider family preferences and economic factors.

2. Limit milk intake to 2–3 glasses per day if a balanced diet is available.

3. Discuss progress of self-feeding.

4. Discuss parents' questions.

B. Physical care

1. Review parental management of illnesses occurring since previous visit.

2. Discuss parents' questions.

C. Behavioral and psychosocial environment

1. Discuss adjustment of family to baby's negativism, and possible frustration of parents' expectations of baby.

2. Discuss discipline and limit setting. Encourage parents to use substitution and positive reinforcement rather than physical punishment.

3. Discuss management of separation from mother.

4. Discuss toilet training and variations in normal patterns.

5. Discuss sleep problems (e.g., night terrors, desire to sleep in parents' room).

6. Discuss parents' questions.

D. **Stimulation.** See Infant and Child Stimulation Guidelines, pp. 39–45.

E. **Safety and Environment.** Review hazards and precautions discussed at previous visits (see Nine-Month Clinic Visit, **VI.E**, p. 18).

F. **Other topics,** based on parents' concerns.

VII. Follow-Up

In 6 months, or sooner if necessary.

Two-Year Clinic Visit

I. Provider

Nurse practitioner.

II. History

Interval medical history.

III. Examination

A. Measurements (record on growth chart):

1. Weight.

2. Length.

3. Head circumference.

B. Complete physical examination.

IV. Procedures*

A. **Immunizations.** Review immunization records.

B. **Developmental appraisal.**

C. **Hearing screening.**

1. Does baby point to at least one part of the body (eyes, feet, etc.) when you ask, without seeing your lips?

2. Does baby point to the right picture when asked, without seeing your lips, "Where's the cat [dog, man, horse, etc.]?"

3. Does baby give you a toy or put an object on a table or chair when asked, without seeing your lips?

Note: Baby may pass this test by observation of examiner or report of parent. Since this test evaluates more than just hearing function, failure requires further evaluation of other aspects of development as well.

D. **Language screening.** Ask parent what words the child uses regularly to denote specific objects, persons, or actions. This procedure is passed if parent reports child has three words other than *Dada* and *Mama*. Words do not have to be intelligible, but they must be specific.

V. Dental Care

A. Examine teeth.

B. Give supplemental fluoride, if necessary (see Two-Week Visit, **V**, p. 8).

C. Discuss rationale for avoiding frequent snacks or sugar-containing foods.

---

*See Use of Health Maintenance Flow Sheet, pp. 1–5, for details.

    D. Remind parents to clean teeth with toothbrush or gauze pad twice a day.

    E. Refer to dental services before age 3, even if teeth appear normal.

VI. Counseling

    A. **Nutrition**

        1. Review diet. Counsel again, if necessary, on importance of basic food groups and of avoiding nonnutritious sugared commercial foods, and of limiting milk intake to 2–3 glasses per day if a balanced diet is available. Consider family preferences and economic factors.

        2. Discuss progress of self-feeding.

        3. Discuss parents' questions.

    B. **Physical care**

        1. Review parental management of illnesses occurring since previous visit.

        2. Discuss parents' questions.

    C. **Behavioral and psychosocial environment**

        1. Discuss parents' concepts of normal behavior and limits. Discuss the fact that child understands "No" before inner controls are available to obey.

        2. Discuss discipline and limit setting and use of substitution and positive reinforcement instead of physical punishment.

        3. Discuss beginning of toilet training. Encourage independence in toileting when day control is achieved.

        4. Discuss management of separation from mother.

        5. Discuss sleep problems.

        6. Discuss parents' questions.

    D. **Stimulation.** See Infant and Child Stimulation Guidelines, pp. 39–45.

    E. **Safety and environment.** Advise parents on the following safety practices:

        1. Lock doors where danger of falling exists (e.g., cellar stairs).

        2. Lock up sharp or electrical tools.

        3. Check driveway, while outside automobile, before backing up.

        4. Lock all car doors.

        5. Never leave child unrestrained in cargo section of station wagon.

        6. Put matches out of reach.

        7. See also Nine-Month Clinic Visit, **VI.E**, p. 18.

VII. Follow-Up

In 1 year, or sooner if necessary.

THREE-YEAR CLINIC VISIT

I. Provider

Nurse practitioner.

II. History

A. Interval medical history.

B. Review and revision of family and social history.

III. Examination

A. Measurements (record on growth chart):

    1. Weight.

    2. Length.

B. Complete physical examination.

IV. Procedures*

A. **Tuberculin skin test.** Depends on prevalence of tuberculosis in the population.

B. **Blood pressure.** (Normal is less than 120/70 mm Hg in the supine position.)

C. **Developmental appraisal.**

D. **Hearing screening.**

E. **Vision screening.**

F. **Language screening.** This test is passed if child makes sentences of three or more words and speech is intelligible to strangers.

V. Dental Care

A. Examine teeth.

B. Give supplemental fluoride, if necessary.

C. Discuss rationale for avoiding frequent snacks or sugar-containing foods.

D. Remind parents to brush teeth twice a day with anticariogenic toothpaste.

E. Refer if patient was not seen by dental service within the previous year.

VI. Counseling

A. **Nutrition**

    1. Review diet. Counsel again, if necessary, on importance of basic food groups and of avoiding nonnutritious sugared commercial foods, and of limiting milk intake to 2–3 glasses per day if a balanced diet is available. Consider family preferences and economic factors.

---

*See Use of Health Maintenance Flow Sheet, pp. 1–5, for details.

2. Discuss possibility of periods of decreased appetite.

3. Explain that eating patterns are influenced by other family members.

4. Discuss parents' questions.

B. **Physical care**

1. Review parental management of illnesses occurring since previous visit.

2. Discuss parents' questions.

C. **Behavioral and psychosocial environment**

1. Discuss balance between need for independence and realistic discipline, guidance, and limits.

2. Discuss need for social interaction with peers.

3. Discuss normal early childhood fears (e.g., bodily injury), imagination (which is different from lying), and curiosity.

4. Discuss value and characteristics of a good nursery school and day care. Assist family in identifying a program, if desired.

5. Discuss sibling rivalry if new baby is due or has arrived.

6. Discuss normal lapses in bladder and bowel control. Issue is not to be made of these with child.

7. Discuss parents' questions.

D. **Sex education** (age 3–5 years)

1. Explore parents' concept of normal psychosexual development in preschool child.

2. Discuss sexual identity and common questions asked by children, including masturbation and sexual curiosity about other children's anatomy.

E. **Stimulation.** See Infant and Child Stimulation Guidelines, pp. 39–45.

F. **Safety and Environment.** Advise parents on the following safety practices:

1. Lock doors where danger of falling exists (e.g., cellar).

2. Place screens or guards over windows.

3. Place guards in front of all space heaters, heating stoves, and radiators.

4. Lock up sharp or electrical tools and firearms.

5. Lock up poisons and medications (review the use of syrup of ipecac as described in Chapter 2, Ingestions and Poisonings: Pediatric, **VI.E**, p. 80).

6. Teach child to watch out for moving automobiles in driveways and streets.

7. Use special young child's car seat for automobile. Shoulder belt may be used. Never leave child unrestrained in cargo section of station wagon.

8. Lock all car doors.

9. Never allow child to swim or wade in water without adult supervision.

10. Teach child to avoid engaging strangers.

G. **Other topics.** To be based on parents' concerns.

VII. Follow-Up

In 1 year, or sooner if necessary.

FIVE-YEAR CLINIC VISIT

I. Provider

Nurse practitioner.

II. History

A. Interval medical history, including complete review of systems.

B. Review and revision of family and social history.

III. Examination

A. Measurements (record on growth chart):

1. Weight.

2. Length.

B. Complete physical examination.

IV. Procedures*

A. Immunizations, after reviewing contraindications and discussing side effects.

1. Diphtheria-pertussis-tetanus vaccine.

2. Oral polio vaccine (trivalent).

3. Measles-mumps-rubella vaccine. (It is an acceptable alternative to give this vaccine booster at entry into junior high or middle school (i.e., 11 or 12 years of age.)

B. Tuberculin skin test, depending on the prevalence of tuberculosis in the population.

C. Hematocrit determination (normal is 33% or greater).

D. Urine culture (girls only); (optional).

E. Blood pressure (normal is less than 120/70 mm Hg in the supine position).

F. Developmental appraisal.

G. Hearing screening.

H. Vision screening.

I. Language screening. This test is failed if child does any of the following:

---

*See Use of Health Maintenance Flow Sheet, pp. 1–5, for details.

1. Often substitutes easy for difficult sounds (e.g., *wabbit*).
2. Constantly drops word endings.
3. Stutters or stammers.
4. Speaks in a monotonous voice.
5. Speaks in a voice that is excessively loud or inaudible.
6. Speaks with hypernasality or hyponasality.

V. Dental care

A. Examine teeth.

B. If water supply has less than 0.3 ppm of fluoride, prescribe 1 tablet per day of sodium fluoride (Luride Lozi-Tabs, which releases 1 mg of fluoride per tablet). If water supply has 0.3–0.7 ppm of fluoride, prescribe one-half tablet per day of sodium fluoride.

C. Discuss rationale for avoiding frequent snacks of sugar-containing foods.

D. Remind patient to brush teeth twice a day with anticariogenic toothpaste.

E. Refer if patient was not seen by dental service within previous year.

VI. Counseling (age 5–8 years)

A. Nutrition

1. Discuss parents' anxieties about eating problems. Remind them to encourage child's independence, that is, have nutritious foods available but allow child to choose amount and kind of food for his own plate. Reassure parents with growth chart if they are concerned about adequate intake.
2. Emphasize importance of breakfast, especially when child is going to school all day.
3. Discuss nutritious after-school snacks.
4. Encourage parents not to focus on strict table manners. Mealtime should be enjoyable for family.
5. Discuss parents' questions.

B. Physical care

1. Review parental management of illnesses occurring since previous visit.
2. Discuss importance of adequate sleep and consistent sleep routine.
3. Discuss teaching child personal hygiene.
4. Discuss parents' questions.

C. Behavior and psychosocial environment

1. Discuss preparing child for separation and independence associated with attending school. Assess parental concerns.
2. Discuss importance of regular school attendance.

3. Discuss importance of parent-teacher relationship and periodic meetings.

4. Discuss importance of peer acceptance and need for praise.

5. Discuss the worries and fears common in young school-age children (e.g., death, competition with peers, parental marital conflict, need to achieve). Discuss signs of excessive stress and availability of health care provider for counseling, if needed.

6. Discuss parents' expectations of child (e.g., chores, self-discipline, handling of anger). Are they realistic?

7. Discuss potential problems with teacher after obtaining parental permission.

D. Sex education

1. Explore parents' preparedness for potential questions.

2. Encourage parents to be aware of the scope of sex education programs in school.

E. Stimulation. Parents should be encouraged to do the following:

1. Converse with child regularly. Listen to child and encourage expression of thoughts.

2. Read to child and have child read to them.

3. Be sure child can dress completely.

4. Provide pencil, crayons, paper, paints, and scissors.

5. Show interest in child's schoolwork and provide encouragement.

6. Teach child responsible use of money.

7. Review television-viewing habits. Encourage balanced selective viewing of educational and entertaining programs.

F. Safety and environment. Parents should be encouraged to do the following:

1. Teach child to watch for moving automobiles, especially at intersections. Teach traffic signals and rules.

2. Teach bicycle techniques, traffic rules for bicycles, and warn of danger from automobiles.

3. Teach child swimming skills. Never allow child to swim without adult supervision.

4. Discuss fire prevention in the home with the child.

5. Lock up firearms.

6. Do not allow dangerous tools to be used without supervision.

7. Have child and entire family use seat belts for automobile safety. Lock all car doors. Do not allow child to ride in cargo section of station wagon.

8. Remind child to avoid engaging strangers.

9. Discuss with child the risks of tobacco and illicit drug use.

G. Other topics, based on parents' concerns.

VIII. Follow-Up

In 3 years, or sooner if necessary.

EIGHT-YEAR CLINIC VISIT

I. Provider

Nurse practitioner.

II. History

A. Interval medical history, including complete review of systems.

B. Review and revision of family and social history.

III. Examination

A. Measurements (record on growth chart):

1. Weight.

2. Height.

B. Complete physical examination.

IV. Procedures*

A. Review of immunization record.

B. **Blood pressure.** (Normal is less than 120/70 mm Hg in the supine position.)

C. **Hearing screening.**

D. **Vision screening.**

E. **Urine culture.** (Girls only; optional.)

V. Dental Care

A. Examine teeth.

B. Give supplemental fluoride, if necessary (see Five-Year Clinic Visit, **V.B**, p. 28).

C. Discuss rationale for avoiding frequent snacks of sugar-containing foods.

D. Remind patients to brush teeth twice a day with anticariogenic toothpaste and to floss once a day.

E. Refer to dental service if patient was not seen within the previous year.

VI. Counseling

(age 8–11 years)

A. **Nutrition**

1. Review diet. Counsel again, if necessary, on importance of

---

*See Use of Health Maintenance Flow Sheet, pp. 1–5, for details.

basic food groups and of avoiding nonnutritious sugared commercial foods. Consider family preferences and economic factors.

2. Emphasize importance of breakfast, especially when child is going to school all day.

3. Discuss nutritious after-school snacks.

4. Discuss parents' questions.

B. **Physical care**

1. Review parental management of illnesses occurring since previous visit.

2. Discuss importance of adequate sleep.

3. Discuss parents' questions.

C. **Behavioral and psychosocial environment**

1. Discuss school adjustment and progress with child and parents.

2. Discuss problems with teacher after obtaining parental permission.

3. Discuss importance of parent–teacher relationship and periodic meetings.

4. Explore peer relationships and involvement in group activities (e.g., scouts, religious groups, summer camp, summer recreational programs).

5. Discuss child's interpersonal relationships with siblings and with parents.

6. Discuss parents' and child's attitudes toward responsibilities (e.g., chores, neatness, monetary allowance).

7. Pursue child's as well as parents' concerns.

D. **Sex education**

1. Discuss parents' response to questions raised by child since last visit.

2. Encourage parents to be aware of the scope of sex education programs in school and to complement it as appropriate.

3. Discuss possibility of menarche before next visit and parents' plans for discussion with daughter.

4. Discuss parents' concerns.

E. **Stimulation.** Parents should be encouraged to do the following:

1. Converse with child regularly. Listen to child and encourage expression of thoughts.

2. Show interest in child's schoolwork and provide encouragement.

3. Provide child with quiet area and as much privacy as possible.

4. Encourage application of skills learned at school, including the following:

       a. Reading—encourage use of the library.

       b. Mathematics—assist child in planning use of money.

       c. Art, music, woodworking—provide child with simple equipment as desired.

     5. Review television-viewing habits. Encourage balanced selective viewing of educational and entertaining programs.

  F. Safety and environment. Parents should be encouraged to do the following:

     1. Teach child rules of pedestrian and cycling safety.

     2. Encourage development of swimming, water, and boating safety skills. Never allow child to swim without adult supervision.

     3. Discuss fire prevention in the home and use of telephone for emergencies.

     4. Lock up firearms.

     5. Do not allow electrical tools to be used without supervision.

     6. Have child and entire family use seat belts for automobile safety. Lock all car doors.

     7. Remind child to avoid engaging strangers.

     8. Continue discussion with child about the risks of tobacco and illicit drug use.

  G. Other topics. To be based on parent's concerns.

VII. Follow-Up

In 3 years, or sooner if necessary.

ELEVEN-YEAR CLINIC VISIT

I. Provider

Nurse practitioner.

II. History

  A. Interval medical history, including complete review of systems.

  B. Review and revision of family and social history.

III. Examination

  A. Measurements (record on growth chart):

     1. Weight.

     2. Height.

  B. Complete physical examination.

IV. Procedures*

---

*See Use of Health Maintenance Flow Sheet, pp. 1–5, for details.

A. **Immunizations**

1. Review immunization record.
2. Measles–mumps–rubella vaccine booster if not provided at first preschool visit or later.

B. **Tuberculin skin test.** Depends on the prevalence of tuberculosis in the population.

C. **Blood pressure.** (Normal is less than 140/80 mm Hg in the supine position.)

D. Hearing screening.

E. Vision screening.

V. Dental Care

A. Examine teeth.

B. Give supplemental fluoride, if necessary (see Five-Year Clinic Visit, **V.B**, p. 28).

C. Discuss rationale for avoiding frequent snacks or sugar-containing foods.

D. Remind patients to brush teeth twice a day with anticariogenic toothpaste and to floss once a day.

E. Refer if patient was not seen by dental service within the previous year.

VI. Counseling

A. **Nutrition**

1. Review diet. Counsel parents and child, if necessary, on importance of basic food groups and of avoiding nonnutritious sugared commercial foods. Consider family preferences and economic factors.
2. Emphasize importance of breakfast, especially when child is going to school all day.
3. Discuss nutritious after-school snacks.
4. Discuss parents' and child's questions.

B. **Physical care**

1. Review parental management of illnesses occurring since previous visit.
2. Discuss importance of adequate sleep and exercise.
3. Discuss with patient physical changes associated with puberty and the wide variation in time of onset.
4. Discuss skin care relative to acne.
5. Discuss parents' and child's questions.

C. **Behavioral and psychosocial environment**

1. Discuss school adjustment and progress with child and parents. Assess degree of parental involvement and concern.

2. Discuss problems with school personnel after obtaining parental permission.

3. Discuss importance of parent–teacher relationship and periodic meetings.

4. Discuss attitudes of parents and child toward school, achievement, and long-range plans. Are they realistic?

5. Explore peer relationships and involvement in group activities (e.g., scouts, YMCA or YWCA, religious groups, summer camp, summer recreational programs).

6. Discuss with parents normal increased desire for independence combined with need for consistent limits and someone who will *listen* to child's concerns.

7. Discuss child's interpersonal relationships with siblings and with parents.

8. Discuss parents' and child's attitudes toward responsibilities (e.g., chores, neatness, monetary allowance).

9. Assess and discuss patient's and parents' attitudes toward alcohol, tobacco, and drugs. Counsel when appropriate.

10. Pursue child's as well as parents' concerns.

D. **Sex education**

1. Discuss parents' response to questions raised by child since last visit.

2. Discuss child's understanding of menarche and parents' plans for discussion with daughter.

3. Discuss variable increase in interest in opposite sex.

4. Discuss with parents the normal child's concerns and need for sex education, especially girls who mature early. Counsel patient as needed and desired by parents in mechanisms of pregnancy and high-risk relationships. Plan another visit for counseling in this area before next health maintenance visit (age 13), if appropriate. Emphasize to patient and parents your availability.

E. **Safety and environment.** Parents should be encouraged to do the following:

1. Reinforce the rules of pedestrian and cycling safety.

2. Encourage development of swimming, water, and boating safety skills. Never allow child to swim alone.

3. Discuss fire prevention in the home and use of telephone for emergencies.

4. If firearms are available, instruct child in safe use.

5. Have child and entire family use seat belts for automobile safety. Lock all car doors.

6. Remind child of potential dangers of engaging strangers.

7. Continue discussion with child about the risks of tobacco and illicit drug use. Add a note of caution about riding in automobiles driven by someone using alcohol or other drugs.

F. **Other topics.** To be based on parents' concerns.

VII. Follow-Up

In 2 years, or sooner if necessary.

THIRTEEN- AND FIFTEEN-YEAR CLINIC VISITS

I. Provider

Nurse practitioner.

II. History

A. Interval medical history, including complete review of systems.

B. Review and revision of family and social history.

III. Examination

A. Measurements (record on growth chart):

1. Weight.

2. Height.

B. Complete physical examination.

IV. Procedures*

A. **Immunizations**

1. Review immunization record.

2. Tetanus–diphtheria toxoid (adult type Td), if 10 years have elapsed since previous booster.

B. **Tuberculin skin test.** To be given at age 15, depending on the prevalence of tuberculosis in the population.

C. **Hematocrit determination.** To be given at age 13 (normal greater than 33%).

D. **Blood pressure.** (Normal is less than 140/80 mm Hg for males and less than 140/85 mm Hg for females in the supine position.)

E. Hearing screening.

F. Vision screening.

V. Dental Care

A. Examine teeth

B. Discuss rationale for avoiding frequent snacks or sugar-containing foods.

---

*See Use of Health Maintenance Flow Sheet, pp. 1–5, for details.

    C. Remind patients to brush teeth twice a day with anticariogenic toothpaste and to floss once a day.

    D. Refer if patient was not seen by dental service within the previous year.

VI. Counseling

    A. **Nutrition**

        1. Review diet. Counsel patient and parents again, if necessary, on importance of basic food groups. Consider family preferences and economic factors.

        2. Emphasize importance of breakfast, especially when the patient is going to school all day.

        3. Discuss nutritious after-school snacks.

        4. Discuss patient's and parents' questions.

    B. **Physical care**

        1. Review home management of illnesses occurring since previous visit.

        2. Discuss importance of adequate sleep and exercise.

        3. Discuss patient's and parents' questions about physical changes associated with puberty.

        4. Discuss skin care relative to acne.

        5. Discuss patient's and parents' questions.

    C. **Behavioral and psychosocial environment**

        1. Discuss school adjustment and progress with patient and parents.

        2. Discuss problems with school personnel after obtaining parental permission.

        3. Emphasize practical importance of school relative to careers and employment, if necessary.

        4. Explore peer relationships and involvement in group activities.

        5. Discuss with parents how to achieve a balance between adolescent's appropriate desire for independence and need for consistent, fair limits and someone who will listen to concerns.

        6. Discuss with patient and parents interpersonal relationships with siblings and with parents (individual interview, or joint conference with parents, if desired by patient).

        7. Discuss with parents the adolescent's need for occasional privacy.

        8. Discuss with patient concerns about body image and being different (e.g., acne, tallness, fatness, shortness, delayed puberty).

        9. Assess and discuss patient's and parents' attitudes toward alcohol, tobacco, and drugs. Counsel as appropriate.

    D. **Sex education.** Extent of counseling at a particular visit will depend on patient's maturity, experience, and stage of development. Special visits with teenager for counseling in this area should be scheduled at appropriate times during adolescence.

1. Discuss patient's relationship with opposite sex and his or her concerns.
2. Assess patient's understanding of anatomy and physiology of reproduction.
3. Assess the immediacy of patient's need for contraceptive information and specific management. Discuss with patient the approach to be taken with parents.
4. Discuss with patient the responsibility that both male and female have for sexual activity and contraception.
5. Discuss venereal disease, including HIV.
6. Discuss patient's and parents' questions.

E. **Safety and environment.** Encourage the following:

1. Enrollment in driver-education course.
2. Use of seat belts for automobile safety.
3. Development of swimming, water, and boating safety skills. Never swim alone.
4. Safe use of firearms, if these are available.

F. **Other topics.** To be based on patients' and parents' concerns.

VII. Follow-Up

In 2 years or sooner, as needed.

SEVENTEEN-YEAR CLINIC VISIT

I. Provider

Nurse practitioner.

II. History

A. Interval medical history, including complete review of systems.
B. Review and revision of family and social history.

III. Examination

A. Measurements (record on growth chart):
   1. Weight.
   2. Height.
B. Complete physical examination.

IV. Procedures*

A. **Immunizations**
   1. Review immunization record.
   2. Tetanus–diphtheria toxoid (adult type Td), if 10 years have elapsed since previous booster.

---

*See Use of Health Maintenance Flow Sheet, pp. 1–5, for details.

B. **Blood pressure.** (Normal is less than 140/90 mm Hg in the supine position.)

C. Hearing screening.

D. Vision screening.

V. Dental care

A. Examine teeth.

B. Discuss rationale for avoiding frequent snacks or sugar-containing foods.

C. Remind patients to brush teeth twice a day and to floss once a day.

D. Refer if patient was not seen by dental service within the previous year.

VI. Counseling

A. **Nutrition**

1. Review diet. Counsel on importance of basic food groups. Consider family preferences and economic factors.

2. Emphasize importance of breakfast.

B. **Physical care**

1. Review home management of illnesses occurring since previous visit.

2. Discuss importance of adequate sleep and regular exercise.

3. Discuss patient's questions.

C. **Behavioral and psychosocial environment**

1. Discuss school adjustment and progress.

2. Discuss future career and education plans.

3. Discuss relationship with opposite sex and his or her concerns.

4. Discuss interpersonal relationship with parents (individual interview, and joint conference with parents if desired by patient).

5. Assess and discuss patient's attitudes toward alcohol, tobacco, and drugs. Counsel as appropriate.

D. **Sex education**

1. Discuss patient's concerns about relationship with opposite sex.

2. Discuss contraception and responsibility of both male and female.

3. Discuss venereal disease.

E. **Safety and environment.** Encourage the following:

1. Enrollment in driver-education course. If patient is already driving, emphasize the great risk of injury and death associated with poor driving habits. Review the association of alcohol with automobile accidents.

2. Discuss use of seat belts for automobile safety. Review statistics establishing their value.

3. Discuss development of swimming, water, and boating safety skills. Emphasize that one should never swim alone.

F. **Other topics.** To be based on the patient's concern.

VII. Follow-Up

In 3 years, or sooner if needed. If provider does not care for adults, arrange referral at this visit.

◢ INFANT AND CHILD STIMULATION GUIDELINES

BIRTH TO SIX MONTHS

I. Language and Personal–Social Development

A. Talk and sing to the baby even though he cannot understand what you say.

B. Repeat the noises he makes.

C. While he is awake, place him where he can see and hear what is going on.

II. Visual, Auditory, and Tactile Stimulation

A. **Hang pictures on the wall or crib.** Put them where the baby can see them. Cut pictures from magazines or use pictures that older children bring home from school.

B. **Hang dangling toys above the baby:**

   1. Attach ribbon, bright cloth, colored paper, ball, shiny spoon, painted spools, measuring spoons, or rubber jar rings to a string or coat hanger and hang it across the crib.

   2. Make a mobile. Cut a circle from cardboard or a plastic bleach bottle. Using thread, tie on colorful cutouts from boxes (e.g., circles, birds, butterflies). Hang the mobile from a light fixture or the ceiling over the crib.

C. **Make rattles (noisemakers).** Fill small cardboard boxes, plastic salt shakers, or soft drink cans with large stones, bottle caps, poker chips, large buttons, or spools, and tape the end shut. (Use large objects that the baby cannot swallow just in case the rattle comes apart).

D. **Make soft, cuddly toys.** Cut two pieces of cloth (old towel) in pattern, sew together and stuff with rags, nylons, cotton batting, facial tissues, or toilet paper, or stuff an old sock or glove.

E. **Put the child on a blanket on the floor.** Let baby see more of the world around him and have an opportunity to exercise his muscles.

SIX TO TWELVE MONTHS

I. Language and Personal–Social Development

A. **Talk to him.** Tell him what you are doing to or with him even though he does not understand.

B. **Point to objects and people** and name them over and over.

C. **Play games.** For example, patty cake, peek-a-boo, where is John-ny's nose?

D. **Have him in the room with you while he is awake.** Let him crawl on the floor and explore or put him in a walker.

E. **Let him see himself in the mirror.** Talk to him while he is looking in the mirror—"Look at baby's nose," "Here is Johnny's mouth."

II. Visual, Auditory, and Tactile Stimulation

A. **Provide soft, cuddly toys.**

B. **Make noisemakers:**

1. Make a drum out of an empty oatmeal box and give the child a stick with which to bang on it.

2. Fill containers of different shapes with previously mentioned articles (see Birth to Six Months, **II.C**).

C. **Give him objects to handle and explore.** (Objects that are unbreakable and too large to be swallowed.)

1. Let him play with a rolling pin, large spoons, boxes (cereal, shoe, berry, match), bowls, pots, pans, cans, baking tins (cake, pie, muffin), plastic cups, screw-top plastic bottles, coffee pot, bandage cans.

2. Present a variety of textures (hard, soft, fuzzy, smooth), sponges, different types of material (velvet, imitation fur, cotton, wool) by making a ball out of different textured materials and stuffing it with cotton, rags or pantyhose.

D. **Provide fill-and-dump toys.** Use a container with a large open-ing (e.g., milk carton, coffee can, oatmeal box) and gather small objects to place in the container and dump out (e.g., spools, mea-suring spoons, clothespins, corks, poker chips).

E. **Put baby's favorite toy in a paper bag.** Have him find it.

ONE TO THREE YEARS

I. Language Development

A. **Talk to the child.** Listen with interest to what he has to say. Use complete thoughts—not "Pick it up," but "Pick up the ball from under the table."

B. **Read to him.** Also, tell him stories.

C. **Have him tell you stories.** For example, stories about pictures in books or magazines.

D. **Make a picture book.** Cut out large pieces of paper bag for the cover and pages. Fold them in half and tie them together with string or yarn. Paste pictures in the book from magazines, cereal boxes, or newspapers.

E. **Name parts of his body.** Also, name pictures of people. Have him name objects.

    F. Let him look in a mirror and point out his facial features and body parts.

    G. Play singing games For example, "Ring Around the Rosy," "Row, Row, Row Your Boat").

    H. Play telephone with him.

    I. Play with puppets. Have a conversation using puppets.

        1. Paper bag puppets. Fill a small bag with cotton or crumpled newspaper; insert a stick or pencil; tie a string around the stuffed area; and stick-paint, draw, or color a face on the bag.

        2. Potato puppets. Insert a stick in a small potato. Create facial features by painting the surface of the potato.

        3. Potato finger puppets. Make by cutting a small hole in the bottom of the potato and slipping the potato over one's finger.

        4. Old-glove puppets. Cut off the fingers and thumb of a glove and stuff them with cotton, nylons, or old rags. The thumb becomes the head and body of the puppet, and two fingers become the arms when sewn to the thumb section. Bind the head and waist sections off with string or yarn. Decorate with pieces of material, yarn, and ribbon.

II. Personal–Social Development

    A. Toys. Let the child play with dolls and stuffed animals.

    B. Take him on trips. To the store, to a neighbor's house. Ride in a car or bus to the park and zoo. Point to and name people, objects, and animals.

    C. Play games. For example, hide and seek.

    D. Role playing. Allow the child to experiment with dressing up and with adult role playing.

        1. Give the child mother's or father's old hats, dresses, suits, shoes, purses, and wallets.

        2. Make hats and masks out of paper bags or paper plates. Make dresses out of blankets or materials.

        3. Let the child use cooking utensils, house-cleaning equipment, and safe tools.

        4. Make a house by putting a blanket over a high table.

III. Gross Motor Development

    A. Push-pull toys

        1. Attach a string to a large box and fill it with light-weight objects.

        2. Make a train by tying boxes (shoe boxes, milk cartons, salt boxes) together with heavy string and attaching a pull string.

    B. Cardboard tunnel to crawl through. Cut ends off large cardboard boxes and attach several boxes together to make a tunnel.

    C. Climbing stairs.

D. **Walking board.** Rest a board 1 foot wide by 3 feet long on bricks. Encourage the child to walk forward, backward, sideways, and jump down. As the child's coordination improves, decrease the width of the board.

E. **Throwing and catching a ball or bean bag.** Make a large ball out of two pieces of cloth sewn together and stuffed with rags, cotton, or nylons.

F. **Sand play.** (Using unbreakable things.)
1. Use an inner tube as an outside frame for a sandbox and fill the inside area with sand.
2. Give the child spoons, cans, bowls, cups, sieves, and funnels to fill and dump.
3. Cut a bleach bottle in half. Use bottom for a pail (make a handle out of heavy string); use the top for a funnel.

G. **Water play.** Use a large tub outdoors or the sink or bathtub indoors. Give the child unbreakable containers, sponges, cork, bar of soap.

H. **Riding a tricycle.**

IV. Fine Motor Development

A. **Fill-and-dump toys.** As the child's coordination improves, decrease the size of the container and the opening (e.g., plastic milk bottle, small jars and cans) and give him smaller objects to put into the container (e.g., buttons, bottle caps, peas, beans, macaroni).

B. **Sorting activity.** Give the child three containers and bottle caps, buttons, and beans; have him put all the caps in one container, buttons in another, and beans in the other. Later, use the sections of an egg carton.

C. **Stacking toys.** Build a pyramid with different-sized boxes or cans, the largest on the bottom and the smallest on top.

D. **Nesting toys.** Use graduated-sized boxes, bowls, pots, pans, or cups that fit inside one another. Start by using three sizes.

E. **Clothespins and a coffee can or loaf pan.** Have the child put the clothespins on the edge of the can. This can also be used as a sorting activity; paint the pins different colors and have child sort them by color.

F. **Blocks.** Make different-sized blocks from boxes and wood scraps. Cut off the tops of two thoroughly washed milk or cream cartons and push them together. Show the child how to build. Have him copy what you build.

G. **Stringing objects.** Use old shoelaces or heavy string and spools of different sizes. As coordination improves, give the child smaller objects (macaroni and beads).

H. **Puzzles.** Make your own by pasting pictures from magazines onto cardboard and cutting it into pieces. Start with simple pictures of one object and cut into three to five large pieces. With an older child, use a more complex picture and five to ten small pieces.

I. **Large pencil or crayon.** Have the child copy a line or simple shape you make. Allow him to draw whatever he wishes. Use this time to start teaching colors. Use paper bags or cut-up cardboard boxes to draw on.

THREE TO FIVE YEARS

I. Language Development

A. **Talk to the child.** use complete thoughts and ideas. Listen to him. Encourage him to tell you what he did during the day by asking questions.

B. **Read to him.** Or tell him stories.

C. **Play singing games.** For example, "Here We Go Round the Mulberry Bush," "This Is the Way We Wash Our Clothes."

D. **Encourage him to make up stories.** For example, stories about pictures in books and magazines ("Once upon a time . . . ").

E. **Play with puppets.**

II. Personal–Social Development

A. **Dressing.** Show him how.

B. **Small tasks.** Give him things to do around the house (e.g., set table, help clear table, sweep floor, pick up toys).

C. **Allow him to experiment with dressing up and adult role playing.**

1. Let him use old clothes, cooking utensils, house-cleaning equipment, and safe tools.

2. Put chairs together to play train or bus.

3. Make a house under a table.

4. Use paper bags decorated with colored paper, ribbon, or paint to make hats.

5. Use paper bags to make hats and masks.

D. **Grow plants in cans.**

E. **Encourage him to play outdoor games with peers** (e.g., red rover, hide-and-seek).

III. Gross Motor Development

A. **Cardboard tunnel.**

B. **Walking board.** Use a board about 4 inches wide.

C. **Sand play.** Encourage child to build creatively (e.g., make cities).

D. **Water play.** Let child enjoy washing dishes or clothes.

E. **Throwing, catching, and batting a ball.** Use a small rubber or semihard ball.

F. **Throwing a bean bag at a target.** Fill an old sock with beans and sew the end shut (reinforce by sewing it several times). Make a target out of a cardboard box folded like an inverted V (tent-shaped); attach a heavy string to each side to stabilize it. Cut a hole in one side of the target and paint or color a clown's face around the hole.

G. **Rope ladder.** Make a ladder out of rope and attach it to a low branch of a tree for the child to climb.

H. **Playing jump rope and hopscotch** (start between 5 and 6 years of age).

I. **Riding a tricycle and bicycle.**

IV. **Fine Motor Development**

A. **Fill-and-dump toys.**

B. **Stacking toys.** Increase the number and use smaller objects to be stacked (e.g., spools).

C. **Nesting toys.** Increase the number and sizes of objects to be nested.

D. **Sorting activity.** Give the child many objects and ask him to sort them according to color, shape or function. For example, give the child an egg carton or small cans and colored buttons and have him sort according to color.

E. **Blocks.** Give him blocks of different sizes and encourage him to build more complicated structures (e.g., houses, farms, forts).

F. **Stringing objects.** String macaroni or straws cut into small pieces. Make necklaces and bracelets and paint them bright colors.

G. **Puzzles.** Make more complicated puzzles, using detailed pictures cut into 8 to 20 pieces.

H. **Pencils and crayons.** Use paper bags or cut-up cardboard boxes to draw on. Draw a simple picture and have him color it. Draw simple forms (circles, squares, cross) and have the child copy them. Encourage the child to draw his own pictures.

I. **Finger Painting**

1. Use the want-ad section of the newspaper (because it has small, all-over print) or shelf paper for painting paper.

2. Old shirts or blouses make good smocks.

3. Recipe for paint:

   1½ cups laundry starch

   1 quart boiling water

   1½ cups soap flakes

   Few drops food coloring

   1½ cup talcum powder (optional)

   Mix starch with enough cold water to make a paste, add boiling water, and stir until clear and glossy. Add talcum. Cool mixture. Add soap flakes, and stir until evenly distributed. Mixture should be thick. Add a few drops of food coloring. Pour into jar and cover. Store in a cool place.

J. **Clay or play dough**
   1. Show the child how to make objects and animals.
   2. Recipe for play dough:

   1 part flour

   1 part salt

   1 part water

   Mix together to a soft consistency. Will keep 3–4 days if wrapped in wax paper and stored in the refrigerator.

K. **Collages**
   1. Paste bits of cotton, cloth, colorful yarn, ribbon, paper, calendars, catalogues, magazines, or pipe cleaners to a piece of cardboard to create a picture. Hang in a place for people to admire.
   2. Paste recipe: To a handful of flour add water, a little at a time, until mixture is gooey (should be quite thick so it will not run all over the page). Add a pinch of salt.

L. **Sewing cards.** Draw a design or picture on a piece of cardboard. Punch holes along the line. Give the child an old shoelace or large needle and yarn to sew with, along the outline.

M. **Child's blunt scissors**
   1. Show child how to hold and use scissors.
   2. Give him a long strip of paper ¼ inch wide marked with thick lines at 1-inch intervals. Have him cut off sections with one snip.
   3. When he is older give him wider strips sectioned off in large pieces that require several strokes of the scissors.
   4. Have the child practice cutting curves. When this is mastered, he can cut circles and other objects.
   5. Have him cut zig-zag strips, which become crowns, mountains, Christmas trees.
   6. Draw large, simple geometric shapes and have him cut them out.

N. **Materials for construction.** Give the child wood scraps and nails and help him build things.

▲ PERIODIC HEALTH SCREENING: ADULT

I. Value of the Periodic Health Assessment

The periodic screening and examination of well adults remains controversial and continues to be changed as each test is critically evaluated. What is considered an adequate age-related assessment today is a far cry from the high water mark of the sixties. As we more critically look at screening tests, few fulfill the criteria of a useful screening procedure: (a) The disease sought is an important problem for which there is a treatment; (b) there is a latent asymptomatic or early symptomatic period during which a screening test is positive; (c) the screening test is available at a reasonable cost and has adequate specificity and sensitivity.

Nonetheless, it has been the experience of most programs that a periodic meeting between patient and health care provider is beneficial. In keeping with this conclusion, we recommend an age-related assessment that includes the most widely recognized screening procedures plus health education about important health issues. Assessment reflects current thinking about screening procedures; and includes health education and inquiry about health habits. The preventive health services may be administered during a visit for an acute problem.

II. Conditions of Screening

A. Cardiovascular Disease

1. **Cholesterol.** Asymptomatic middle-aged males with high cholesterol levels have been shown to have lower rates of myocardial infarction and death from coronary disease after cholesterol reduction; females and older males may obtain the same benefit, but clinical trials have not been completed in these groups.

   a. The National Cholesterol Education Program recommends that all American adults have their cholesterol measured every 5 years. Other expert panels recommend an approach that targets somewhat higher risk groups; for example, the Toronto Working Group recommends screening men above 35 years of age and women above 45 years of age.

   b. According to the National Cholesterol Education Program, treatment decisions regarding elevated serum lipid should be based on an average of at least two LDL cholesterol levels. Diet treatment is recommended for an LDL cholesterol above 160 mg/dL or above 130 mg/dL if there are two or more risk factors. Total cholesterol may be elevated because of a high HDL cholesterol which would not necessarily mean an increased risk. If total cholesterol is above 240 mg/dL and there are two or more risk factors, LDL determination is recommended for treatment decisions. Total cholesterol/HDL ratio is used by some to make decisions regarding treatment (increased risk with a ratio greater than 5); however, the National Cholesterol Education Group recommends that decisions be made on LDL cholesterol alone.

   c. For patients with known CHD (prior MI, angina, or disease on angiography) a more aggressive approach to lipid lowering is warranted. As angiographic studies have shown, there is less progression and more regression of disease among patients receiving intensive lipid lowering interventions when compared with controls. Many experts suggest an LDL goal of less than 100 mg/dL for these patients.

   d. Recheck cholesterol levels at 3 and 6 months; consider drug therapy if there is no significant improvement after 6 months.

e. Consult physician for institution of drug therapy if the target goal is not reached after 6 months, if the initial LDL cholesterol is above 190 mg/dL, or if the patient has high LDL cholesterol and has known CHD.

f. Discuss exercise. As a general rule, all patients being given advice about cholesterol should have an exercise program as part of their regimen. Exercise can promote weight loss and is often associated with a reduction in LDL cholesterol and an increase in HDL cholesterol.

2. **Hypertension.** Check at least once a year, but most practices measure at every office visit. See Chapter 7 for treatment of hypertension.

3. **Smoking.** Inquire about smoking habits from every patient. See below for smoking cessation.

4. **Stress.** Assess at each visit for levels of stress.

5. **Exercise.** Assess levels of exercise; if not exercising suggest gradually increasing exercise. Simple walking, swimming, or gardening for 30 minutes a day is often adequate.

B. **Cancer Screening**

1. **Cervical Cancer.** The Papanicolaou or Pap smear is an effective means for finding early cervical cancer. The frequency of screening and the women to be screened are still somewhat controversial; however, more than 90% of the reduction in risk can be obtained by screening patients at risk every 3 years with little additional benefit from more frequent screening. Patients at low risk are women over 65 years of age who have had multiple negative results, women who have had total hysterectomies and have no cervix, and women who are not engaged in sexual activity at all. These women may not need to be screened at all.

    a. Women to be screened with a Pap smear using a cytobrush: All sexually active women at least once every three years, women with no previous Pap smears, and women who have had a subtotal hysterectomy and therefore still have a cervix.

    b. Higher risk women (women with multiple sexual partners or with recent abnormal Pap smears) should be special targets for screening.

2. **Breast Cancer.** Mammography and clinical breast examination (CBE) can reduce mortality in women between 50 and 74 years of age; there is general agreement that women between 50 and 75 years of age should be screened every 1–2 years. It is harder to justify screening before 50 years of age, both because mammography is a poorer screening tool in premenopausal women and the natural history of cancer in younger women is not well understood. After 75 years of age screening should be

based on life expectancy. There is no evidence that the base-line mammogram at some arbitrary age such as 40 is an effective screening tool.

   a. Women to be screened:

      (1) Annual mammography and CBE in women aged 50–74 years of age.

      (2) Earlier screening beginning at age 40 in women with first degree relatives with breast cancer (e.g., mother, sister, or daughter), if the relative got breast cancer before age 50.

      (3) Annual CBE beginning at age 40.

      (4) It is important to remember that:

         (a) Breast self-examination cannot replace mammography and clinical breast examination as breast cancer screening.

         (b) A dominant lump on clinical breast examination is abnormal and should be referred even if the mammogram is negative.

3. Colorectal Cancer. The primary methods of screening are annual fecal occult blood testing and flexible sigmoidoscopy every 5–10 years.

   a. Patients 50 years of age and older should be screened annually with fecal occult blood testing and every 5–10 years with a flexible sigmoidoscopy. To do the fecal occult blood test properly, patients should be given Hemoccult cards and instructed not to eat or take red meat, aspirin, nonsteroidal anti-inflammatory drugs, and vitamin C for three days. Fresh stool from three consecutive bowel movements should be spread on the windows of each card as described on the Hemoccult instructions and returned for developing within 2 days. Recent evidence suggests that a drop of water should be added to the smear before developing. Any blue color on any window should be considered a positive test.

   b. Patients at higher risk may need to be screened more aggressively. These include patients with:

      (1) First degree relatives with colorectal cancer.

      (2) Personal history of endometrial, ovarian, or breast cancer.

      (3) Previous diagnosis of inflammatory bowel disease.

      (4) History of adenomatous polyp or colon cancer.

      (5) A family history of familial polyposis who are over 19.

4. Prostate Cancer. Digital rectal examination has not proved to be of benefit in finding treatable cancers and tumor markers such as prostatic-specific antigen are not sufficiently specific to be effective screening tools. This is a very controversial area; many practices will still perform Digital Prostate examinations on all males over 50, and others may choose to measure PSA. If examinations are done (it is acceptable not to screen at all), all patients with an asymmetrical, indurated, or nodular prostate and those with an elevated PSA should be referred to a physician.

C. **Screening for Other Problems** A number of other tests are routinely considered for inclusion in an annual or periodic assessment. Among those frequently listed are

1. **Glaucoma screening.** Not recommended in primary care settings.

2. **Thyroid function testing.** Not recommended for routine testing, but should be ordered especially in older women with a high level of suspicion.

3. **Visual acuity testing.** Should be done annually in patients over 65. Those with vision worse than 20/40 in either eye should be referred.

4. **Hearing testing.** Should be done in patients over 65 every 5 years using a hand-held audiometer or a simple screening questionnaire such as the Hearing Handicap in the Elderly (HHIE). Those with a 40-dB or greater hearing loss at 1000 or 2000 Hz in either ear should be referred.

5. **Tuberculosis.** Tuberculosis screening is suggested in the following high-risk groups who have not previously been treated or had a positive result on the Mantoux test:

    a. Persons with human immunodeficiency virus (HIV) infection, or other medical conditions that have been reported to increase the risk of tuberculosis (e.g., diabetes mellitus, gastrectomy, chronic renal failure, high-dose corticosteroid therapy, malignancies).

    b. Close contacts of persons with newly diagnosed infectious tuberculosis.

    c. Intravenous drug users known to be HIV-seronegative.

    d. Persons with possible old tuberculosis on chest films.

    e. People who come to the United States from high-prevalence countries.

    f. Medically underserved low-income groups.

    g. Residents of nursing homes. Those patients who have a negative test (<10 mm of induration) should have a repeat test with the same dose one week after the original test.

    h. Residents of correctional institutions.

    i. Children and adolescents.

    j. Health care workers.

    Repeat testing at 6- to 24-month intervals should be carried out in persons at continued risk of exposure to active tuberculosis.

6. **Screening for HIV.** All patients at high risk for HIV disease should be offered HIV testing. This would include IV drug

abusers, homosexual males, males and females with multiple partners, partners of known HIV-positive patients, and patients with other sexually transmitted diseases. In addition, testing should be done whenever a patient requests it, even if one is not able to identify significant risk factors.

In all cases, patients must give informed consent before testing is done and must be given counseling and appropriate further evaluation and treatment if results are positive. Case reporting and follow-up of contacts is important, but should be done in a manner consistent with local laws and convention, always showing respect for patient confidentiality and sensitivity to the many social issues HIV disease raises.

▲ IMMUNIZATIONS*

A. **DPT.** All adults who have not had primary immunizations should have a series of three tetanus–diphtheria toxoid (Td) intramuscular injections, the second injection at 4–8 weeks and the third at 6–12 months. Booster injections should be given every 10 years. See Minor Wounds for management of acute injuries.

B. **Polio.** Routine primary polio vaccination is not recommended for those 18 years old and over residing in the United States. Immunization is recommended for certain adults at greater risk—travelers to certain developing countries or health care workers at risk of exposure.

C. **Influenza vaccine.** Influenza vaccine is recommended annually for individuals at increased risk of adverse consequences from infection of the lower respiratory tract. Groups with conditions predisposing to such risk include:

1. Groups at greater risk:

   a. Adults and children with chronic disorders of the cardiovascular (e.g. congestive heart failure and angina pectoris) or pulmonary (e.g. chronic obstructive pulmonary disease) systems that required regular medical follow-up or hospitalization during the previous year.

   b. Residents of nursing homes and other chronic care facilities.

2. Groups at moderate risk:

   a. Otherwise healthy persons 65 years of age or older

   b. Adults and children with chronic metabolic disease (including diabetes mellitus), sickle cell disease, renal dysfunction,

---

*Based on Recommendations in MMWR, Update on Adult Immunization, Vol. 40 (DDHS Publication No. RR12, Nov. 15, 1991).

alcohol abuse, cirrhosis, anemia, immunosuppression (human immune deficiency virus [HIV] infection) or asthma requiring regular follow-up or hospitalization in the past year.

   c. Children on long-term aspirin treatment who may be at risk for Reye syndrome.

  3. Groups potentially capable of nosocomial transmission to high-risk persons:

   a. Medical personnel

   b. Providers of care to high-risk people in the home setting (family members, visiting nurses, volunteer workers).

D. Pneumococcal vaccine. Pneumococcal vaccine contains capsular polysaccharides from the 23 most commonly encountered types of pneumococci, replacing the 14-valent vaccine. Patients who have previously received the 14-valent vaccine get little increased benefit from the 23-valent vaccine and should not be revaccinated with the 23-valent vaccine, but a booster shot may be considered at 6 years for patients at greatest risk, e.g., those with asplenia. Immunization is recommended for all individuals over 65 years old, and for anyone with increased risk for pneumonococcal disease or its complication. The latter group includes:

  1. Adults with chronic illnesses, especially cardiovascular disease and chronic pulmonary diseases, who sustain increased morbidity with respiratory infections.

  2. Adults with chronic illnesses specifically associated with an increased risk for pneumonococcal disease or its complications. These include splenic dysfunction or anatomic asplenia, Hodgkin's disease, multiple myeloma, cirrhosis, alcoholism, renal failure, CSF leaks, HIV infection, organ transplant, and conditions associated with immunosuppression.

E. Mumps vaccine. Mumps vaccine, 0.5 cc of live attenuated virus, should be given subcutaneously to adults born after 1956 who do not have documentation of previous infection, prior immunization, or serology of previous infection.

F. Measles vaccine. Measles vaccine is indicated in all adults born after 1956 who do not have a documentation of immunity; also all those who had inactivated measles virus vaccine between 1964 and 1967 and those who had only one injection should be reimmunized. See Ch 16, Measles: Pediatric and Adult.

7. Rubella titer and vaccine. See Rubella, Chapter 16. Live attenuated virus vaccine should be given 0.5 cc subcutaneously in a single injection to the following groups:

  1. Women of child-bearing age. Routine serology on all patients without certain knowledge of the disease is very expensive. Administration of the vaccine to non-pregnant females with no history of immunization is justified without serologic testing.

2. College students.

3. Health care workers.

H. Hepatitis B vaccine. Genetically engineered hepatitis B vaccine is now available, but costly. The vaccine should be given in three 1 cc doses, with the second and third doses coming at 1 and 6 months. There are few side effects of the vaccine and the genetic engineering removes the risk of contamination with other viruses; however, because yeast is used in the preparation of the vaccine people allergic to yeast should use the plasma-derived vaccine. High risk groups that should be immunized are as follows:

1. Health care workers and public safety workers at risk for exposure to blood.

2. Clients and staff of institutions for the developmentally disabled.

3. Hemodialysis patients.

4. Recipients of certain blood products, e.g., clotting factors.

5. Household contacts and sex partners of HBV carriers.

6. Adoptees from countries where hepatitis B virus infection is endemic.

7. International travelers who are staying longer than 6 months in a country with a high incidence of infection or those staying a shorter time in a country with a high or intermediate risk, but who will be engaging in a risky behavior.

8. Injecting drug users.

9. Sexually active homosexual or bisexual men.

10. Sexually active heterosexual men and women who have recently acquired a sexually transmitted disease, are prostitutes, or who have had more than one sex partner in the past 6 months.

11. In-mates of long-term correctional institutions.

The timing of booster injections has not been worked out and they are not recommended.

▲ COUNSELING AND PATIENT EDUCATION

A large number of potential problems fall under this rubric, but the following subjects seem reasonable targets for periodic review: smoking cessation (see below), prevention of injuries, dietary fat content, exercise, birth control (see Chapter 14), prevention of sexually transmitted diseases (see Chapters 9 and 14), and advanced directives.

A. Smoking Cessation. Health can be adversely affected by either direct smoking or by passive smoking, both side stream and exhaled smoke. Studies suggest that one year quit rates can be significantly raised by increasing the intensity of the office program. A smoking history should be obtained on every patient and interest in quitting determined. For patients interested in stopping establish:

1. **Motivation.** Reinforce motivation by citing social, financial, and medical advantages of not smoking. Also, give personal and family reasons for stopping. Provide those not yet prepared to stop with information to help them stop.

2. **Obstacles to smoking cessation.**

    a. Addiction to nicotine. This is suggested by a history of smoking within 60 minutes of arising, smoking more than 25 cigarettes a day, and symptoms of withdrawal when the patient is under conditions that prohibit smoking.

    b. Fear of obesity.

    c. Previous failed attempts.

3. **Treatment plan.**

    a. Set a quit date. A quit date usually should be set with some lead time (2 weeks is usually sufficient) that allows the patient to prepare for the project. Patients should prepare to quit completely; efforts to cut down are rarely successful. The proposed date should be free of stress and may commemorate some important date for the patient.

    b. Follow-up within 2 weeks to reinforce success or to discuss difficulties.

    c. Prescribe nicotine gum or transdermal patches to prevent withdrawal symptoms in dependent patients. Do not use replacement therapy if the patient may continue smoking. Replacement therapy is used to help patients get started and to get over the initial psychological problems and pharmacological withdrawal. It should never be used as an indefinite maintenance for patients using replacement therapy to help them cut down. Consult physician before beginning therapy.

        (1) Nicotine Gum: 2 or 4 mg:

            (a) Begin with 2 mg.

            (b) Chew gum slowly.

            (c) Park gum along the buccal mucosa.

            (d) Repeat sequence when there is an urge to smoke. Each piece of gum may last 30 minutes.

            (e) Try 4-mg gum if the patient requires more than 20 pieces of gum in a day.

        (2) Transdermal nicotine patches: 7, 14, and 21 mg:

            (a) Begin at 21 mg and continue for 4 weeks.

            (b) Taper to 14 mg patches for 4 weeks.

            (c) Complete 3 months at 7 mg for 4 weeks.

Table 1-3
Guidelines for Adult Screening

Procedure	Women < 50	50–64	>65	Men < 50	50–64	>65
Screening						
Cholesterol	Once	Every 5 yrs	Every 5 yrs	Once	Every 5 yrs	Every 5 yrs
Fecal bld.	—	Annually	Annually	—	Annually	Annually
Sigmoidoscopy	—	Every 5–10 yrs	Every 5–10 yrs	—	Every 5–10 yrs	Every 5–10 yrs
CBE	Annually after 40	Annually	Annually			
Mammography		Every 1–2 yrs	Every 1–2 yrs to 75			
Pap	Every 3 yrs if sex active	Every 3 yrs if sex active	Every 3 yrs to 75			
Vision						
Hearing		Every 5 yrs	Annually		Every 5 yrs	Annually
Immunizations						
Td	Every 10 yrs	Every 10 yrs	Every 10 yrs	Every 10 yrs	Every 10 yrs	Every 10 yrs
Influenzae	Pat. at risk (annually)	Pat. at risk (annually)	Annually	Pat. at risk (annually)	Pat. at risk (annually)	Annually
Pneumococcal	Pat. at risk (once)	Pat. at risk (once)	Once	Pat. at risk (once)	Pat. at risk (once)	Once
Annual Counseling						
Smoking	+	+	+	+	+	+
Exercise	+	+	+	+	+	+
Diet	+	+		+		
Ca			+			
Fat		+	+		+	+
Depression			+			+
ETOH/Driving	+	+	+	+	+	+

54

2

Emergencies

▲ ANAPHYLAXIS: PEDIATRIC AND ADULT

I. Definition

A hypersensitivity reaction usually occurring within seconds to minutes after exposure to an antigen. The reaction ranges from mild, self-limited symptoms to rapid death.

II. Etiology

Agents commonly associated with anaphylaxis include the following. This list is not exhaustive.

A. **Antibiotics** (especially penicillin and its semisynthetic derivatives).

B. **Biologicals** (nonhuman sera, gamma globulin, vaccines).

C. **Local anesthetics.**

D. **Aspirin.**

E. **Hymenoptera stings** (bee, yellow jacket, wasp, and hornet).

F. **Allergic extracts** (skin-testing and treatment solutions).

G. **Foods** (especially eggs, nuts, and shellfish).

Patient Care Guidelines for Nurse Practitioners, 4th ed. by Axalla J. Hoole, C. Glenn Pickard, Jr., Ruth M. Ouimette, Jacob A. Lohr, and Robert A. Greenberg. Copyright © 1995 by J. B. Lippincott Company.

H. Intravenous narcotics (heroin).

Note: Generally, agents administered parenterally are more likely to result in life-threatening or fatal anaphylactic reactions than those ingested orally or administered topically to mucous membranes. Medications administered orally, such as aspirin or penicillin, however, have been associated with fatal reactions.

III. Clinical Features

Anaphylaxis is usually characterized by some or all of the following sequence of signs and symptoms. The more quickly symptoms develop after the initiating stimulus, the more intense the reaction.

A. Generalized flush.

B. Urticaria.

C. Paroxysmal coughing.

D. Severe anxiety.

E. Dyspnea.

F. Wheezing.

G. Orthopnea.

H. Vomiting.

I. Cyanosis.

J. Shock.

IV. Laboratory Studies

None.

V. Differential Diagnosis

The development of symptoms and signs within minutes after contact with an antigen, especially a parenterally administered antigen, makes the diagnosis of anaphylaxis almost certain. An anxiety reaction to an injection might produce some of the symptoms, but consideration of that diagnosis should not result in more than momentary delay in instituting treatment for anaphylaxis.

VI. Treatment

A. Prevention

1. Before administering or prescribing any medication, inquire carefully for a history of reactions.

Note: Anaphylactoid reactions can occur without prior known sensitization.

2. Minimize the use of biologic products (e.g., horse antiserum, unnecessary boosters of tetanus toxoid).

3. After receiving an agent capable of inducing anaphylaxis (e.g., injection of penicillin, allergy vaccine) the patient should be required to remain in the clinic for at least 30 minutes.

4. If a patient is allergic to insect venom, he should be counseled to wear a medical alert bracelet; not to go barefoot; to avoid fields of flowers, ripe fruit, bright-colored clothing, and perfume during warm weather; and to carry a kit containing epinephrine and a syringe for injection.

B. **Immediate treatment.** Symptoms beginning within 15 minutes after administration of the inciting agent require the most expedient management.

1. **Tourniquet.** If an injection has been given into an extremity, a tourniquet should immediately be applied proximal to the site to obstruct venous return from the injection.

2. **Aqueous epinephrine 1:1000**

   a. **Pediatric dose.** 0.01 mL per kg (0.005 mL per lb); maximum single dose, 0.3 mL.

   b. **Adult dose.** 0.3–0.5 mL.

   c. Inject dose (**a** or **b**) subcutaneously into the upper arm and massage area. Repeat same dose in 5 minutes if necessary.

   d. Also inject same dose (**a** or **b**) one time below the tourniquet around the site of the offending injection or sting to decrease absorption of antigen.

3. **Aqueous epinephrine 1:10,000** (1 mL of 1:1000 diluted with 9 mL of IV fluid) should be given intravenously *(if patient is in shock).*

   a. **Pediatric dose.** 0.1 mL per kg (0.05 mL per lb); maximum dose 3 mL.

   b. **Adult dose.** 3–5 mL.

4. **Airway.** Maintain airway and administer oxygen by mask. Hypoxia can result from hypotension and upper airway edema.

5. **Intravenous therapy.** Start an intravenous infusion and be prepared to administer the following supportive therapy if patient fails to respond to initial therapy or is in shock when first seen. *Steps 1–4 above should always be done first.*

   a. **Shock.** Give intravenous fluid (normal saline solution or lactated Ringer's solutions) *rapidly* to support blood pressure. In anaphylaxis, shock results from vasodilation and subsequent inadequate plasma volume.

      (1) **Pediatric dose.** 20 mL per kg (10 mL per lb) over 15–30 minutes, then slow to 10 mL per kg (5 mL per lb) per hour.

      (2) **Adult dose.** 1000 mL per 15–30 minutes.

   b. **Bronchospasm.** Give aminophylline solution intravenously *after shock is controlled.*

(1) **Pediatric and adult dose.** 6 mg per kg (3 mg per lb) diluted in 100–200 mL of IV fluid over 10–20 minutes; maximum dose, 500 mg. Inject slowly, not more rapidly than 25 mg/min.

(2) **Reduce dose of aminophylline if patient has received recent theophylline therapy.**

6. **Solumedrol** as an intravenous bolus may prevent delayed effects or be useful in severe bronchospasm; consult physician.

7. **Record.** Maintain a flow sheet with time, vital signs, and medications administered.

8. **Consultation.** Contact physician for further therapeutic guidance, but do not leave the patient alone.

VII. Complications

A. **Upper airway obstruction.** Pharyngeal, uvular, or laryngeal edema, or any combination of these, can develop acutely, especially in children. Observe pharynx frequently. Be prepared to insert oral or endotracheal airway.

B. **Lower airway obstruction.** Bronchospasm in children may be so severe that decreased tidal volume makes wheezing inaudible.

C. **Hypotension.** Frequent pulse and blood pressure determinations should be done.

D. **Cardiac arrhythmias.** Arrhythmias may arise owing to hypoxia, especially in adults.

E. **Aspiration of gastric contents.** In children, vomiting often accompanies anaphylaxis.

F. **Hypoxic seizures.**

G. **Cardiac arrest.**

VIII. Consultation–Referral

After instituting immediate therapy (**VI.B**), contact physician for further therapy and disposition.

IX. Follow-Up

A. An allergy label should be placed on the front cover of the patient's medical record.

B. If the reaction was to an insect sting, the patient should be referred for desensitization. Follow-up should be done to ensure that desensitization is instituted and that preventive measures (**VI.A.4**) are being taken.

C. Patients at risk for recurrent Anaphylaxis (insect hypersensitivity) should have and be instructed in the use of epinephrine injectable (EA-Pen or Ana-Kit).

▲ ANIMAL BITES: PEDIATRIC AND ADULT

I. Definition and Etiology

Bites of any animal, provoked or unprovoked, excluding snakes (see Snake Bites: Pediatric and Adult).

II. Clinical Features

A. **Symptoms.** Few, other than pain at the site of bite.

B. **Signs.** Puncture wounds or lacerations.

III. Laboratory Studies

Culture of infected bites.

IV. Differential Diagnosis

The chief concern is the possibility of rabies in the offending animal. Unprovoked bites must be treated with more suspicion than bites from teased or taunted animals. Bites from wild animals should be treated as rabid unless the animal is found to be free of rabies.

A. Any mammal may carry rabies.

B. The dog is no longer the chief carrier in the United States; other animals, such as skunks, foxes, raccoons, and bats now account for almost 85% of animal rabies annually.

C. Bite: the virus is contained in the saliva of the infected animal and transmitted to the wound by the teeth penetrating the skin; thus, claw scratches do not transmit virus. Nonbite: contamination of open wounds and mucous membranes, or abrasion with saliva from an infected animal.

D. Rabbits, squirrels, chipmunks, rats, and mice are seldom infective.

E. Properly vaccinated animals have only a slight chance of developing the disease.

V. Treatment

A. Wash the wound immediately with copious amounts of soap and water. Then carefully wash away all traces of soap and wash with Zephiran (benzalkonium chloride) solution (Zephiran is inactivated by soap). Alcohol, 40–70%, or povidone-iodine solution may be substituted for Zephiran.

B. **Control bleeding.**

C. **Tetanus prophylaxis** in wound management (see Table 2-1.)*

D. **Rabies prophylaxis.** Consult physician; therapy only after consultation. There appear to be benefits from beginning therapy as soon as possible if a risk of rabies is present.

---

*See MMWR, Update on Adult Immunization, Vol. 40 (DHHS Publication, No. RR12, (Nov. 15, 1991), pp. 63–64.

TABLE 2-1

SUMMARY GUIDE TO TETANUS PROPHYLAXIS*
IN ROUTINE WOUND MANAGEMENT, UNITED STATES

	CLEAN, MINOR WOUNDS		ALL OTHER WOUNDS†	
	Td§	TIG	Td§	TIG
Uncertain or <3	Yes	No	Yes	Yes
>3**	No††	No	No§§	No

*Refer also to text on specific vaccines or toxoids for contraindications, precautions, dosages, side effects, adverse reactions, and special considerations, important details are in the text and in the ACIP recommendations on diphtheria, tetanus, and pertussis (DTP) (MMWR 1991:40[RR-10]).

†Such as, but not limited to: wounds contaminated with dirt, feces, and saliva; puncture wounds; avulsions; and wounds resulting from missiles, crushing, burns, and frostbite.

§Td = Tetanus and diphtheria toxoids, adsorbed (for adult use). For children <7 years old, DTP (DT, if pertussis vaccine is contraindicated) is preferred to tetanus toxoid alone. For persons ≥7 years old, Td is preferred to tetanus toxoid alone. TIG = Tetanus immune globulin.

**If only three doses of fluid toxoid have been received, a fourth dose of toxoid, preferably an adsorbed toxoid, should be given.

††Yes, >10 years since last dose.

§§Yes, >5 years since last dose. (More frequent boosters are not needed and can accentuate side effects.)

VI. Complications

A. Infection at wound site.

B. Rarely, tetanus.

C. Rabies.

VII. Consultation–Referral

A. All bites in which there is reasonable suspicion of rabies.

B. All large or dirty bites for instructions, wound management, and rabies and tetanus prophylaxis.

IX. Follow-Up

As recommended by consultant.

▲ SNAKE BITES: PEDIATRIC AND ADULT

I. Definition

Snake bites can be classified as those caused by:

A. Nonpoisonous snakes.

B. Poisonous snakes but with no envenomation (injection of venom).

C. Poisonous snakes with envenomation.

II. Etiology

(snakes native to the United States)

A. Pit vipers

1. Varieties

   a. **Rattlesnakes.** Several different rattlesnakes are found in the continental United States with a pattern of distribution such that all areas of the country have one or more species.

   b. **Copperhead moccasin.** This snake is found in the southern United States, especially in the highlands.

   c. **Water, or cottonmouth, moccasin.** This snake is found in southern swamps, rivers, and ponds.

2. **Description**

   a. All have **triangular heads.**

   b. All have **pits** between each eye and nostril.

   c. All have **elliptical** (rather than round) **pupils.**

   d. **Other features.** Rattlesnakes usually have rattles on the ends of their tails. Water moccasins have white mouths.

3. **Severity.** Rattlesnake bites generally are more serious than those of other species because of the amount and potency of venom injected by its bite.

B. Eastern coral snake

1. **Location.** Florida, coastal Georgia, and the coastal Carolinas.

2. **Description.** This is a small red and black striped snake with yellow rings separating red from black. Its nose is black, and it does not have a noticeable neck or a spade-shaped or triangular head. It may be confused with the nonpoisonous scarlet king snake, which does not have a black nose.

3. **Severity.** Venom is very toxic and affects the nervous system. Fortunately, the snake is shy and rarely bites.

III. Clinical Features of Pit Viper Bites

A. Symptoms (with envenomation)

1. Pain at site of bite.

2. Paresthesias of affected part, scalp, tongue, perioral region.

3. General weakness.

4. Faintness and dizziness.

5. Nausea, vomiting, and diarrhea.

Note: Eastern coral snakes cause almost no local symptoms, and systemic symptoms are slow to develop.

B. **Signs**
1. **General** (if severe envenomation)
a. Hypotension.
b. Sweating.
c. Muscle vesiculation.
2. **Local**
a. Puncture wound.
b. Swelling and edema.
c. Erythema.
d. Ecchymoses.
C. **Gradation of wounds**
1. **Grade 0** (no envenomation). Minimal pain and less than 1 inch of surrounding edema and erythema. *No* systemic involvement. Approximately 20% of pit viper bites produce Grade 0 (no envenomation) reactions.
2. **Grade 1** (minimal envenomation). Severe pain, and 1–5 inches of surrounding edema and erythema in the first 12 hours after the bite. No systemic involvement.
3. **Grade 2** (moderate envenomation). Severe pain, 6–12 inches of surrounding edema and erythema in past 12 hours. Systemic symptoms (e.g., nausea, vomiting, giddiness, shock, prosis, weakness, abnormal reflexes) occasionally present.
4. **Grade 3** (severe envenomation). Severe pain and greater than 12 inches of surrounding edema and erythema in first 12 hours. Systemic symptoms and coagulation defects present.
5. **Grade 4** (very severe envenomation). Severe pain, edema of entire extremity, and generalized petechiae and ecchymoses. Systemic symptoms appear rapidly.

IV. **Laboratory Diagnosis**
None is necessary before consultation with physician.

V. **Differential Diagnosis**
A. Poisonous versus nonpoisonous snake.
B. Envenomation versus nonenvenomation. (Pit vipers may not envenomate, particularly if the snake has just eaten or struck another object.) Usually symptoms will appear within 10–20 minutes of the bite. If the wound is more than 1 hour old and there is no local pain or tenderness, then envenomation has probably not occurred. If edema and erythema have not occurred in 4 hours, then it is generally safe to assume that envenomation has not occurred.

VI. **Treatment**
A. **All snake bites** (including those of nonpoisonous snakes)

1. Clean wound with an antiseptic solution, such as benzalkonium chloride (Zephiran) or povidone-iodine (Betadine) or with soap and water.

2. Carry out tetanus prophylaxis, depending on immunization status (see Animal Bites: Pediatric and Adult, **V.C.**, p.59).

B. **Pit viper bites**

1. **Bites seen within 1 hour.** If specific therapy is not available in less than 1 hour, administer first aid for Grades 1–4 bites seen within 1 hour and suspected of being made by a poisonous snake.

    a. Apply a tourniquet above the site of the bite. The tourniquet should be applied just tightly enough to impede lymphatic flow. A different technique for impeding the absorption and spread of the venom consists of placing a firm dressing such as folded gauze or a clean handkerchief over the bite site; with Ace bandage tightly wrap the area of the bite as well as proximal to the bite.

    b. Make a single longitudinal incision 1/8–1/4 inch in length through the fang marks and about 1/4 inch deep or as deep as the fang mark. Apply mechanical suction over the incision for at least 15 minutes.

2. **Bites seen after 1 hour.** Steps **1a** and **b** are no longer helpful and should not be done.

    a. Keep patient quiet and lying down.

    b. Do *not* pack extremity in ice or ice water.

    c. Do *not* give patient alcohol.

    d. Monitor blood pressure, pulse, and respiratory rate every half hour.

    e. Be prepared to treat shock.

3. **Specific therapy.** Consult physician for all snake bites. There is good evidence that prompt local excision of the poisonous snake bite wound can remove large amounts of venom and reduce the need for antivenin, particularly for bites by the copperhead. If the decision to give antivenin has been made, first evaluate for sensitivity, and then proceed promptly to administration, because delay decreases the effectiveness.

    a. **Evaluating for sensitivity.**

    Antivenin (Crotalidae) is in horse serum and can cause immediate anaphylaxis and a delayed serum sickness reaction. Appropriate measures to guard against a severe allergic reaction must be taken:

    (1) A careful history of previous allergic reactions or illnesses such as hives, asthma, or drug reaction should be obtained. Specific questions about prior exposure to

horse serum and/or allergic reaction to horse serum or horses should be asked.

(2) A skin test should be performed as below prior to the injection of antivenin regardless of the history as obtained above. Inject 0.02–0.03 mL of 1:10 dilution of antivenin intracutaneously. A control test using sodium chloride injection USP may be used in another site.

If the history for allergy and the skin test are negative, one may proceed with caution to infuse the antivenin IV. If the history and skin tests are positive, one must carefully weigh the presumed need for antivenin vs. the likelihood of a severe, perhaps fatal anaphylactic reaction. Techniques for dealing with allergic patients are included in the package insert and in the PDR. A syringe of aqueous epinephrine (1:1000 dilution) should be readily available at all times when using antivenin in case of severe allergic reaction.

b. **Dosage and route of administration.** Antivenin should be given by IV drip. To administer, prepare a 1:1 to 1:10 dilution of the reconstituted antivenin in sodium chloride for injection USP or 5% Dextrose Injection USP.

(1) **Grade 0.** No antivenin.

(2) **Grade 1.** 2–4 vials (20–40 mL) antivenin (Crotalidae) polyvalent* IV.

(3) **Grade 2.** 5–9 vials (50–90 mL) antivenin IV. Do sensitivity test first (see **a**).

(4) **Grade 3.** 10–15 vials (100–150 mL) antivenin IV. Do sensitivity test first (see **a**).

(5) **Grade 4.** Greater than 15 vials (Greater than 150 mL).

C. **Coral snake bites**

1. Any person who is bitten by a coral snake and who has a break in the skin from teeth or fangs should be referred to a physician and observed for 48 hours.

2. If there are fang marks, wash the lesion and apply a tourniquet until consultation can be obtained.

3. Refer to physician and obtain North American coral snake antivenin.*

VII. Complications

A. Respiratory depression.

---

*Wyeth Lab, P.O. Box 8299, Philadelphia PA 19101.

    B. Cardiovascular collapse.

    C. Coma.

    D. Local necrosis.

    E. Infection of wound.

    F. Joint disability.

    G. Loss of digits or extremity.

VIII. Consultation–Referral

Consult physician for management of all snake bites.

IX. Follow-Up

All persons receiving antivenin should be told of the possible symptoms of serum sickness (malaise, arthralgia, urticaria, swelling of lymph nodes, fever). Should any of these develop (usually within 8–12 days), patient should return.

▲ Minor Burns: Pediatric and Adult

I. Definition

Thermal injuries to the skin, which may be

    A. **First degree.** Erythema only.

    B. **Second degree (partial thickness).** Blister formation with or without peeling and weeping.

    C. **Third degree (full thickness).** Early on, may have charred or whitish appearance and areas of anesthesia.

II. Etiology

Contact with any heat source. The degree of damage depends on the duration of exposure and the source of heat. Scalds generally cause second-degree burns, whereas flame or hot metal may cause third-degree burns.

III. Clinical features

    A. **Symptoms.** Usually only pain. Severe burns with nerve damage may be less painful than first- or second-degree burns.

    B. **Signs.** See I.

IV. Laboratory Studies

None.

V. Differential Diagnosis

Consider abuse or neglect in pediatric age group and in the elderly or mentally retarded.

VI. Treatment

    A. **First-degree burn**

    1. Plunge affected area into cold water for several minutes, if less than 45 minutes have elapsed since burn injury.

    2. Clean gently with soap and water.

    3. No dressings are necessary.

B. Second-degree burn

    1. Plunge affected area into cold water for several minutes, if less than 45 minutes have elapsed since burn injury.

    2. Clean gently with soap and water.

    3. Leave blisters intact but may perform simple debridement of open blisters.

    4. Cover burned area with silver sulfadiazine 1% cream (Silvadene) nonadherent gauze, and bulky dry sterile dressing.

    5. Carry out tetanus prophylaxis; see Animal Bites: Pediatric and Adult, **V.C.**, p. 59.

C. Third degree burn. Refer to physician in all cases.

VII. Complications

    A. Bacterial infection.

    B. Progression of second to third degree, if infection develops.

VIII. Consultation–Referral

    A. All third-degree burns including those that may only partially involve the burned area.

    B. Extensive second-degree burns that involve an area greater than that covered by examiner's hand.

    C. Facial burns.

    D. Any suspicion of child abuse or neglect.

IX. Follow-Up

    A. **First-degree burn.** None.

    B. **Second-degree burn**

        1. Have the patient return in 2 days for dressing change.

        2. Have the patient return every 1–2 days thereafter until epithelialization occurs without infection.

▲ CARDIAC ARREST: PEDIATRIC AND ADULT

I. Definition

The cessation of effective cardiac function due to either a failure of electrical excitation (cardiac standstill) or an arrhythmia that does not permit effective ventricular contraction (e.g., ventricular fibrillation).

II. Etiology

Cardiac arrest may be associated with any severe illness, but in an ambulatory setting it usually occurs in persons with acute or chronic cardiac or respiratory disease, that is, arteriosclerotic heart disease with or without myocardial infarction or chronic obstructive pulmonary disease. In children, cardiac arrest is much more likely to be caused by hypoxia (with or without airway obstruction) or shock/hypovolemia due to other causes.

III. Clinical Features

A. **Symptoms.** Associated with underlying disease.

B. **Signs**

1. Absent pulses and blood pressure. (See also Shock: Pediatric and Adult, pp. 83–87.)

2. Unconsciousness.

3. Absent or gasping respirations.

4. Cyanosis.

IV. Laboratory Studies

There is no need for laboratory tests other than blood gases and pH during the acute episode surrounding a cardiac arrest.

V. Differential Diagnosis

See II.

VI. Treatment

Ultimately, treatment depends on etiology; initially, however, there are certain things that must be done once it has been determined that there is no perfusion and that heartbeat is either absent or irregular and ineffective. If a physician is not present and the patient is a candidate for resuscitation, the nurse practitioner should begin the following measures with assistance from other clinical personnel and notify physician.

A. **Notify physician and activate EMS system.**

B. **Airway measures**

1. Examine the airway for foreign objects.

TABLE 2-2

SUGGESTED VENTILATION/STERNAL COMPRESSION RATES IN CHILDREN

	12 MOS	1–8 YRS	OVER 8 YRS
Site of compression	midsternal	lower third of sternum	lower third of sternum
Rate of compression	at least 100 min.	100/min	80–100/min
Rate of ventilation*	20/min	20/min	12/min

*This is the minimal rate of ventilation. Hyperventilation is often useful.

2. Pull jaw forward and tilt neck. A mouthpiece that holds the tongue forward may be useful. In cases involving trauma to the neck or head, use a modified jaw thrust.

3. Begin mouth-to-mouth resuscitation, or if available use an Ambu bag.

4. Attach oxygen to Ambu bag as soon as it becomes available.

5. Suction secretions present in the mouth and throat frequently.

6. See Table 2-2 for proper rate of ventilation.

7. A nasogastric tube is usually helpful to prevent vomiting.

C. External cardiac massage*

1. If patient is lying on couch or other soft surface, place board under his or her back. If no board is available, quickly transfer patient to floor.

2. Place hands on lower sternum (midsternum in a young child) so that downward pressure will compress the heart between the sternum and the spinal column. For adults arms should be relatively stiff so that pressure is applied from the shoulder through the heels of the hands.

3. Begin cardiac massage. See Table 2-2 for rate.

4. External massage should generate a pulse. Evaluate success by palpating a large artery, such as the femoral or brachial artery.

D. **Place an intravenous line**

1. Use one of the following fluids to keep the IV line open for medication:

   a. 0.9% saline solution.

   or

   b. Lactated Ringer's solution.

   or

   c. Any available standard IV solution.

2. Begin flow sheet to record drug administration and vital signs.

3. Sodium bicarbonate is not routinely used and should not be administered at this time.

E. **Obtain initial ECG**

1. **No electrical activity.** Confirm asystole in 2 leads. Administer epinephrine (see Table 2-3). Alternative treatment is used if standard Rx fails.

---

*Guidelines for Cardiopulmonary Resuscitation and Emergency Cardiac Care. Emergency Committee and Subcommittee, American Heart Association. JAMA 268(16): 2171–2275, Oct. 28, 1992.

TABLE 2-3

RECOMMENDED DOSES OF EPINEPHRINE IN ADULTS AND CHILDREN

	INTRAVENOUS	ENDOTRACHEAL
Adult		
Standard therapy	1 mg (10 mL of 1:10,000 solution)	2 mg (2 mL of 1:1,000 solution)
Alternative therapy	2–5 mg	Double the dose
	Repeat every 3–5 minutes	
or	1 mg–3 mg–5-mg push,	
	3 minutes apart	
or	0.1 mg/kg	
	Repeat every 3–5 minutes	
Pediatric		
Standard therapy	0.01 mg/kg (1:10,000)	0.1 mg/kg (1:1,000)
	followed by	followed by
	0.1 mg/kg (1:10,000)	0.2 mg/kg (1:1,000)
Alternative therapy	0.2 mg/kg (1:10,000)	Double the dose
	Repeat every 3–5 minutes	

2. **Ventricular fibrillation.** Begin defibrillation at 2–3 watt-seconds/kg in children, 200 watt-seconds in adults, if the following conditions apply:

   a. No pulse or heartbeat is detectable.

   b. An airway has been established and oxygen therapy begun.

   c. A blow to the sternum has not generated a heartbeat.

   d. Ventricular fibrillation is likely or is seen on ECG. If initial defibrillation is ineffective, increase voltage to 300 watt-seconds in adults and double the voltage in children and repeat defibrillation up to 2 times for the first round.

F. **Treatment without defibrillation.** If there is no defibrillator available or no one present trained in its use, maintain assisted respiration and external cardiac massage (see **B** through **D** above).

   1. **No electrical activity.** Administer epinephrine (see Table 2-3). Alternative therapy is used if standard therapy fails.

   2. **Electrical activity without palpable pulse** (electromechanical dissociation).

      a. Continue CPR.

      b. Epinephrine (see Table 2-3).

      c. Consider sodium bicarbonate, 1 mEq/kg and repeat half original dose every 10 minutes.

3. **Ventricular fibrillation.** Although in this situation chemical intervention is rarely effective, one may try the following:

   a. Lidocaine, 1.5 mg/kg directly into IV line over 2–4 minutes (use IV lidocaine labeled for cardiac arrhythmias, which has no preservatives); 1 mg/kg IV bolus for children.

   b. If initial dose of lidocaine does not stop fibrillation, repeat in 10–15 minutes.

   c. Bretylium 5 mg/kg bolus (500 mg in adult). May double dose in 10 minutes.

G. **Final steps.** Continue resuscitation until heartbeat and adequate respiration are restored. The patient then should be transferred to a hospital as soon as a vehicle with support equipment is available. Discontinue resuscitation only after consultation with a physician.

VII. Complications

A. Central nervous system damage from hypoxia.

B. Renal tubular necrosis.

C. Adult respiratory distress syndrome (shock lung).

VIII. Consultation–Referral

All patients, after lifesaving measures have been initiated.

IX. Follow-Up

Varies with each patient.

▲ CONVULSIONS: PEDIATRIC

I. Definition

Tonic or clonic muscular contractions, or both, usually associated with unconsciousness. They are expressions of abnormal electrical discharge of neurons in the central nervous system (CNS).

A. The terms *convulsions, seizures, epilepsy,* and *fits* may be used synonymously by patients.

B. This definition applies to major motor convulsions only. Any unexplained, episodic alteration of consciousness could represent a seizure or abnormal electrical discharge in the CNS.

II. Etiology

(list is not exhaustive)

A. **Neonatal period**

   1. Anoxic CNS injury.

   2. Birth trauma.

   3. CNS infection.

   4. Hypoglycemia.

    5. Hypocalcemia.

    6. Congenital abnormalities of the CNS.

B. Infancy

    1. Febrile convulsions.

    2. CNS infection.

    3. Residual damage from prenatal or perinatal causes.

    4. CNS trauma.

    5. Ingestion of drugs or poisons.

    6. Ischemia or anoxia, such as breath-holding spells.

C. Childhood

    1. Idiopathic and familial epilepsy.

    2. Residual damage from prenatal or perinatal causes.

    3. CNS infection.

    4. Ingestion of drugs or poisons.

    5. CNS trauma.

    6. Glomerulonephritis.

    7. Brain masses.

III. Clinical Features

(depend to some extent on age and etiology)

A. Symptoms

    1. Sometimes, short prodrome of irritability, anorexia, headache and lethargy.

    2. Symptoms characterizing underlying disorder.

B. Signs (usual sequential evolution; may be great variation, however, depending in part on underlying disorder)

    1. Usually, abrupt onset of tonic muscular contraction.

    2. Tonic spasm often occurring simultaneously with loss of consciousness.

    3. Facial pallor, often followed by erythema and then cyanosis, depending on length of tonic spasm of respiratory muscles.

    4. Eyeballs rolled upward or to one side.

    5. Head hyperextended or turned to one side. Contorted expression caused by contraction of facial muscles.

    6. Abdominal and chest muscles in tonic spasm, often accompanied by urination and occasionally by defecation.

    7. Clonic phase (rhythmic contraction of muscles), localized or generalized, and lasting for a variable period of time.

    8. Often, sleep or lethargy.

IV. Laboratory Studies

After consultation. Tests depend on suspected underlying cause. (Save blood for glucose determination, or do Dextrostix before giving glucose.)

V. Differential Diagnosis

A. Tremulousness associated with high fever or chills or both.

B. Hypoglycemia can cause both behavior disturbances and convulsions.

C. Breath-holding spell causing unconsciousness. Occasionally breath-holding spell can lead to enough anoxia to cause a convulsion.

D. Syncope can at times precipitate a brief tonic/clonic seizure.

VI. Treatment

In the great majority of cases, convulsions are self-limited and cease before treatment is instituted. Occasionally, more harm is done by overtreatment than by observation.

A. General measures

1. Maintain a clear airway by turning the patient on one side with head low to encourage gravitational drainage of secretions and vomitus and to prevent aspiration. Suction when necessary.

2. Give oxygen.

3. Position the patient so as to prevent injury by falling or knocking against objects.

4. Do *not* try to pry clenched jaws apart to place an object between teeth.

5. Observe and be able to describe the duration and focal elements of the convulsion, which include:

   a. Unusual behavior before the convulsion.

   b. Movements of one part or side of the body early or late in the convulsion.

   c. Persistent weakness of one part of the body after the convulsion has occurred.

B. Specific therapy

1. **History.** Obtain a brief history sufficient to discover any etiologic disorder that will respond to specific therapy, for example:

   a. Insulin-induced hypoglycemia.

   b. Intracranial hemorrhage caused by head trauma.

   c. Hyponatremia from treatment of prolonged diarrhea by non-sodium-containing fluids.

   d. High fever prior to convulsion.

2. Lorazepam (or diazepam if lorazepam is not available) should be used under the following circumstances (see Table 2-4):

   a. A convulsion has lasted more than 10 minutes.

   or

TABLE 2-4

ANTICONVULSANT DOSES

Lorazepam 0.05–01 mg/kg IM or PR up to 4 mg maximum. May repeat same dose in 15 minutes up to a total dose of 0.2 mg/kg or 8 mg maximum.

Valium 0.5 mg/kg PR up to 10 mg maximum.

---

     b. Three or more separate convulsions have occurred in the preceding 30 minutes.

   3. **Transfer of patient.** If a physician consultation is not available at the time lorazepam or diazepam (Valium) is given, transfer the patient, accompanied by trained personnel, to a facility where a physician is available.

VII. Complications

  A. Aspiration of vomitus causing pneumonitis or lung abscess.

  B. Prolonged anoxia causing CNS injury.

  C. Traumatic injury during convulsion.

  D. Complications of the underlying disorder.

  E. Cardiorespiratory depression caused by anticonvulsants.

VIII. Consultation–Referral

A physician should be consulted concerning all convulsing patients, even if convulsions stop spontaneously before patient arrives in the clinic. Therapy may be started while the consultant is being contacted.

IX. Follow-Up

As recommended by consultant.

▲ CONVULSIONS: ADULT

I. Definition

Clonic or tonic muscular contractions, or both, usually associated with unconsciousness. Contractions are often accompanied by salivation and followed by incontinence.

II. Etiology

  A. Idiopathic epilepsy

    1. Initial onset may occur in adulthood but most frequently happens in childhood and puberty.

    2. Seizure in a known epileptic.

  B. Drug withdrawal (most commonly barbiturates).

  C. Alcohol withdrawal. Usually short-lived and occurring as one seizure or repeated seizures within a space of a few hours during the first several days after withdrawal.

D. **Hypoglycemia.** The effects of hypoglycemia on CNS range from inappropriate behavior to confusion to coma.

E. **Hypertensive encephalopathy.**

F. **Cardiac arrhythmia.** Seizures associated with arrhythmias are usually short-lived and generally have only the tonic component.

G. **Expanding brain lesion.**

III. **Clinical Features**

A. **Symptoms**

1. History of

   a. Epilepsy.

   b. Use of insulin or oral hypoglycemic agents.

   c. Hypertension.

   d. Alcohol or drug abuse.

   e. Situational problems and emotional stress, particularly in young females.

2. No obvious cause.

3. Classic cry at beginning of seizure.

B. **Signs** (usual sequential evolution; may be great variation, however, depending in part on underlying disorder).

1. Usually, abrupt onset of tonic muscular contraction.

2. Tonic spasm often occurring simultaneously with loss of consciousness.

3. Facial pallor, often followed by erythema and then cyanosis, depending on length of tonic spasm of respiratory muscles.

4. Eyeballs rolled upward or to one side.

5. Head hyperextended or turned to one side. Contorted expression caused by contraction of facial muscles.

6. Incontinence, abdominal and chest muscles in tonic spasm, often accompanied by urination and occasionally by defecation.

7. Clonic phase (rhythmic contraction of muscles), localized or generalized, and lasting for a variable period of time.

8. Usually, postictal confusion, sleep or lethargy.

IV. **Laboratory Studies**

Not necessary in the case of an actively convulsing patient.

V. **Differential Diagnosis**

A. See II.

B. Occasionally an hysterical patient may mimic movements of a convulsion.

C. Simple vasovagal syncope may produce brief episodes of tonic or clonic movement.

VI. Treatment

A. **History of a seizure.** Refer to physician for:

1. Diagnosis.

or

2. Regulation of drugs, if seizure was in a known epileptic.

B. **Active convulsion.** Nurse practitioners should not attempt to treat convulsions alone, unless there is no alternative. The following are guidelines for treating adults until transfer or consultation is obtained. Most seizures are self-limited and often stop during evaluation. Occasionally more harm is done by overtreatment than by observation.

1. **General measures**

   a. Maintain a clear airway by turning the patient on one side with head low to encourage gravity drainage of secretions and vomitus and to prevent aspiration. Suction when necessary.

   b. Give oxygen for cyanosis.

   c. Position the patient so as to prevent injury by falling or knocking against objects.

   d. Do *not* try to pry clenched jaws apart to place an object between teeth.

   e. Observe and be able to describe the duration and focal elements of the convulsion (see Convulsions: Pediatric, **VI.A.5**, p. 72).

   f. Monitor respirations, blood pressure, temperature, and pulse.

B. **Specific therapy**

1. If after above assessment, patient is still having seizure:

   a. Start IV infusion.

   b. Give 20 mL of 50% glucose IV.

2. If no response in 5 minutes, give up to 10 mg of diazepam (Valium) IV over 3–5 minutes.

Note: Phenytoin takes sufficiently long for effective therapeutic action that it is not used initially to terminate seizures. Acute initiation of phenytoin therapy requires a loading dose and should *not* be done without physician consultation.

VII. Complications

A. Status epilepticus.

B. Aspiration.

C. Traumatic injury during convulsion.

D. Complications of the underlying disorder.

VIII. Consultation–Referral

Consult on all seizures, but therapy may be started.

IX. Follow-Up

Individualize for patient or cause of seizure.

▲ MINOR HEAD INJURIES: PEDIATRIC AND ADULT

I. Definition

Trauma to the head that does *not* result in any alteration of cerebral function.

II. Etiology

A blow to the head occurring in any of a host of circumstances in which either an object strikes the skull or the skull strikes an object.

III. Clinical Features

The nurse practitioner should manage *only* those patients having minor head injuries as defined by the following positive and negative symptoms and signs:

A. Symptoms
   1. *No* loss of consciousness at time of injury.
   2. *No* alteration in sensorium from the time of injury until the patient is seen and evaluated.
   3. *No* nausea or vomiting.
   4. *No* focal neurologic symptoms.
   5. Sometimes, minimally to moderately severe headache.

B. Signs
   1. Normal vital signs.
   2. *No* palpable defect on examination of the skull.
   3. Sometimes, localized area of tenderness over the skull.
   4. *No* discharge from the ears.
   5. *No* discharge from the nose.
   6. *No* blood behind tympanic membranes.
   7. Full consciousness, alertness, and orientation to time, person, and place.
   8. Intact cranial nerves.
   9. *No* weakness on motor testing.
   10. *No* demonstrable sensory loss.
   11. Intact and symmetric reflexes.
   12. Flexor plantar response.

IV. Laboratory and Other Studies

None indicated in minor head injury.

V. Differential Diagnosis

Minor head injury (see III) must be differentiated from all other head injuries.

VI. Treatment

Careful observation. The patient *may* be allowed to go home if:

A. There is a competent person who will assume responsibility for observing the patient carefully.

B. Detailed written instructions as to the nature of the observations to be made are provided. Figure 2-1 is an example of the type of written instructions to be given to the patient's family.

VII. Complications

Even a minor head injury can result in severe complications, such as subdural or epidural hematoma, and can result in rapid deterioration of the patient's neurologic status and severe disability or death. Thus, serial observations are warranted several hours post event.

VIII. Consultation–Referral

All head injuries that do not fit the definition of a minor head injury according to these guidelines.

IX. Follow-Up

See **VI** and Figure 2-1.

▲ INGESTIONS AND POISONINGS: PEDIATRIC

I. Definition

A. Ingestion or absorption of any nonfoodstuff.

B. Accidental ingestion of a medicine.

II. Etiology

Almost every substance has probably been ingested by children. Commonly ingested toxic substances include acetaminophen, iron tablets, petroleum products, psychotropic drugs (antidepressants, tranquilizers) and aspirin.

III. Clinical Features

Ingestions are most common under 5 years of age.

A. History

1. The ingestion is often witnessed, or an empty container is found where the child could have ingested its contents.

2. Ingestions are more likely to occur during periods of disruption or stress in the household.

3. Someone in the household may be on drug therapy or using illicit drugs.

FIGURE 2-1

FIGURE 2-1

INSTRUCTIONS FOR HOME OBSERVATION OF A PATIENT AFTER HEAD INJURY

OBSERVATION AFTER HEAD INJURY

The patient should be checked every 2 hours for the first 24 hours after the injury. If he is asleep, he should be awakened. If any of the following signs are noted, please call the nurse practitioner (NP) immediately or return the patient to the clinic as soon as possible.

1. Patient unusually sleepy or hard to wake up.
2. Patient mentally confused. Does not know who he is or where he is. Does not recognize familiar people or places.
3. Patient very restless, disturbed, or agitated. Being upset is normal after an accident, but when a patient becomes very nervous and excited after having been quiet and calm, it is important to report it.
4. Nausea and vomiting (complains of being "sick to my stomach" or is throwing up).
5. Severe headache.
6. Difference in the size of the pupils of the eyes. The pupil is the round, dark part of the center of the eye. Normally, pupils are both the same size.
7. Weakness of the arms or legs. This sign is especially important if it is only on one side of the body.
8. Fits, seizures, or convulsions.
9. Drainage of fluid from the ears or nose.

GUIDELINES FOR CARE AT HOME

1. The patient may move around and be up as much as he desires.
2. He may eat or drink anything, except *no* alcoholic beverages.
3. If the patient takes medicines regularly, he should be advised by a physician about taking these medicines after head injury.
4. For mild headache, the patient should lie flat until the headache goes away.

_____

NP or MD

I understand the above instructions.

_____

Signed

_____

Relationship to patient

_____

Date

4. Accidental ingestion or other accidents may have occurred in the past.

5. Child under 1 year of age may be receiving an excessive dose of medication.

6. Any ingestion in a developmentally normal school-age child may be a suicide attempt, and this possibility should be pursued.

B. **Symptoms and signs**

1. Symptoms and signs are likely to be absent if the ingestion is discovered or suspected soon after it occurred. Many ingested substances have low toxicity and will produce no symptoms or signs.

2. Poisonings and overdosage of medicines can cause a great variety of symptoms and signs, often simulating natural diseases. Consider poisoning especially under the following circumstances:

   a. History suggests (see **A**).

   b. Patient aged 1–4 years.

   c. Very sudden onset of symptoms.

   d. Abnormal odor to breath or clothes.

   e. Unexplained findings, especially unconsciousness in any patient.

IV. Laboratory Studies

As suggested by consultant, save vomitus, gastric contents, empty containers, and urine.

V. Differential Diagnosis

A. **Nonaccidental ingestion**

1. Suicide attempt in child over 5 years of age.

2. Child abuse or neglect.

B. **Natural diseases** (depending on symptoms and signs).

VI. Treatment

A. **Prevention.** Advise parents on the following preventive measures:

1. Label all containers with contents.

2. Keep medicines in safety-cap containers. Always replace cap after use.

3. Lock all medicines and poisons away and out of reach of children.

4. Do not store nondrinkable or nonedible substances in drink or food containers.

5. Keep syrup of ipecac in the house.

6. Caution parents about the risks of ingestions during disruptive periods in the household (e.g., moving, house painting, emotionally stressful situations).

B. **Telephone calls about ingestion**

1. Try to determine what and how much was ingested and when it was ingested.

2. Ask that the remainder of the ingested substance and its container be brought with the patient to the clinic or emergency department. If uncertain what might have been ingested, have all potentially ingested materials that are available in the household brought with the patient (e.g., medications).

3. *If no contraindications to vomiting exist* (see **E.2**), vomiting may be induced before leaving home or on the way to the clinic to decrease potential toxicity. Syrup of ipecac should be available in every household as part of health maintenance procedures and may be given by parents to induce vomiting (see **E.1** for dosage).

C. **General supportive therapy (as needed)**

1. **Maintenance of airway**

   a. Suction of secretions.

   b. Head turned to side and lower than stomach to avoid aspiration of vomitus.

   c. Jaw thrust, head tilt, oral airway.

2. **Cardiopulmonary resuscitation**

3. **Control of convulsions** (see Convulsions: Pediatric, **VI.** pp. 72–73.)

4. **Treatment of shock.** Start administering intravenous fluids (normal saline solution or Ringer's solution) in a dose of 20 mL per kg of body weight (10 mL per lb) over 15–30 minutes.

D. **Consultation.** Seek consultation, especially from poison control center, before further therapy if consultant is immediately available.

E. **Induction of emesis.** If consultant is not immediately available and ingestion is suspected, induce emesis with syrup of ipecac, if not contraindicated. (Do not wait for symptoms to develop.)

1. **Dose of syrup of ipecac** to induce emesis, if no contraindications are present (see **E.2**).

   a. **Six months to one year of age.** 10 mL (2 teaspoons) followed by at least 4–6 ounces of clear liquid.

   b. **One to five years of age.** 15 mL (1 tablespoon) followed by at least 6–8 ounces of clear liquid.

   c. **Over 5 years of age.** 30 mL (2 tablespoons) followed by at least 8–12 ounces of clear liquid.

   Note: If child does not vomit after 20 minutes, the same dose may be repeated once.

2. **Contraindications**

   a. **Unconsciousness** or diminished level of consciousness.

   b. **Convulsions.**

c. **Ingestion of corrosives** (strong alkali or acid) such as toilet bowl cleaners and drain cleaners (lye, Drano, Liquid PlumR, Saniflush). This may be suspected if burns are present on the lips or tongue or in the mouth, or there is pain on swallowing.

d. **Ingestion of petroleum products** (e.g., kerosene, gasoline, furniture polish, cleaning fluid, paint thinner). May be suspected by odor on the breath or clothes or by odor of the container. This is a relative, not absolute, contraindication. For example, a petroleum product may be the solvent for an extremely toxic substance. Contact the poison control center for further guidance.

e. **Other.** Ipecac should generally not be used for ingestions of tricyclic antidepressants such as amitriptyline (Elavil and others), imipramine (Tofranil and others) or nortriptyline (Aventyl and others). It should not be used for ingestion of anti-emetic medications or for non-toxic substances.

VII. Complications

These vary depending on the substance and amount to which the patient was exposed.

VIII. Consultation-Referral

All patients with established or suspected ingestion or poisoning.

IX. Follow-Up

As suggested by consultant.

▲ OVERDOSE OF SEDATIVE, HYPNOTIC, OR OPIATE DRUGS: ADULT

I. Definition

Alterations in the sensorium usually progressing to coma as a result of the accidental or intentional ingestion or injection of large quantities of any one of various central nervous system depressants.

II. Etiology

Barbiturates, opiates, phenothiazine tranquilizers, and benzodiazepams, and similar agents. The agent may be taken intentionally in a suicide attempt or accidentally, as in the injection of an unusually potent "street" drug, such as heroin.

III. Clinical Features

A. Symptoms

1. Alteration of consciousness is present and usually progresses rapidly to coma.

2. Respiratory depression is common, including progression to apnea.

3. A history obtained from those who bring the patient to the clinic often is essential in establishing the diagnosis. It is often helpful to have the patient's pill bottles or other drug containers brought to the clinic.

B. Signs

1. Varying levels of coma are present.
2. Pupils often pinpoint in opiate overdose.
3. Needle tracks may be present on arms at sites of previous IV injections of heroin.
4. Spontaneous respirations are absent.

IV. Laboratory Studies

None indicated in acute situation.

V. Differential Diagnosis

A. **Trauma.**

B. **Cerebrovascular disease** (including all forms of strokes).

C. **Severe metabolic derangements** (including diabetic ketoacidosis, hypoglycemia, and severe uremia).

VI. Treatment

A. Clear and maintain open airway.

B. Maintain respirations. Assisted ventilation by means of mouth-to-mouth respiration or an Ambu bag may be necessary.

C. Start IV infusion of dextrose in water. Give 50 mL of 50% glucose if hypoglycemia is suspected.

D. Carry out gastric lavage if drug ingestion is suspected.

E. Opiate overdose. Give naloxone HCl (Narcan), 0.4–2 mg IV if opiate overdose is suggested by the history or physical findings. An initial dose of 1 mg is frequently used. Additional doses may be administered at 2–3 minute intervals. Most patients with suspected opiate overdose have some response after 2 mg but some patients, particularly those suspected of overdosing with pentazocine (Talwin), may require more than 2 mg. If no response is observed after 10 mg has been administered, question the diagnosis of narcotic-induced toxicity.

F. Benzodiazepam overdose. If benzodiazepam overdose is suspected, give flumazenil (Anexate) 0.2 mg IV over 30 seconds. If the desired response is not obtained after waiting an additional 30 seconds, a dose of 0.3 mg IV over 30 seconds can be given. Additional doses of 0.5 mg IV given over 30 seconds can be given at 1 minute intervals to a total cumulative dose of 3.0 mg.

VII. Complications

None in acute situation.

VIII. Consultation–Referral

    A. Immediate telephone consultation for all patients.

    B. Referral as soon as patient is stabilized and adequate help is available (preferably an ambulance or rescue squad).

IX. Follow-Up

Close psychiatric management if overdose is a suicide attempt.

▲ SHOCK: PEDIATRIC AND ADULT

I. Definition

A clinical state of inadequate tissue perfusion, often characterized by hypotension and manifested by a clinical syndrome described in III.

II. Etiology

    A. **Hypovolemia.** Loss of blood or other body fluid (e.g., bleeding, diarrhea, vomiting, and excessive perspiration).

    B. **Cardiogenic disorders.** Myocardial dysfunction includes infarction, arrhythmias.

    C. **Sepsis.** Often from gram-negative organisms.

    D. **Anaphylaxis.**

    E. **Drugs and toxins.** For example, opiates, barbiturates, and hypotensive agents.

    F. **Heat prostration.**

    G. **Hypoglycemia.**

    H. **Hypoxia/asphyxia.**

III. Clinical Features

    A. **Symptoms**

        1. **General.** Patient manifests anxiousness, dizziness, lightheadedness, confusion, stupor, nausea, vomiting.

        2. **Specific** (related to etiology).

            a. **Hypovolemia.** Early in the sequence of events leading to hypovolemic shock, the patient may be syncopal on standing because of orthostatic hypotension. Patient may have a history of severe diarrhea and vomiting or inadequate fluid intake while working outside in hot weather.

            b. **Cardiogenic shock.** The characteristic pain of myocardial infarction may predominate and may be accompanied by diaphoresis.

            c. **Sepsis**

                (1) **Infants.** Poor feeding, lethargy, and fever or hypothermia.

        (2) **Older children and adults.** Fever or hypothermia, chills, lethargy, sweating. (Septic shock is seen especially with urinary tract infections in the elderly or in patients with indwelling catheters.)

    d. **Anaphylaxis.** Insect sting and drug injection are the most common causes.

    e. **Drug.** Patients usually are stuporous or in coma with barbiturate overdose. Hypotensive agents initially cause orthostatic hypotension.

B. **Signs**

  1. **General**

    a. Delayed capillary refill.

    b. Hypotension. (When shock is from volume depletion, the first manifestation may be orthostatic hypotension.) Blood pressure is not a sensitive indicator of shock in children. Hypotension in children suggests severe decompensated shock.

    c. Tachycardia.

    d. Cool, moist skin, poor capillary refill, cyanosis.

    e. Weak, thready pulse.

    f. Sweating.

    g. Pallor.

    h. Decreased urine output.

  2. **Specific** (related to etiology)

    a. **Hypovolemia**

      (1) **Bleeding**

        (a) **External.** Usually obvious, but large quantities of blood may be sequestered in the thigh from fracture of the femur.

        (b) **Internal.** Usually due to trauma; bleeding peptic ulcer manifested by hematemesis or coffee ground vomitus and melena; intraperitoneal bleeding (e.g., from a ruptured ectopic pregnancy) often manifest as a rigid, tender abdomen.

      (2) **Dehydration.** Decreased skin turgor, dry mouth, and sunken eyes.

    b. **Cardiogenic shock**

      (1) Findings may be only those cited in **B.1** that are related to lowered cardiac output.

      (2) Signs and symptoms of congestive heart failure may be present.

c. **Sepsis.** Patient usually is febrile, although elderly people, neonates, and patients with gram-negative sepsis may be afebrile or hypothermic. The patient may have signs related to underlying urinary tract infection, meningitis, etc.

d. **Anaphylaxis**

(1) **Bronchospasm.** Wheezes, increased expiratory phase may be present.

(2) **Urticaria or angioedema** are sometimes present.

(3) **Laryngeal edema** (inspiratory stridor)

e. **Drug.** Patients who have taken enough opiates or barbiturates to cause shock are usually stuporous or in coma.

IV. Laboratory Studies

Always check blood glucose (BG stick or Dextrostix). In the initial assessment of shock there is very little need for most laboratory tests, but if the cause is obscure, hematocrit and blood sugar determinations may be helpful. Do not wait for results before starting treatment. For later blood studies, see **VI.I.**

V. Differential Diagnosis

See **II.**

VI. Treatment

A physician should be consulted about the treatment of all patients. Emergency measures, however, should be started *while* the physician is being contacted.

A. Call for help from other clinic personnel and notify physician.

B. Take vital signs. Start a flow sheet and evaluate vital signs every 5 minutes after IV infusion (see **F**) has been started.

C. Assess the airway (as in any emergency):

1. Remove vomitus, if present.

2. Pull jaw forward and tilt neck (if there is no trauma involving the neck).

3. If laryngospasm is present (upper airway obstruction without foreign body or infection), treat patient as for anaphylactic shock; see Anaphylaxis: Pediatric and Adult, **VI.B,** pp. 57–58.

D. Check breathing (auscultate the chest):

1. If there are wheezes, consider anaphylaxis as well as pulmonary edema from heart failure.

2. Assist ventilation with Ambu bag and mask if necessary.

E. Check cardiac status:

1. Palpate a major vessel.

2. Quickly auscultate the heart.

F. Start an IV infusion:

1. **Fluid.** Use lactated Ringer's or normal saline solution.

2. **Rate**

   a. **Adult.** Run IV as rapidly as possible up to approximately 20–30 mL per minute in the first 30 minutes (except for cardiogenic shock [see **J.5**]).

   b. **Pediatric.** See Anaphylaxis: Pediatric and Adult, **VI.B.5.a.(1)**, p. 57.

G. Obtain a quick medical history:

1. **Underlying diseases**

   a. Heart disease.

   b. Allergy to insect or medication.

   c. Bleeding disorder.

   d. Diabetes mellitus.

   e. Chronic urinary tract infection.

2. **Current history**

   a. Insect sting.

   b. Drug injection or ingestion.

   c. Symptoms (vomiting, diarrhea) or signs (fever).

   d. Exposure to infection, heat, toxin, trauma.

   e. Symptoms of urinary tract infection.

   f. Time course.

H. Do a quick physical examination:

1. **Skin.** Petechiae or purpura (occasionally associated with sepsis).

2. **Neck.** Rigidity (meningitis).

3. **Chest.** Wheezing, rales (anaphylaxis, pneumonia, sepsis, congestive heart failure).

4. **Heart.** Arrhythmias, murmurs.

5. **Abdomen**

   a. Size of liver.

   b. Abdominal rigidity (peritonitis).

   c. Flank pain.

   d. Prostatic tenderness.

   e. Stool for occult blood.

   f. Vomitus for blood.

I. Draw blood for:

1. Glucose.

2. Blood culture.

3. Complete blood count differential and platelet count.

4. Electrolytes.

5. Blood urea nitrogen.

6. Future use (hold).

J. Start specific treatment:

1. **Bleeding or hypovolemia.** IV fluids have been started, which is initially sufficient and lifesaving until help can be obtained.

2. **Anaphylaxis.** See Anaphylaxis: Pediatric and Adult, VI.B, pp. 57–58.

3. **Hypoglycemia.** 20 mL of 50% dextrose (2 mL/kg of 25% solution for children) should be given IV, without waiting for results of blood glucose test.

4. **Sepsis.** IV fluids should be sufficient until help can be obtained.

5. **Cardiogenic shock.** If shock and pulmonary edema are present in a setting that suggests myocardial infarction, IV fluid should not be pushed, but an open IV line is essential in administering the drugs necessary to treat this condition after consultation.

VII. Complications

A. Complications of the **etiologic** problem.

B. Complications of shock (generally **end-organ destruction**).

1. **Brain.** Ischemia, leaving neurologic deficits.

2. **Kidney.** Acute tubular necrosis.

3. **Lungs.** Adult respiratory distress syndrome (ARDS, shock lung).

VIII. Consultation–Referral

All patients require immediate consultation.

IX. Follow-Up

Varies with individual patient.

▲ SMALL OPEN WOUNDS: PEDIATRIC AND ADULT

I. Definition

Lacerations that:

A. Are *not* located on the face.

B. Do *not* penetrate the subcutaneous tissue.

C. Are *not* associated with functional disturbance, that is, not involving tendons, ligaments, vessels, or nerves.

D. Have *not* been made by a grossly contaminated object.

E. Are small and sufficiently clean so that the edges can be easily

approximated using adhesives or cutaneous sutures. Approxima-
tion must be carried out without trimming tissue or placing undue
tension on the suture line.

II. Etiology

Any of innumerable objects that could sever the skin.

III. Clinical Features

See I.

IV. Laboratory Studies

Culture infected wounds.

V. Treatment

A. Wounds that do not require sutures

1. The primary consideration is to keep the wound clean and dry:
   a. Clean with warm water and soap, making sure that dirt and foreign bodies have been removed.
   b. Cover with a loose bandage that will keep out dirt and protect the wound from trauma.
   c. If wound is clean and easily approximated, steri strips may be used.
2. If there is inflammation, the wound should be soaked and washed with soap and water for 15–20 minutes 3–4 times a day, and a clean dressing should be applied at home each day until healing begins; then, daily soaking and dressing are sufficient. Do not use steri strips.
3. Tetanus prophylaxis; see Animal Bites: Pediatric and Adult, V.C, p. 59.

B. Wounds that require sutures

1. Do not suture wounds if they are more than 6 hours old, as risk of infection increases with time.
2. Clean the wound with warm water and soap.
3. Irrigate the wound with sterile saline solution.
4. Anesthetize the wound with 1%–2% lidocaine (Xylocaine).
5. Palpate or probe the wound for foreign objects, such as glass.
6. Generally, make sutures on the extremities with 4-0 or nylon; a larger suture material , such as 2-0 nylon, may be used on the soles of the feet.
7. Keep the sutured wound dry and covered with a clean, dry dressing for several days, changing the dressing after the first 24 hours.
8. Remove sutures on the basis of the location of the wound:
   a. Head and trunk (5–7 days).

        b. Extremities (7–10 days).

        c. Soles and palms (10–14 days).

     9. Tetanus prophylaxis; see Animal Bites: Pediatric and Adult, **V.C**, p. 59.

VI. Complications

    A. Infection.

    B. Reopening of the wound.

    C. Hematoma in the wound.

VII. Consultation–Referral

    A. Infected wounds.

    B. Fever or chills or other evidence of systemic infection.

    C. Facial wounds.

    D. Wounds penetrating subcutaneous tissue.

    E. Wounds associated with functional disturbance.

    F. Wounds that cannot be easily cleansed.

    G. Wounds with macerated edges that cannot be easily approximated.

VII. Follow-Up

    A. Return visit for suture removal (see **V.B.8**).

    B. Return visit for complications (describe to patient).

3

DISORDERS OF THE SKIN

▲ ACNE: PEDIATRIC AND ADULT

I. Definition

Comedones (blackheads, whiteheads), pimples, and tender, red bumps (cysts) on the face, chest or back, or a combination of these, usually in adolescence or early adulthood.

II. Etiology

Increased activity of sebaceous glands, with obstruction leading to rupture of the glands. Steroids or phenytoin sodium (Dilantin) may produce eruptions in which pustules predominate and comedones are absent.

III. Clinical Features

A. Symptoms

  1. Lesions may be painful.

  2. Climate (heat and humidity) often can be identified as a precipitating factor.

  3. Psychologic consequences of the condition may be present.

Patient Care Guidelines for Nurse Practitioners, 4th ed. by Axalla J. Hoole, C. Glenn Pickard, Jr., Ruth M. Ouimette, Jacob A. Lohr, and Robert A. Greenberg. Copyright © 1995 by J. B. Lippincott Company.

B. **Signs.** Increasing numbers of blackheads, whiteheads, pimples, and tender red bumps on the face, chest, or back are seen, which may lead to pitted scars. One type of lesion may predominate, or all may be present.

IV **Laboratory Studies**

None.

V. **Differential Diagnosis**

A. Pyoderma.

B. Drug eruptions.

VI. **Treatment**

A. **General measures.** Advise the patient to do the following:

1. Keep hands off the face. Avoid picking lesions.

2. Avoid greasy cleansing creams, oils, and cosmetics.

3. Shampoo regularly to treat seborrhea, which often accompanies acne.

4. Expect exacerbations even while under treatment, especially during menses and periods of increased heat and humidity.

5. Eat a normal balanced diet. There is *no* need to avoid chocolate, sodas, or other specific foods.

6. Realize the value of psychological support.

B. **Blackheads, whiteheads, papules, and pimples**

1. General measures (see A).

2. Soaps and astringents:

a. For very mild acne, wash face with water and any soap 3–4 times a day to remove oil film.

b. For more extensive acne, use special cleansers (e.g., Oxy-Wash) instead of regular soap. Reduce frequency if skin becomes irritated. Discontinue if other topical treatments are used.

3. Drying lotions or gels with benzoyl peroxide 5–10% (Benzoyl, Persa-gel, Benzagel, Desquam-X) can be applied 1 or 2 times a day. Reduce frequency if excessive dryness or irritation develops.

4. For acne which is predominantly blackheads and whiteheads, Tretinoin (retin A) may be used.

a. Apply Tretinoin 0.025% cream to dry skin at bedtime. To avoid excessive irritation, begin with use every 2–3 days and increase to daily as tolerated. Caution about sun exposure.

b. Increase to Tretinoin 0.1% cream if necessary, after 2 month trial of lower strength cream.

C. **Pustules and cysts**

1. General measures (see A).

2. Soaps and astringents (see **B.2**).

3. Drying lotions (see **B.3**).

4. Topical antibiotic therapy may be very effective.

   a. Clindamycin 1% solution (Cleocin T), apply twice daily

   or

   b. Erythromycin 1.5%–2% solution (EryDerm, A/T/S, Staticin, Erycette, T-Stat), apply twice daily.

5. Oral antibiotic therapy for moderate to severe disease. (To avoid staining baby's teeth, do not use tetracycline during pregnancy.) Consult physician before starting.

   a. Tetracycline, 250 mg 4 times a day, 1 hour before or 2 hours after meals and at bedtime for 6 weeks. Then decrease to:

   b. Tetracycline, 250 mg 2 times a day, 1 hour before or 2 hours after meals, until the lesions are under good control. Then decrease to:

   c. Tetracycline, 250 mg daily, indefinitely.

   Note: In some case tetracycline may be decreased to 250 mg every other day or discontinued completely in the summer. On the other hand, some patients need a continued dosage of 250 mg 2–3 times a day.

   d. Tetracycline may cause side effects (*Candida* vaginitis, nausea, vomiting, diarrhea). Patients who do not tolerate tetracycline can be treated with similar doses of erythromycin or ampicillin.

VII. Complications

A. Secondary bacterial infection.

B. Excessive dryness of skin due to over vigorous washing and use of lotion.

C. Antibiotic side effects.

D. Psychologic consequences.

VIII. Consultation–Referral

A. Secondary bacterial infection (increasing numbers of pustules or cysts despite oral antibiotic therapy).

B. Resistance to therapy or sudden, persistent worsening after initial improvement.

C. Severe psychologic stress associated with the lesions.

D. Moderate to severe pustular acne requiring oral antibiotics.

IX. Follow-Up

A. **Oral antibiotic treatment**

1. Monthly visits until the acne is under good control and the patient is taking a single daily dose.

2. Semiannual (every 6 months) visits while patient is taking maintenance dose of oral antibiotics.

B. Topical treatment

1. In 8 weeks to assess response.

2. As needed on the basis of the severity of the lesions, the patient's compliance with the regimen, and his or her need for psychologic support.

▲ ATOPIC DERMATITIS (ECZEMA): PEDIATRIC AND ADULT

I. Definition

A chronic inflammatory disease of the skin characterized by pruritus and tending to occur in patients with an allergic diathesis. Onset is commonly in infancy after age 2 months. There is often a family history of asthma, allergic rhinitis, and/or eczema.

II. Etiology

Unknown. Manifestations are usually secondary to pruritus and scratching of the sensitive skin. The following may initiate and aggravate the itching and inflammation:

A. Dry skin (cold weather).

B. Perspiration (hot, humid weather).

C. Certain foods (orange or tomato juice) on contact with the skin.

D. Irritating clothing (wool, silk, nylon, rayon).

E. Certain soaps (Ivory, deodorant soaps), detergents or cosmetics.

F. Emotional stress.

III. Clinical Features

A. Symptoms

1. Pruritus.

2. Restlessness, hyperactivity, difficulty going to sleep.

3. Concomitant symptoms of asthma and allergic rhinitis (about 50% of cases).

B. Signs

1. **Infancy**

   a. Rough, erythematous, papular, and occasionally vesicular or scaling eruption, which frequently progresses to weeping and crusting.

   b. Onset usually after 2 months of age.

   c. Located commonly on cheeks, scalp, postauricular area, neck, and flexural surface of forearms and legs; occasionally on trunk and diaper area.

    d. Definite alteration between quiescent periods and exacerbations, usually seasonal.

    e. Frequent rubbing of involved areas by infant.

    f. In most patients, resolution of the condition prior to the age of 30 years.

  2. Childhood

    a. Less weeping and crusting and more dry, papular, scaling eruption with hypopigmentation.

    b. Intensely pruritic and excoriated lesions.

    c. Located commonly on flexor surfaces of wrists and on antecubital and popliteal areas.

  3. Adolescence and adulthood

    a. Dry, thickened skin, with accentuation of normal lines and folds; often hyperpigmentation.

    b. Located commonly on flexor areas of extremities, eyelids, back of neck, and dorsum of hands and feet.

IV Laboratory Studies

None.

V. Differential Diagnosis

  A. Seborrheic dermatitis (sometimes impossible to differentiate in infancy).

  B. Fungal infections of the skin.

  C. Contact dermatitis (e.g., poison ivy).

  D. Irritant dermatitis (e.g., diaper dermatitis).

  E. Rare systemic diseases of infancy associated with an atopic dermatitis type of rash (e.g., phenylketonuria. Wiskott-Aldrich syndrome, histiocytosis X, acrodermatitis enteropathica).

VI. Treatment

  A. Patient should avoid factors that initiate pruritus and irritate skin. Advise patient to:

    1. Spend time outdoors in warm weather. Humidify home in winter if heating system dries air.

    2. Prevent dry skin by:

      a. Minimizing duration of soap exposure during bathing. Exposure to water is beneficial. Use a mild soap (e.g., Neutrogena, Tone, Caress, Dove, Gentle Touch).

      b. Applying agents that seal water into the skin after it is moistened by a bath or shower (e.g., Alpha-Keri, Domol, Nivea, Aquaphor, Eucerin, petrolatum)

    3. Use tepid-to-warm water for brief baths or showers. Hot water causes pruritus.

4. Use soft cotton clothing and bedding. Avoid wool, starched, or rough clothing.

5. Place a cotton pad under the bed sheets to further separate an infant from a plastic mattress.

6. Keep fingernails short.

B. Therapy for active dermatitis:

1. If lesions are weeping or crusted, patient can apply soft cloth compresses of clear water at room temperature for 15 minutes 4 times a day for softening and débridement of crust and control of exudative reactions and pruritus.

2. After an acute, exudative phase has been controlled patient should apply a corticosteroid to the affected area.

a. Hydrocortisone (1%) in Eucerin cream is applied 4–6 times a day. Other low-potency steroid creams may be used: e.g., Hytone, Westcort, Locoid, Cutivate).

b. The importance of frequent application of a small amount, gently massaged into the affected area, must be emphasized.

3. Patient can use an antihistamine for antipruritic and sedative effect (see Tables 3-1 and 3-2 for dosage).

4. Secondary bacterial infection (beta-hemolytic streptococcal or staphylococcal) is common and must be treated before atopic dermatitis can be controlled. Consult physician.

VII. Complications

A. **Secondary bacterial infection** (beta-hemolytic streptococcal or staphylococcal).

B. **Secondary viral infection** (vaccinia or herpes simplex). Generalized vesiculopustular lesions develop; the patient can become seriously ill.

TABLE 3-1

ORAL DOSAGE OF DIPHENHYDRAMINE HCl (BENADRYL) AS AN ANTIPRURITIC AND SEDATIVE

DRUG FORM	BODY WEIGHT	DOSE	FREQUENCY
Benadryl elixir	8–10 kg (18–22 lb)	5.0 mL	
(12.5 mg/5 mL[a]	10–15 kg (22–23 lb)	7.5 mL	
	15–20 kg (33–44 lb)	10.0 mL	3 or 4 times
	20–30 kg (44–66 lb)	15.0 mL	a day
or			
Benadryl capsules	15–25 kg (33–55 lb)	1 capsule	
(25 mg/capsule)	Over 25 kg (over 55 lb)	2 capsules	

[a]*Caution:* May cause drowsiness.

TABLE 3-2

ORAL DOSAGE OF HYDROXYZINE HCL (ATARAX, VISTARIL) AS AN ANTIPRURITIC AND SEDATIVE

DRUG FORM	BODY WEIGHT	DOSE	FREQUENCY
Hydroxyzine syrup[a]	8–10 kg (18–22 lbs.)	2.5 mL	
(Atarax) 10 mg/5 mL[b]	10–15 kg (22–23 lbs.)	3.5 mL	
	15–20 kg (33–44 lbs.)	5.0 mL	
	20–30 kg (44–66 lbs.)	7.5 mL	3 or 4
or			times
Hydroxyzine tablets[a]	20–23 kg (44–66 lbs.)	1 tablet	a day
(Atarax) 10 mg/tablet	30–50 kg (66–110 lbs.)	2 tablets	
or			
Hydroxyzine tablets[a]	>50kg (110 lbs)	1 tablet	
(Atarax) 25 mg/tablet			

[a]Caution: May cause drowsiness.
[b]*Caution:* Hydroxyzine *suspension* (Vistaril) is 25 mg per 5 mL.

Note: Patients with atopic dermatitis and persons with whom they have close contact should *not* be vaccinated against smallpox.

VIII. Consultation–Referral
A. Secondary bacterial infection.
B. Failure to respond to treatment within 2 weeks.

IX. Follow-Up
Return visit in 1 week, and periodically as needed.

▲ DIAPER DERMATITIS

I. Definition
Inflammation of the skin within the area usually covered by the diaper. It can be caused and aggravated by many factors acting separately or in combination, and a variety of morphologic changes can result.

II. Etiology
A. Contact irritants
  1. Urine irritation is probably caused by ammonia and other breakdown products.
    a. Diaper is not changed frequently enough.
    b. Occlusive plastic pants, plastic liner or disposable diapers allow moisture and warmth to irritate and macerate skin.
  2. Stool

      a. Diaper is not changed frequently enough.

      b. Perineum is not cleaned thoroughly after defecation.

      c. Diarrhea (including that secondary to administration of oral antibiotics).

   3. Chemicals. Detergents and soaps.

   4. Discharge (from vulvovaginitis).

B. Infection

   1. Bacterial. This is usually a secondary irritating colonization by a variety of organisms. Sometimes small staphylococcal furuncles are present.

   2. Fungal. *Candida albicans* organisms also may cause what is usually a secondary infection. It may be associated with oral candidiasis (thrush). Broad-spectrum antibiotic therapy (e.g., ampicillin) may lead to candidiasis. Occasionally an infant acquires the infection from the contaminated hands of an adult with vaginal candidiasis.

   3. Viral. Vaccinia lesions may spread to the area of dermatitis.

C. Underlying skin disorder exaggerating the effects of contact irritation and infection.

   1. Seborrheic dermatitis.

   2. Atopic dermatitis.

III. Clinical Features

A. Symptoms

   1. Sometimes, none.

   2. Pruritus.

   3. Irritability.

B. Signs

   1. Erythema is present, especially on the buttocks, genitalia, and lower abdomen.

   2. Erythematous papules, vesicles, and pustules as well as superficial ulcerations are present.

   3. Affected area may be moist and exudative.

   4. During healing of moderate to severe dermatitis, skin may be dry and scaly.

   5. *Candida* characteristically produces diffuse erythema that may be moist with satellite papules and pustules outside the margin of the erythema. The patient may also have oral candidiasis.

IV. Laboratory Studies

Potassium hydroxide preparation of pustule contents or scraping of affected area, if candidiasis is suspected and morphology is not typical.

V. Differential Diagnosis

None.

VI. Treatment

Advise patient to do the following:

A. General treatment and prevention

1. Keep diaper area dry and free from urine and stool:
   a. Change diapers frequently.
   b. Wash contaminated area with warm water at each diaper change. Use mild, nonperfumed, nonmedicated soap sparingly to avoid irritation.
   c. Allow air to circulate under diaper:
      (1) Use only one layer of diaper pinned loosely.
      (2) Do not put plastic pants over diaper.
      (3) Expose involved areas as much as possible to air.
      (4) Consider use of newer disposable diapers that draw moisture away from skin.
2. Clean diapers well:
   a. Rinse thoroughly to remove soap.
   b. In the final rinse use a disinfectant (benzalkonium chloride [Zephiran] solution, 4 tablespoons per quart of water, or Diaparene).

B. Mild inflammation (noncandidal)

1. Follow general hygiene (see A).
2. Apply bland ointment after each diaper change (e.g., petrolatum, lanolin and petrolatum [A and D Ointment], Diaparene, Desitin).

C. Moderate to severe inflammation (noncandidal)

1. Follow general hygiene (see A).
2. For severe inflammation and weeping, apply aluminum acetate (Burow's) solution compresses for 20 minutes 3 times a day for 3–5 days only.
3. If there is no weeping, apply 1% hydrocortisone cream 4 times a day.

D. Candidiasis

1. Use good general hygiene (see A).
2. Apply nystatin (Mycostatin) cream liberally to affected area 3 times a day.

   or

   miconazole 2% (Micatin) or clotrimazole 1% (Lotrimin) to affected areas twice a day.

   or

Apply Mycolog ointment (a combination of nystatin and tri-amicinolone) to affected area 2 or 3 times a day.

or

for stubborn cases, apply Lotrisone cream 2 or 3 times daily. (This medication should not be used for more than 2 weeks at any one time.)

3. If oral candidiasis is present or dermatitis is severe or recurring, use nystatin (Mycostatin) oral suspension (100,000 units per milliliter) in a dosage of 2 mL orally 4 times a day for 1 week (1 mL in each side of mouth, not in the back of the throat, so that the medication is in contact with oral lesions as long as possible). It may be helpful to rub a portion of the dose on oral lesions with a cotton swab.

4. Examine mother for oral candidal vaginitis if infant has recurrent candidal diaper dermatitis.

VII. Complications

A. Spread to contiguous areas of abdomen and thighs.

B. Severe secondary bacterial infection.

VIII. Consultation–Referral

Failure to respond to treatment within 1 week.

IX. Follow-Up

Return visit in 1 week if there is no improvement.

▲ SEBORRHEIC DERMATITIS: PEDIATRIC AND ADULT

I. Definition

Oily, scaling condition affecting areas with large numbers of sebaceous glands (scalp, ears, central face, sternal area, and rarely, axillae and inguinal areas).

II. Etiology

Unknown (possibly genetic predisposition).

III. Clinical Features

A. Symptoms

1. Usually pruritus or flaking, or both.

2. Sometimes, no symptoms other than visible flaking ("dandruff").

B. Signs

1. Usually, symmetric scaly eruption, often starting in scalp (cradle cap in infants).

2. May progress to

a. Eyebrows.

    b. Eyelids (scales around base of eyelashes).

    c. Nasolabial and postauricular folds, external auditory canal.

    d. Presternal area.

    e. Axillae and groin (rare).

    f. Diaper area in infants.

  3. Greasy scales, oily hair.

  4. Occasional association with acne.

  5. In infants, usually short-lived course without recurrence; in adults, tendency to persist or recur.

IV. Laboratory Studies

Potassium hydroxide preparation is negative in pure seborrhea; perform when diagnosis is in doubt or associated *Candida* infection is suspected.

V. Differential Diagnosis

  A. Tinea capitis or corporis.

  B. Psoriasis.

  C. Contact dermatitis.

  D. Candidiasis.

  E. Atopic dermatitis.

VI. Treatment

Advise patient on the following measures:

  A. Adults

    1. Mild cases involving primarily the scalp

      a. Use any nonprescription dandruff shampoo containing selenium sulfide (e.g., Selsun Blue) or zinc pyrithione (e.g., Head & Shoulders, Sebulon) every 2–3 days (less often after symptoms subside). Lather, massage, and rinse well. Repeat sequence; leave second lather on scalp 6–10 minutes.

      b. If desired, use 2% sulfur and 2% salicylic acid cream twice a day on the skin.

      c. For more stubborn cases, use ketoconazole (Nizoral) shampoo twice weekly.

    2. Severe cases

      a. Use one of these tar-containing shampoos every 1–3 days:

        (1) Sebutone.

        (2) Vanseb-T.

        (3) Ionil-T.

        (4) Pentrax.

        (5) T-Gel.

      b. Apply 2% sulfur and 2% salicylic acid cream twice a day to affected areas.

   c. Apply a cortisone-containing lotion (Scalpicin) to:
      (1) Scalp—twice a day for 10 days, then once a day for 7 days, then periodically as needed.
      (2) Other areas—once a day for 7–10 days, then as needed. Once the rash on the scalp is controlled, eruptions usually disappear from the face and ears.

B. **Children**
   1. **Scalp**
      a. **Mild cases.** Use any nonprescription shampoo. Lather, massage scalp with brush (soft brush for infant), and rinse well. Repeat sequence. Shampoo every other day until scales are gone, then twice a week.
      b. **Extensive or thick scaling (cradle cap)**
         (1) Use 2% sulfur and 2% salicylic acid shampoo (e.g., Sebulex). Lather, massage scalp with brush (soft brush for infant), and rinse well. Repeat sequence. Shampoo for next 2 days, then twice a week until scales are gone.
         (2) Use any nonprescription shampoo, with scalp massage, twice a week to prevent build-up of scales after using sulfur and salicylic acid shampoo treatment.
   2. **Skin** (oily skin with nonerythematous papules, as found on face and near hairline of infants)
      a. Wash twice a day with mild soap and water.
      b. Do not oil skin.
      c. Provide reassurance.
      d. 0.5% hydrocortisone cream once daily.

C. **Erythema and scaling**
   1. Examine potassium hydroxide preparation of scales if the affected area is moist and in diaper or intertriginous areas, to rule out candidiasis.
   2. Apply 1% hydrocortisone cream 2–4 times a day until dermatitis clears.

VII. **Complications**
   A. Secondary bacterial infection (usually beta-hemolytic streptococcal or staphylococcal).
   B. Candidal infection, especially in intertriginous, moist areas. Infection is more likely in obese patients.
   C. Contact dermatitis from medicated shampoo or lotion.

VIII. **Consultation–Referral**
   A. Secondary bacterial infection.
   B. No response to treatment.

IX. Follow-Up.

Return visit in 1 week if there is no improvement.

▲ FOLLICULITIS, FURUNCLES (BOILS), CARBUNCLES: PEDIATRIC AND ADULT

I. Definition

A. **Folliculitis.** A localized infection of a hair follicle, in areas of concentrated hair (e.g., axilla), multiple infected follicles may be present.

B. **Furuncle.** A large, deep follicular infection with one drainage point.

C. **Carbuncle.** A large coalescence of furuncles with several drainage points, most commonly occurring in the back of the neck, the back, and thighs.

II. Etiology

Staphylococcus aureus. Preceding cutaneous trauma or lesion, immunologic deficiencies, diabetes, and nasal colonization with a virulent strain all predispose to infections.

III. Clinical Features

A. **Symptom.** Pain. Tenderness, localized swelling.

B. **Signs**

1. Lesions vary in size from erythematous papules to large nodules with one or more drainage points.

2. Lesions are extremely tender, erythematous, and surrounded by inflammation.

3. Lesions initially are firm, but centers progress to become fluctuant.

4. Regional lymphadenitis may be present.

IV. Laboratory Studies

There is no need to culture routinely in a patient without complicating disease or recurrences.

V. Differential Diagnosis

A. Impetigo.

B. Foreign objects, with associated infection.

C. Insect bites.

VI. Treatment

A. **Folliculitis.** Tell the patient to wash affected area with antibacterial soap and water and apply warm compresses for 20 minutes 2–4 times a day.

B. **Furuncles and carbuncles**

1. Tell the patient to apply warm compresses for 20 minutes 2–4 times a day until fluctuant and ready for drainage.
2. When fluctuant, have patient return for incision and drainage (after physician consultation).
3. Pack cavity with iodoform or sterile gauze.

VII. Complications
A. Usually, very few.
B. Recurrences.
C. Bacteremia, with metastatic infection.

VIII. Consultation–Referral
A. Carbuncles.
B. Fever.
C. Cellulitis or furuncles on the face.

IX. Follow-Up
A. **Folliculitis.** Return visit if lesions do not clear within a week.
B. **Furuncle.** Return visit every other day until ready for drainage, then in 48 hours for dressing change. Further follow-up depends on the size of the lesion.

▲ HERPES SIMPLEX: PEDIATRIC AND ADULT

I. Definition
A vesicular eruption of skin and mucous membranes appearing in usually two distinct clinical syndromes.
A. **Herpes simplex labialis** ("of the lip") appears most often in children in its primary form and in adults in a less severe, recurrent form.
B. **Herpes simplex progenitalis** appears as a primary and recurrent problem in sexually active persons.

II. Etiology
Two similar but antigenically different strains of herpesvirus hominis:
A. **Type 1** usually affects skin and mucous membranes above the umbilicus.
B. **Type 2** usually affects skin and mucous membranes below the umbilicus. After the primary infection, the virus remains latent in nerve cells that are in the area of the original lesions. (This is true of both types 1 and 2.)

Note: The difference in distribution between types 1 and 2 has become less distinct in recent years.

III. Clinical Features
A. Type 1

1. **Primary infection (acute gingivostomatitis)** appears in persons not previously infected by the virus, usually children. The initial infection may be subclinical and asymptomatic or may appear as below.

   a. **Symptoms**

      (1) Soreness of the lips, mouth, and/or salivation.

      (2) Fever (as high as 105 °F in children).

      (3) Malaise.

      (4) Course of 1–3 weeks.

   b. **Signs**

      (1) Vesicular eruption of gingival mucosa or lips.

      (2) Breaking of vesicles, with grayish ulcerations.

      (3) Inflammation and swelling of gums or lips and, sometimes, bleeding.

      (4) Usually, enlarged, tender submandibular lymph nodes.

      (5) Fever (as high as 105 °F in children).

      (6) Infrequently, only tonsillar lesions.

2. **Recurrent infection**

   a. **Symptoms**

      (1) Burning and pain in affected area.

      (2) Generally, no systemic symptoms unless associated with another disease.

      (3) Reactivating factors, such as physical trauma, sunlight, fever.

      (4) Course of about 10–14 days.

   b. **Signs.** Vesicles and ulcers, usually around vermilion border of lips.

B. **Type 2**

1. **Primary infection**

   a. **Symptoms**

      (1) Incubation period of 3–7 days.

      (2) Mild to severe discomfort.

      (3) Sometimes, prodrome of mild paresthesia or burning.

      (4) Later, continuous vulval or penile pain, which may be severe.

      (5) Dysuria and, occasionally, urinary retention.

      (6) Tenderness of infected area.

      (7) Sometimes, dyspareunia.

      (8) Fever, headache, malaise.

(9) Course of 2–4 weeks.
  b. **Signs**
    (1) Indurated papules or vesicles surrounded by erythema, which often coalesce to form large ulcers.
    (2) Location—vulva, genitocrural folds, perianal skin, vaginal and cervical mucosa in females, and urethral meatus and penis in males.
    (3) Maceration in moist areas.
    (4) With extensive involvement, edema is present.
    (5) Inguinal lymphadenopathy.
    (6) Low-grade fever.
    (7) Sometimes, urethral discharge in males.
    (8) A cluster of blisters or round erosions in the genital area (the most common clinical picture at the time the patient seeks medical attention).
  2. Recurrent infection
  a. **Symptoms**
    (1) Symptoms are similar to those of the primary infection but usually less severe.
    (2) Reactivation of the latent virus may be related to fever, premenstrual tension, vigorous sexual activity.
  b. **Signs**
    (1) Lesions are found in the same location as the primary infection.
    (2) Signs tend to be less severe than those of primary infection.
    (3) Early lesions are vesicles, which rupture and tend to ulcerate.
IV. Laboratory Studies
  Diagnosis is usually made on the basis of clinical syndrome. Specific viral cultures, however, are now available to confirm the diagnosis.
V. Differential Diagnosis
  A. Primary infection with herpesvirus type 1 may produce a generalized eruption that resembles chickenpox.
  B. Coxsackie and ECHO viruses cause herpangina, with papules, vesicles, and ulcers on the anterior tonsillar pillars, tonsils, soft palate, pharynx, and posterior buccal mucosa. If herpes simplex lesions begin posteriorly, as they occasionally do, they may be confused with herpangina.
  C. Lesions localized to the tonsils and pharynx may be confused with pharyngitis or tonsillitis of bacterial (most commonly streptococcal), viral, or mycoplasmal origin.

VI. Treatment

Advise patient on the following measures:

A. Type 1

1. **Primary infection**

   a. **General measures**

   (1) Take acetaminophen (Tylenol) or aspirin (adults) for pain or fever; see Chapter 5, Upper Respiratory Tract Infection (Common Cold): Pediatric and Adult, **VI.C**, Table 5-5, p. 156, for dosage.

   (2) Use saline solution as mouthwash or for gargling.

   (3) Apply topical anesthetic, such as viscous lidocaine, to lesions as necessary.

   (4) Avoid contact with certain patients (see **VII.D**).

   (5) Maintain adequate fluid intake (especially children) to prevent dehydration. Use bland liquids (not citrus juices or carbonated drinks). Use straws to avoid lip, tongue and gum lesions.

   b. **Specific measures.** Oral acyclovir (consult physician).

2. **Recurrence**

   a. **General measures**

   (1) Apply a local drying or soothing agent (e.g., Blistex or Debrox) 3–4 times a day.

   (2) Avoid contact with certain patients (see **VII.D**).

   b. **Specific measures.** Oral acyclovir (consult physician).

B. Type 2

1. **Primary infection**

   a. **General measures**

   (1) Take acetaminophen (Tylenol) or aspirin (see pp. 156–157).

   (2) Take sitz baths in tepid water as often as necessary.

   (3) Use a topical anesthetic, such as dibucaine HCl (Nupercaine), if pain is intense. Generally, however, topical anesthetics are to be avoided because of the potential for allergic reactions.

   (4) Avoid contact with certain patients (see **VII.D**).

   (5) Avoid sexual intercourse until lesions heal.

   b. **Specific measures.** Oral acyclovir 200 mg 5 times daily for 10 days (consult physician).

   or

   In mild cases, apply acyclovir 5% ointment 4–5 times daily.

2. **Recurrent infection.** Intermittent or chronic suppressive ther-

apy with oral acyclovir (Zovirax) may be indicated in recurrent episodes. Consult physician.

VII. Complications

A. Involvement of other parts of the body:

1. Conjunctivitis.

2. Keratitis.

3. Generalized vesicular eruption.

B. Secondary bacterial infection (beta-hemolytic streptococcal or staphylococcal, or both) of skin lesions.

C. Dehydration in infants and younger children with gingivostomatitis and poor fluid intake.

D. Spread to patients at risk of developing disseminated and severe herpes simplex. Isolate from the following:

1. Patients with open skin lesions, such as burns and dermatitis.

2. Newborns.

3. Patients on immunosuppressive therapy.

VIII. Consultation–Referral

A. Conjunctivitis.

B. Keratitis.

C. Persistent headache and vomiting, photophobia, convulsions, or neurologic findings suggestive of encephalitis.

D. Infection in late pregnancy because of risk to newborn, in whom fatal disseminated disease can develop.

E. Severe primary infection (type 1 or 2).

F. Very poor oral fluid intake (usually in infants and younger children).

G. Secondary bacterial infection.

IX. Follow-Up

Return visit in 1 week if no improvement or if any of the following develops:

A. Eye symptoms.

B. Secondary bacterial infection.

C. Inadequate fluid intake.

▲ HERPES ZOSTER (SHINGLES): PEDIATRIC AND ADULT

I. Definition

Usually, a unilateral vesicular eruption distributed along the dermatome of an infected nerve root. It is known to be due to reactivation of the varicella (chicken pox) virus.

II. Etiology

A. Herpes zoster is caused by a virus as above.

B. Certain patients, particularly those with altered immune responses, have an increased tendency toward development of herpes zoster. They include:

1. Patients with lymphomas, especially Hodgkin's disease.

2. Patients on corticosteroids.

3. Patients on other immunosuppressive agents.

4. Patients with disseminated malignancies.

5. Elderly.

6. HIV (see Chapter 16, The Asymptomatic HIV-Infected Adult, pp. 363–365).

III. Clinical Features

A. Symptoms

1. Fever.

2. Pain, occasionally quite severe, along a dermatome. (Pain may begin as long as 3–5 days before the rash begins.) Children may not have pain.

B. Signs

1. Eruption begins with red macules; progresses sequentially to papules, vesicles, pustules, and crusts; and resolves over 2–4 weeks.

2. Vesicles appear in clumps over the first week.

3. Involvement is unilateral.

4. Pain and eruption follow a dermatomic pattern.

5. The thoracic and cervical nerve roots are most often affected.

IV. Laboratory Studies

Tzanck prep is available in some labs.

V. Differential Diagnosis

A. **Pain appearing before rash.** Diagnosis is difficult in this situation, and the differential diagnosis must include any cause of pain localized to the area in question. (After rash develops, the distribution and appearance of herpes zoster are typical).

B. Impetigo

C. Herpes simplex

VI. Treatment

Advise patient on the following measures:

A. General therapy

1. Take acetaminophen (Tylenol) or aspirin for fever or pain; see Chapter 5, Upper Respiratory Tract Infection (Common Cold): Pediatric and Adult, **VI.C**, Table 5-5, pp. 156–157, for dosage.

2. If needed, use a narcotic for pain. Consult physician.

3. Use cool water or aluminum acetate (Burow's) solution soaks for vesicles or crusts. Apply calamine lotion.

4. Avoid contact with patients listed in **II.B**.

B. **Specific therapy.** Oral and intravenous Zovirax therapy (consult physician).

VII. Complications

A. **Dissemination**

1. Occurs in more than 50% of patients with Hodgkin's disease.

2. Rarely occurs in patients without underlying immunologic problems.

B. **Bacterial superinfection**

C. **Postherpetic neuralgia** (continued pain in dermatome site after rash has disappeared). Occurs more frequently in persons over 50.

VII. Consultation–Referral

A. Any patient on steroids or other immunosuppressive drugs or over 50.

B. Coexisting Hodgkin's disease or other malignancy.

C. Symptoms persisting beyond 2 weeks.

D. Bacterial superinfection.

E. Involvement of tip of nose that suggests risk for ocular involvement.

F. Ocular involvement.

IX. Follow-Up

Return visit if there is no improvement within 2 weeks.

▲ IMPETIGO: PEDIATRIC AND ADULT

I. Definition

A condition involving the superficial layers of the skin characterized by seropurulent vesicles surrounded by an erythematous base.

II. Etiology and Epidemiology

A. Impetigo is caused by either group: beta-hemolytic streptococci, or coagulase-positive staphylococci. Occasionally, both organisms may be found.

B. It may be spread by direct contact with infected persons and possibly by insects, or it may be secondary to infections of the upper respiratory tract.

C. Incubation period is 2–10 days.

D. The untreated patient is contagious until the lesions are healed; treatment shortens the period of contagiousness.

E. Impetigo may be a complication of insect bites, abrasions, or dermatitis.

F. Peak incidence is in late summer and early fall.

G. Impetigo is most common in infants and children.

III. Clinical Features

A. **Symptoms**

1. Constitutional symptoms are unusual unless lesions are widespread.

2. Itching is common.

B. **Signs**

1. Superficial vesicles are present, containing serous fluid that becomes purulent and surrounded by areas of erythema.

2. Pustules rupture, dry centrally, and form a honey-colored crust.

3. Lesions vary in size from a few millimeters to several centimeters.

IV.   Laboratory Studies

If the diagnosis is in doubt, culture fluid from an intact vesicle or pustule or the base of a lesion after the crust is removed.

V. Differential Diagnosis

A. Noninfected insect bites.

B. Herpes simplex.

C. Chickenpox.

D. Other vesicular or ulcerating skin lesions.

VI. Treatment

A. Advise the patient to do the following:

1. Soak and then gently scrub lesions with warm water and soap three times a day to soften and remove crusts. Be careful not to spread infection to family members by contaminated clothes and towels.

2. Trim fingernails to prevent further spread.

B. Use antibiotic therapy for all patients with more than a few lesions: there is some debate among authorities about the use of antibiotics for treatment of patients with one or two small lesions. However, mupirocin (Bactroban) applied topically is efficacious in patients with a small number of lesions. (Antibiotic therapy will promote healing, decreasing the period of contagiousness and therefore the spread of impetigo.) It is not known whether early treatment of streptococcal impetigo will decrease the incidence of secondary nephritis. Because of increasing incidence of staphylococcus, some prefer to use an antibiotic effective against both staphylococcus and streptococcus.

1. Benzathine penicillin G (Bicillin, long-acting). (Ask whether

patient is allergic to penicillin.)

a. Patients weighing less than 25 kg (55 lb)—one IM injection of 600,000 units.

b. Patients weighing more than 25 kg (55 lb)—one IM injection of 1,200,000 units.

Note: Patients should be observed by health care provider for at least 20 minutes after receiving an injection.

or

2. Oral penicillin (children and adults)—penicillin V, 250 mg 3 times a day for 10 days. (Ask whether patient is allergic to penicillin.)

or

3. If patient is allergic to penicillin, use erythromycin as directed in Table 3-3.

C. In cases where lesions are predominantly bullous, staphylococcus aureus is almost always the etiologic agent and should be treated with: erythromycin (40–50 mg/kg/d divided into 4 doses), or dicloxacillin (12–25 mg/kg/d divided into 4 doses), or cephalexin (25–50 mg/kg/d in 3 doses—this preparation is more palatable for children).

D. Treat all people in close contact with patient, who have impetiginous lesions, as soon as possible to avoid reinfection and further spread.

TABLE 3-3

ORAL DOSAGE OF ERYTHROMYCIN ETHYL SUCCINATE SUSPENSION (200 MG PER 5 ML)

BODY WEIGHT	DOSE	FREQUENCY
6–9 kg (13–20 lb)	160 mg (4 mL)	
9–12 kg (20–26 lb)	240 mg (6 mL)	
12–16 kg (26–35 lb)	320 mg (8 mL)	
16–20 kg (35–44 lb)	400 mg (10 mL)	2 times day
20–24 kg (44–53 lb)	480 mg (12 mL)	for 10 days
24–28 kg (53–62 lb)[a]	560 mg (14 mL)	
28–32 kg (62–70 lb)[a]	640 mg (16 mL)	
Over 32 kg (over70 lb)[a]	800 mg (20 mL)	

[a]Patients weighing over 25 kg (over 55 lbs) may be given erythromycin base tablets (250 mg per tablet), 500 mg (2 tablets) twice a day for 10 days taken 1 hour before meals.

Note: If abdominal discomfort develops, divide dose in half and give 4 times a day.

VII. Complications

A. Acute glomerulonephritis may follow infection if the strain of streptococcus is nephritogenic.

B. Acute rheumatic fever is rarely a complication.

VIII. Consultation–Referral

A. Failure to resolve.

B. Presence of acute glomerulonephritis in the community.

IX. Follow-Up

A. Clinic visit if no improvement within 1 week.

B. Clinic visit for persons in close contact with the patient, who have impetiginous lesions, as soon as possible.

▲ CANDIDIASIS: ADULT

I. Definition

An infection of the skin caused by the fungus *Candida albicans.*

II. Etiology

A. *C. albicans*

B. Patients with certain problems (e.g. diabetic, immunosuppression) have predilection for candidal infection.

III. Clinical Features

A. Symptoms

  1. Itching.

  2. Burning pain, particularly with vulval involvement.

  3. Frequent association with diabetes mellitus, particularly involving intertriginous areas and vulva and sometimes becoming confluent with satellite lesions (inguinal creases and scrotum in males).

  4. Occasional association with use of birth control pills

B. Signs

  1. An erythematous macular rash is seen, usually involving intertriginous areas and vulva and sometimes becoming confluent with satellite lesions (inguinal creases and scrotum in males).

  2. Vulval rash, with white, cheesy exudate, is usually associated with candidal vaginitis. Exudate may also appear in intertriginous areas.

IV. Laboratory Studies

A. Potassium hydroxide preparation of the lesion is positive for *Candida.*

B. Culture of organisms should be obtained when the diagnosis is in doubt.

C. The level of urine or blood sugar, or both, should be measured to evaluate possible diabetes mellitus.

V. Differential Diagnosis

A. Seborrheic dermatitis.

B. Other fungal skin infections.

VI. Treatment

A. **Coexisting diabetes.** In a diabetic patient, candidiasis usually *cannot* be controlled or cured until the diabetes is controlled. Therefore, diabetes must be evaluated and properly managed by a physician.

B. **Intertriginous candidiasis.** Use one of the following 2–4 times daily:

1. Miconazole (Micatin) 2% cream,

   or

2. Clotrimazole (Lotrimin, Mycelex) 1% cream,

   or

3. Nystatin (Mycostatin) cream.

4. Lotrisone cream.

C. **Candidal vulvovaginitis.** Advise patient on the following measures:

1. Apply aluminum acetate (Burow's) solution compresses or Mycolog ointment, or both, to vulval lesions twice a day if they are moist or markedly inflamed.

2. Vaginal treatment with: a. Miconazole nitrate 2% (Monistat) vaginal cream, 1 applicator nightly for 3 days; or b. Clotrimazole 1% (Gyne-Lotrimin) vaginal cream or suppositories, 1 dose nightly for 7 days; or c. Miconazole 100 mg vaginal tablets (Monistat-3), 1 tablet nightly for 3 days.

3. Avoid contamination from gastrointestinal tract (instruct patient in proper toiletry).

4. Use Mycostatin oral tablets in resistant cases.

5. In recurrent cases, the male sexual partner may need to be treated for intertriginous candidiasis.

6. For resistant cases, oral ketoconazole (Nizoral) is now available (consult physician).

VII. Complications

Usually none.

VIII. Consultation–Referral

Failure to resolve in 2 weeks.

IX. Follow-Up

Once a week until resolution occurs.

▲ PITYRIASIS ROSEA: PEDIATRIC AND ADULT

I. Definition

A self-limiting, mild, scaly skin eruption occurring primarily in adolescents and young adults and lasting from 3–12 weeks.

II. Etiology

Unknown. (Possibly a hypersensitivity reaction to a viral infection.)

III. Clinical Features

A. Symptoms

1. Pruritus—usually mild, sometimes intense.
2. Occasionally, mild malaise.
3. Occasionally, symptoms of a mild upper respiratory tract infection.

B. Signs

1. The herald patch is the initial lesion in most cases, but it may not be present or may go unnoticed. It presents as a 2–5 cm round or oval scaling erythematous plaque occurring anywhere on body (often misdiagnosed as "ringworm").
2. The herald patch is followed in several days to a week by multiple small 1–2 cm maculopapular lesions that are pale red and round or oval, with a wrinkled surface and peripheral rim of small, fine scales. These lesions occur in crops over the trunk and proximal extremities and tend to occur with their long axis oriented in the direction of the skin cleavage planes parallel to the ribs.

IV. Laboratory Studies

Serologic test for syphilis to rule out secondary syphilis.

V. Differential Diagnosis

A. Secondary syphilis.
B. Seborrhea.
C. Tinea versicolor.

VI. Treatment

Usually, none. Drying lotions (e.g., calamine lotion) may relieve the itching. Oral antihistamines, either diphenhydramine (Benadryl) or hydroxyzine (Atarax, Vistaril), may also be helpful; see Tables 3-1 and 3-2, pp. 95–96, for dosage. Inform the patient that the rash will last several weeks but is self-limited.

VII. Complications

None.

VIII. Consultation–Referral

None.

IX. Follow-Up

Return visit as needed.

▲ CONTACT DERMATITIS DUE TO POISON OAK OR POISON IVY: PEDIATRIC AND ADULT

I. Definition

An acute dermatitis resulting from contact with the resin of poison oak or poison ivy.

II. Etiology

Most cases from contact with the leaves of the plant; however, cases may come from digging in ground that contains the growing plant. An outbreak may also result from contact with the smoke of burning plants, unwashed contaminated clothes, dried (uprooted) plants that still retain resin, or a pet that has had contact with the plant.

III. Clinical Features

A. Pruritic vesicles usually appear on the extremities.

B. Early eruption may be erythematous and raised without vesicles.

C. Linear streaks of erythema or vesicles are usually seen where plant has brushed across skin.

IV. Laboratory Studies

None.

V. Differential Diagnosis

A. Other contact dermatitides.

B. Insect bites.

VI. Treatment

A. Advise patient on the following preventive measures:

 1. Be familiar with the appearance of the plant and how to avoid it.

 2. Wash all clothes worn at the time of contact.

 3. If known exposure occurs in the future, immediately wash contact area with Dawn dish detergent or other similar lipophilic detergents to prevent or minimize clinical symptoms.

B. **General measures.** Tell patient to do the following:

 1. Soak the affected area in saline or aluminum acetate (Burow's) solution if this can be done easily, or use cold compresses for 20 minutes 4–6 times a day. This is the mainstay of therapy.

 2. Apply a drying lotion (e.g., calamine lotion) after each soak or cold compress.

 3. Avoid topical lotions containing antihistamine or benzocaine derivatives. These ingredients add nothing, and may act as allergens.

4. Use an oral antihistamine for sedation and as an antipruritic in moderate to severe cases (see Tables 3-1 and 3-2, pp. 95–96, for dosage).

5. If there is no weeping, apply 1% hydrocortisone cream 4–6 times a day.

6. Use an oral steroid after consultation for severe cases and cases involving the eyes, face, mucous membranes, and genitalia.

VII. Complications

Secondary bacterial infections (see Impetigo: Pediatric and Adult, pp. 109–112).

VIII. Consultation-Referral

A. Widespread involvement or marked discomfort, or both.

B. Involvement of the eyes or other sensitive areas, such as oral mucous membranes and genitalia.

IX. Follow-Up

Return visit in 3 days if there is no improvement.

▲ SCABIES: PEDIATRIC AND ADULT

I. Definition

An intensely pruritic rash caused by the mite *Sarcoptes scabiei.*

II. Etiology

A. The initial lesion is a burrow 1/2–2 cm in length, with a papule or vesicle at its blind end, not associated with itching. After several days, sensitivity to the mite results in severe pruritus followed by punctate excoriations from scratching and impetiginous and eczematous changes at the site of the lesion. A generalized urticarial rash may also develop.

B. The mite is transferred by personal contact, does not live long in clothing or bedding, and is found in association with poor personal hygiene and crowded living conditions, except during epidemics, when it becomes widespread.

III. Clinical Features

A. **Symptom.** Pruritus (most severe at night).

B. **Signs**

1. The characteristic burrow appears as a thin line 1/2–2 cm in length, ending in a papule or vesicle. Unfortunately, this sign is not seen in many patients due to excoriation by the patient.

2. Characteristic locations of lesions:

a. Men

(1) Interdigital folds, wrists (85% of cases).

        (2) Elbows, genitalia, ankles, feet (40% of cases).

   b. Women (in addition to above): palms and nipples.

   c. Children

        (1) Palms.

        (2) Soles.

        (3) Head.

        (4) Neck.

        (5) Legs.

        (6) Buttocks.

   d. Infants: Lesions may be in less typical locations.

  3. Secondary changes:

   a. Excoriation.

   b. Pustules and crusts of secondary bacterial infection.

   c. Eczema with weeping or scaling, or both.

IV. Laboratory Studies

Attempt to isolate the mite by scraping a burrow, papule, or vesicle and placing the specimen in mineral oil (on a slide) and examine microscopically. (Potassium hydroxide preparation is not used, because it destroys the characteristic feces.)

V. Differential Diagnosis

Scabies may take many forms and be confused with:

A. Impetigo.

B. Eczema.

C. Urticaria.

VI. Treatment

Advise patient on these treatment measures:

A. Specific agents

  1. Gamma benzene hexachloride 1% (Kwell), cream or lotion, applied to entire body from the neck down, not just to obvious lesions, with special attention to hands, feet, and intertriginous areas. Keep away from eyes and mucous membranes. Treatment is preceded by a warm soap and water bath using a soft brush and is followed by drying with a towel. Medication is thoroughly removed in 8 hours by a bath similar to the first.

Note: Effects of Kwell on the central nervous system, including convulsions, have been associated with applying the drug too frequently or leaving it on the skin longer than recommended. Therefore, no more than necessary should be prescribed (30 g or 1 oz for an average adult), and patients should be cautioned against overuse.

    or

2. Crotamiton 10% (Eurax) cream, applied to entire body from neck down, as above for Kwell. A second coat should be applied in 24 hours and the patient should bathe 48 hours past the last application. With correct use, crotamiton has very few side effects; slight local irritation occurs occasionally. Crotamiton has antipruritic properties as well as scabicidal effects.

or

3. Permethrin (Elimite cream) is preferred in infants. Directions same as for Kwell above.

B. Hygiene. Clothing, pajamas, sheets and pillowcases should be laundered.

C. Members of the household and sexual contacts with scabies should be treated at the same time.

D. An oral antihistamine, such as diphenhydramine HCl (Benadryl) or hydroxyzine HCl (Atarax, Vistaril) may be helpful to relieve itching (see Tables 3-1 and 3-2 for dosage, pp. 95–96).

VII. Complications

A. Secondary bacterial infection.

B. Eczema.

C. Reaction to gamma benzene hexachloride (Kwell):

1. Dermatitis.

2. CNS toxicity (seen with overdosage).

D. Inappropriate treatment may worsen the infestation when condition has been previously misdiagnosed.

VIII. Consultation–Referral

A. Failure to respond to therapy.

Note: following effective therapy, signs and symptoms may persist for several weeks due to hypersensitivity reaction to the mite, not necessarily to treatment failure.

B. Absence of characteristic burrows or papules.

C. Eczema.

D. Secondary bacterial infection.

IX. Follow-Up

Patient should return if not cured by therapy, or if disease recurs.

▲ TINEA CORPORIS (RINGWORM OF NONHAIRY SKIN): PEDIATRIC AND ADULT

I. Definition

Superficial fungal infection involving the trunk or limbs. (For fungal infection of the feet, see Tinea Pedis [Athlete's Foot]: Pediatric and

Adult.) Refer all fungal infections of the scalp to a physician.)

II. Etiology

Several different fungi.

III. Clinical Features

A. **Symptoms.** Condition may be asymptomatic or pruritic.

B. **Signs**

1. Erythematous, scaling patches (usually one or two) that are round or oval are seen. The lesions start small, then expand outward, with clearing of the eruption in the center of the patch and activity restricted to the border of the lesion (hence the name *ringworm*). The border of the lesion is usually raised and scaly.

2. Lesions are most common on the face and arms.

IV. Laboratory Studies

A. Potassium hydroxide (KOH) preparation of scales from the active border is positive for hyphae. (Scales from the center of a lesion may be negative.)

B. Fungal culture is a more sensitive test but takes 1–2 weeks for results. It need not be done with a typical lesion.

V. Differential Diagnosis

A. **Candidal infection.** This is usually intertriginous and redder than ringworm. It has less tendency toward central clearing, and satellite lesions are present outside the main lesion.

B. **Pityriasis rosea.** The herald patch may mimic ringworm, but it is KOH-negative. Pityriasis lesions also have a more widespread distribution. Look for other pityriasis lesions elsewhere.

C. **Seborrheic dermatitis.** Lesions are usually not round or oval, and they are KOH-negative. When lesions are on the face, differentiation is very difficult. In contrast to seborrheic dermatitis, fungal infections will not clear with topical steroid treatment.

VI. Treatment

If thickening of skin has occurred, treatment with a topical antifungal agent may require 2–3 weeks longer. Instruct patient to apply one of the following twice daily after soap and water washing and thorough drying of the lesion. Continue application for at least 2 weeks.

A. Tolnaftate 1% (Tinactin), cream or solution,

or

B. Miconazole nitrate 2% (Micatin), cream or lotion,

or

C. Clotrimazole 1% (Lotrimin), cream or solution.

VII. Complications

A. Secondary bacterial infection.

B. Allergy to topical antifungal agent.

VIII. Consultation–Referral

A. Severe or widespread infection.

B. Infection of the scalp.

C. Secondary bacterial infection.

D. Failure to respond to treatment.

IX. Follow-Up

Return visit in 2 weeks if there is no significant improvement.

▲ TINEA PEDIS (ATHLETE'S FOOT): PEDIATRIC AND ADULT

I. Definition

A pruritic cracking and peeling eruption of the feet, especially the toe webs.

II. Etiology

Several different fungi.

III. Clinical Features

A. **Symptom.** Intense itching is characteristic but not always present.

B. **Signs**

1. Eruptions usually start between the toes and occasionally spread to the soles or sides or even the tops of the feet.

2. Vesicles are occasionally present.

3. Toenails may be thickened, with debris under the nail.

4. Hands or groin may show evidence of fungal infection.

IV. Laboratory Studies

A. Potassium hydroxide (KOH) preparation of scales or the top of vesicles for typical hyphae is optional.

B. Fungal culture may be positive when the KOH preparation is negative, but need not be done with typical lesions.

V. Differential Diagnosis

A. Contact dermatitis (shoe leather dye, nylon, soap, etc.).

B. Secondary syphilis.

C. Psoriasis.

D. Dyshidrosis.

E. Neurodermatitis.

F. Candidiasis.

G. Bacterial infection.

H. Reiter's disease.

VI. Treatment

Advise patient on the following measures:

A. **General measures**

1. Thoroughly dry interdigital areas after bathing.

2. Use absorbent cotton socks.

3. Change socks at least once a day.

B. **Specific measures**

1. Soak the feet in aluminum acetate (Burow's) solution or tap water 20–30 minutes twice a day if vesicles are present.

   Then

2. Apply an antifungal agent; see Tinea Corporis (Ringworm of Nonhairy Skin): Pediatric and Adult, VI, p. 119.

VII. Complications

A. Secondary bacterial infection.

B. Allergy to topical antifungal agent.

VIII. Consultation–Referral

A. Secondary bacterial infection.

B. No response to topical antifungal agents or worsening of condition after treatment has started.

C. Fungal infection elsewhere on the body.

IX. Follow-Up

Return visit in 1–2 weeks if there is no improvement.

▲ TINEA VERSICOLOR: PEDIATRIC AND ADULT

I. Definition

Benign, recurrent, asymptomatic, superficial fungal infection.

II. Etiology

The fungus *Malassezia furfur* (pityrosporum ovale).

III. Clinical Features

A. **Symptom.** The patient shows concern about his or her appearance, occasionally associated with mild pruritus.

B. **Signs**

1. White, pink, tan, or brown macular spots, patches, or large confluent lesions are present, located mainly on the upper trunk, front and back. The lesions may extend to the abdomen and upper extremities, and less commonly to the neck and face.

2. Light scratching produces fine scales.

3. Infected areas do not tan when exposed to sunlight and appear much lighter than surrounding skin. In winter they may appear darker than surrounding areas.

IV. Laboratory Studies

Potassium hydroxide (KOH) preparation of scales reveals clusters of round spoors, and filaments.

V. Differential Diagnosis

A. Seborrheic dermatitis.

B. Vitiligo.

C. Pityriasis alba, if lesions are on the face.

VI. Treatment

A. **Counseling.** The patient should be told that:

1. Recurrence is very common.

2. The condition is benign even without treatment.

3. Although the infection is eradicated with treatment and scaling stops, the hypopigmented areas will remain until tanned by exposure to the sun or until the surrounding tanned area fades.

B. **Specific measures.** Advise patient on these measures:

1. Bathe or shower in the evening, scrubbing lesions with a stiff brush.

2. Apply selenium sulfide 2.5% (Selsun, Exsel) to entire body (regardless of location of rash) from neck down to knees and wrists avoiding genital area. Allow it to remain for several hours or overnight. Repeat application in 1 week.

3. In severe or frequently recurrent cases, oral ketoconazole 400 mg daily for 2–7 days (consult physician).

VII. Complications

Irritation from selenium sulfide if it is in contact with the eyes or anogenital area.

VIII. Consultation–Referral

No improvement after treatment and after skin color has had an opportunity to return to normal (may take 6–8 weeks).

IX. Follow-Up

Return visit as desired by patient.

▲ URTICARIA (HIVES): PEDIATRIC AND ADULT

I. Definition

Pruritic, red, raised plaques or welts, usually representing an allergic reaction.

II. Etiology

Urticaria is an allergic reaction, usually to drugs (oral and injected), foods, insect bites, inhalants, or injections. Occasionally it is due to an infection (e.g., herpes simplex, upper respiratory tract infection, tooth abscess, urinary tract infection). No cause is found in many cases. In children, no cause can be identified in most cases.

III. Clinical Features

A. **Symptoms.**

   1. Itching (usually intense).

   2. Occasionally, stinging or paresthesia, or edema (especially lips, around eyes, hands and feet).

B. **Signs**

   1. Red, raised plaques or welts with sharp borders are present, usually on the trunk and extremities. They vary in number and size.

   2. Lesions usually fade in less than 12 hours, sometimes in 20–30 minutes. If lesions persist (in the same location) for more than 24 hours, the diagnosis is often erythema multiform or multiple insect bites.

   3. The chest is clear to auscultation, and the patient is not wheezing.

IV. Laboratory Studies

None.

V. Differential Diagnosis

A. Erythema multiforme.

B. Cutaneous manifestation of anaphylaxis.

C. Multiple insect bites.

D. Contact dermatitis.

E. Acute exanthem.

VI. Treatment

A. If clinical features of anaphylaxis are present, institute immediate specific treatment: see Chapter 2, Anaphylaxis: Pediatric and Adult, VI, pp. 56–58.

B. For widespread urticaria and intense pruritus or angioedema, inject aqueous epinephrine, 1:1000, subcutaneously.

   1. **Pediatric dose.** 0.91 mL per kg (0.005 mL per lb); maximum dose, 0.3 mL.

   2. **Adult dose.** 0.3–0.5 mL.

Note: It may be necessary to repeat the dose every 1–2 hours for several doses.

C. Use an oral antihistamine for less severe urticaria and after injection of epinephrine (**see B**).

TABLE 3-4

ORAL DOSAGE OF CHLORPHENIRAMINE MALEATE (CHLOR-TRIMETON)

BODY WEIGHT	DOSE	FREQUENCY
10–20 kg (22–44 lb)	2.5 mL	
20–30 kg (44–66 lb)	5 mL (1/2 tablet)	4 times a day
30–40 kg (66–68 lb)	5–7.5 mL (1/2 tablet)	
Over 40 kg (over 88 lb)	5–10 mL (1/2–1 tablet)	

1. Diphenhydramine HCl (see Table 3-1, p. 95, for dosage).

   or

2. Chlorpheniramine maleate (Chlor-Trimeton) syrup, 2 mg per 5 mL; or tablets, 4 mg per tablet (see Table 3-4 for dosage).

   or

3. Hydroxyzine HCl (Atarax, Vistaril) (see Table 3-2, p. 96, for dosage).

4. Seldane, 60 mg every 12 hours.

D. Search carefully for offending agent and eliminate or avoid it. Inquire about diet history, drug history, insect bites.

E. Provide additional antipruritic effect, if necessary:

   1. Soak in a tub of cool water.

   2. Add colloidal oatmeal (Aveeno) to bath water.

VII. Complications

A. Systemic reaction to allergen (e.g., anaphylaxis or serum sickness).

B. Drowsiness secondary to antihistamine therapy. Patients must be cautioned about activities requiring alertness (e.g., driving motor vehicles).

VIII. Consultation–Referral

A. Evidence of edema of the larynx (hoarseness, inspiratory stridor).

B. Evidence of anaphylaxis (hypotension, tachycardia, paroxysmal coughing, severe anxiety, dyspnea, wheezing, vomiting, cyanosis). Treat immediately as anaphylaxis; see Chapter 2, Anaphylaxis: Pediatric and Adult, **VI**, pp. 56–58.

C. Chronic or recurrent urticaria lasting more than 6 weeks.

IX. Follow-Up

A. The patient should return in 48 hours if lesions persist or new signs or symptoms develop.

B. If urticaria was caused by an insect sting, patient should be referred for hyposensitization.

▲ WARTS: PEDIATRIC AND ADULT

I. Definition

An intradermal papilloma most frequently appearing in three distinct clinical patterns:

  A. Common warts.

  B. Plantar warts.

  C. Venereal warts.

II. Etiology

Human papilloma virus (HPV).

III. Clinical Features

  A. **Common warts**

  1. **Symptoms.** Generally, none, other than annoyance.

  2. **Signs.** Small circular skin-colored to gray-brown papillomas. These often appear on the hand and fingers, but may appear anywhere on the skin or mucous membranes.

  B. **Plantar warts**

  1. **Symptoms.** Plantar warts may cause severe pain with walking or standing.

  2. **Signs.** These warts resemble corns or calluses, with a central nodule containing several punctate spots.

  C. **Venereal warts**

  1. **Symptoms.** Usually, none, but may itch.

  2. **Signs.** Small papillomas are seen on the foreskin and penis in males (particularly those who are uncircumcised) and on the perineum and vaginal mucosa in females.

IV. Laboratory Studies

None.

V. Differential Diagnosis

  A. Corns, calluses.

  B. Melanoma, or other tumor.

  C. Contact dermatitis.

  D. Acute exanthem.

VI. Treatment

  A. **Common warts.** Apply dichloroacetic acid every 1–2 weeks. A crust will form; this should be removed at each visit and the lesion retreated. Alternative treatments involving freezing with liquid nitrogen and other modalities are available (consult physician). Home remedies containing salicylic acid are often curative if treatment is diligently carried out.

B. **Plantar warts**

1. Pare down callus with scalpel and apply dichloroacetic acid as directed in **A.**

   or

2. Apply a salicylic paint (e.g., Wart-Off, Duofilm or Occlusal HP surrounding skin) once or twice daily.

   or

   Apply a 40% salicylic acid plaster.

   a. Cover the callus with plaster and bandage with tape.

   b. Remove in 5–7 days and pare down callus and wart.

   c. Treatment may be repeated, but if tenderness intervenes, wait until it subsides.

C. **Venereal warts.** Apply 20%–25% Podophyllum resin in tincture of benzoin.

1. Coat area around wart with petrolatum to prevent spread of Podophyllum to uninvolved area.

2. Coat warts with Podophyllum mixture.

3. Allow Podophyllum to remain 3–5 hours. (Use a shorter time initially, increasing the length of time with later application.)

4. Instruct patient to take a sitz bath after 3–5 hours.

5. Inform the patient that the lesions may be painful for several days.

6. Repeat the treatment at weekly intervals until warts are gone.

7. Treat any coexisting vaginitis (see guidelines in Chapter 14, pp. 320–321).

8. Home treatment with Condylox is now available (consult physician).

VII. **Complications**

A. Tenderness may occur around treated area.

B. Over-treatment may lead to scarring.

VIII. **Consultation–Referral**

A. Large numbers of warts or large warts (which are best treated by other methods).

B. Resistance to therapy.

C. Venereal warts involving anus.

IX. **Follow-Up**

As often as necessary for treatment.

4

DISORDERS OF THE EYE

▲ CONJUNCTIVITIS: PEDIATRIC AND ADULT

I. Definition

Inflammation of the eyelid or bulbar conjunctiva, or both.

II. Etiology

A. **Bacterial Infection**

1. Streptococcus pneumonia, *Staphylococcus aureus,* hemophilus influenzae, and possibly others.

2. Gonococcus, especially in the first month of life. If the infection is contracted during birth, onset will be at age 3–5 days.

B. **Viral infection**

1. Adenoviruses: adenopharyngeal conjunctivitis (APC) and epidemic keratoconjunctivitis (EKC) are most frequently found. EKC is highly contagious and proper hand washing is especially important to prevent hand-to-eye spread. Towels and tonemeters have been implicated.

2. Associated with an upper respiratory tract infection.

Patient Care Guidelines for Nurse Practitioners, 4th ed. by Axalla J. Hoole, C. Glenn Pickard, Jr., Ruth M. Ouimette, Jacob A. Lohr, and Robert A. Greenberg. Copyright © 1995 by J. B. Lippincott Company.

3. Conjunctivitis with epidemic sore throat, high fever, and preauricular and submandibular adenitis, usually due to an adenovirus.

4. Inclusion blennorrhea, occurring in newborns and during childhood from contaminated swimming pools.

5. Vaccina, herpesvirus hominis type 1 (herpes simplex), herpes zoster. Lesions are usually present on the skin also.

C. **Chlamydial infection**

1. *Chlamydial trachomatis* is a frequent cause of conjunctivitis in neonates and infants. The organism is acquired from an infected mother during the birth process. The infection may spread to the nasopharynx and subsequently to the lungs.

D. **Allergic reaction.** Conjunctivitis is often associated with seasonal allergic rhinitis, which is usually due to pollen allergy.

E. **Foreign body or trauma**

F. **Chemical irritants**

G. **Systemic infection**

1. Measles.

2. Rocky Mountain spotted fever.

3. Kawasaki disease.

III. Clinical Features

A. **Symptoms**

1. Mild irritation.

2. Mild photophobia.

3. Excessive lacrimation.

4. Normal vision.

B. **Signs**

1. Infected conjunctiva.

2. Discharge

   a. Purulent in bacterial infection.

   b. Mucopurulent in viral infection (occasionally becoming secondarily infected with bacteria).

   c. Mucoid and stringy or watery in allergic reaction.

   d. Watery when caused by a foreign body, air pollution, allergy.

3. Sometimes, conjunctival edema.

4. Clear cornea.

5. Pupils are normal in size and react to light.

6. Enlarged preauricular nodes in viral infection.

IV. Laboratory Studies

TABLE 4-1

DIFFERENTIAL DIAGNOSIS OF THREE EYE DISORDERS

PARAMETER	ACUTE CONJUNCTIVITIS	ACUTE IRITIS	ACUTE GLAUCOMA
Pain	Mild discomfort	Moderate pain photophobia	Moderate to severe pain with nausea and vomiting
Vision	Normal	Slightly to moderately blurred	Very blurred
Discharge	Often muco-purulent	Clear	Clear
Cornea	Clear	Clear	Clear
Pupil	Normal	Small and irregular	Mid-dilated and oval
Response to light	Normal	Poor	Poor
Infection	Conjunctival only	Conjunctival and circumcorneal	Moderate to severe conjunctival and circumcorneal

Culture of exudate for gonococcus or chlamydia in first month of life.

V. Differential Diagnosis

A. **Lacrimal duct obstruction.** This is a congenital disorder seen in the first few months of life as overflow tearing and secondary bacterial infection of obstructed duct, with persistent purulent discharge.

B. **Acute iritis** (see Table 4-1) and **iridocyclitis**.

C. **Acute glaucoma** (see Table 4-1).

D. **Blepharitis.**

VI. Treatment

A. **Consultation** on specific cases (see **VIII**).

B. **Allergic conjunctivitis,** if acute and mild, will respond to treatment of accompanying allergic rhinitis: see Chapter 5, Allergic Rhinitis: Pediatric and Adult, pp. 143–146.

C. **Mild conjunctivitis** associated with an upper respiratory tract infection is usually self-limited and need not be treated.

D. **Purulent or micropurulent conjunctivitis**

1. **Cool compresses** may decrease the mild discomfort that is occasionally present.

2. **Antimicrobial drops.** Continue treatment for 1–2 days after

symptoms have resolved. Instruct patient to use either:

a. Sodium sulfacetamide 10% (Sodium Sulamyd) ophthalmic solution; instill 1 or 2 drops in the lower conjunctival sac of the affected eye 4 times a day.

b. Polymyxin B-bacitracin ointment in the lower conjunctival sac of affected eye 4 times a day.

VII. Complications

A. Keratitis and scarring from gonococcus and herpes simplex.

B. Pneumonia from *Chlamydia trachamatis,* in first months of life.

C. Local allergic reaction to neomycin.

VIII. Consultation–Referral

A. Any suspicion of uveitis or glaucoma (see Table 4-1).

B. Cases that might be due to the following:

1. Gonococcus.

2. Vaccinia, herpesvirus hominis, herpes zoster.

3. Foreign body.

4. Chemical irritants, particularly alkali.

C. Infants under 1 month of age.

D. No improvement in 48 hours.

IX. Follow-Up

Return visit if there is no improvement in 48 hours.

▲ HORDEOLUM (STYE): PEDIATRIC AND ADULT

I. Definition

Localized infection of a sebaceous gland along the margin of the eyelid.

II. Etiology

Usually, *Staphylococcus aureus.*

III. Clinical Features

A. **Symptoms**

1. Some pain.

2. No visual disturbances.

B. **Signs**

1. Painful erythematous swelling at the margin of the eyelid.

2. Sometimes, purulent drainage along the lid margin.

IV. Laboratory Studies

None.

V. Differential Diagnosis

   A. Infection in a deeper gland, forming a painful swelling that drains on conjunctional surface of the lid.

   B. Tumors or granulomas (rare).

   C. Chronic hordeolum.

VI. Treatment

   A. Hot compresses applied for 15 minutes 4 times a day.

   B. Follow compresses with antibiotic ointment such as bacitracin or tobraminim.

VII. Complications

   A. Conjunctivitis.

   B. Cellulitis.

VIII. Consultation-Referral

   A. Nonpainful swelling.

   B. Failure to respond to treatment within 3 days.

IX. Follow-Up

   A. As necessary for recurrence or failure to heal completely in 10 days.

   B. Return visit in 3 days if there is no improvement.

▲ CATARACTS: ADULT)

I. Definition and Etiology

Clouding or opacification of the lens of the eye, which, in 90% of the cases, is associated with aging. More common in diabetics. Rarely associated with hypoparathyroidism, myotonic dystrophy, atopic dermatitis, trauma, drugs such as systemic corticosteroids. Cataracts are usually bilateral, but may develop at different rates.

II. Clinical Features

   A. Symptoms. Most commonly, diminution of visual acuity may be described as clouding of vision. Less commonly, patients may report an improvement in distant or near vision ("second sight") due to change in refractive error associated with hardening of the lens.

   B. Signs. Opacity of the lens noted when shining pen light directly into pupil or on ophthalmoscopic examination of eye.

III. Laboratory Studies

None.

IV. Differential Diagnosis

Loss of visual acuity due to other causes such as macular degeneration, diabetic retinopathy.

V. Treatment

The only treatment is surgical removal of the lens and implantation of an intraocular lens in most patients. Ninety-eight percent of pro-cedures are now done as outpatients. This procedure should be con-sidered only when the cataract causes sufficient visual impairment to reduce the ability of the patient to perform routine daily activities.

VI. Consultation–Referral

As soon as cataracts are readily noted on routine examination, the patient should be referred to an ophthalmologist. Referral is useful for detecting coexisting problems, proper refraction, and establishing need and expectation of benefit from surgery. Recent improvement in surgical techniques (particularly intraocular lens implantation) sug-gests that earlier surgical intervention, before severe visual impair-ment develops, is appropriate.

IX. Follow-Up

By ophthalmologist in 6–12 months.

5

DISORDERS OF THE EAR, NOSE, AND THROAT

▲ OTITIS EXTERNA: PEDIATRIC AND ADULT

I. Definition

Infection of the external auditory canal and auricle from a variety of agents occurs following loss of the integrity of the skin. This may be initiated by trauma from scratching, earplugs, bobby pins, and numerous other foreign objects. Maceration may also occur from water trapped in the canal following bathing or swimming.

II. Etiology

A. **Bacteria.** Most commonly, *Pseudomonas* species, *Proetus, Staphylococcus aureus,* and streptococci.

B. Fungi.

III. Clinical Features

A. Symptoms

1. Pain in ear.

2. Occasionally, decrease in hearing or a sensation of obstruction in the ear.

Patient Care Guidelines for Nurse Practitioners, 4th ed. by Axalla J. Hoole, C. Glenn Pickard, Jr., Ruth M. Ouimette, Jacob A. Lohr, and Robert A. Greenberg. Copyright © 1995 by J. B. Lippincott Company.

B. **Signs**

1. Pain is aggravated by movement of the auricle, by pressure on the tragus, or by chewing.

2. The external canal may be partially occluded by edema or discharge.

3. The external canal is usually tender when examined with an otoscope and is injected or erythematous. Exudate may be seen.

4. The tympanic membranes may be normal, injected, or covered with flecks of exudate but do not show signs of otitis media; see Acute Purulent Otitis Media: Pediatric and Adult, p. 135, and Serous Otitis Media: Pediatric and Adult, p. 139.

5. Preauricular or postauricular lymphadenopathy may be present.

6. There is no swelling or pain over mastoid.

IV. **Laboratory Studies**

None.

V. **Differential Diagnosis**

A. **Otitis media.** See Acute Purulent Otitis Media: Pediatric and Adult, p. xx. There may be pus in the external auditory canal in cases of otitis media where perforation of the tympanic membrane has occurred.

B. **Mastoiditis.** Swelling and pain over the mastoid area are associated with an abnormal tympanic membrane.

C. **Chronic dermatitides.** These usually are not painful but may itch chronically and may be associated with cracking and scaling of the auricle and, in some cases, with discharge. There is usually no pain when the auricle or tragus is moved, unless it is secondarily infected. Types of chronic dermatitides include:

1. Seborrhea.

2. Eczema.

3. Psoriasis.

VI. **Treatment**

A. **Prevention.** Advise patient on the following preventive measures:

1. Keep fingers and instruments, including cotton swabs, out of ears; the ear canal does *not* need cleaning.

2. Persistent itching of the external canal warrants medical consultation; do *not* scratch with a foreign object.

B. **Specific therapy.** After gently and thoroughly removing debris from the ear canal by suctioning or by genetic irrigation, give patient the following instructions:

1. Acetaminophen (Tylenol) for all ages or aspirin for adults for pain; See pp. 156–157 for adult doses and Table 5-5, p. 156 for pediatric doses of acetaminophen.

2. Apply heat to ear by warm compresses, hot water bottle, or heating pad.
3. Use ear drops. Medication applied to the external ear canal will not be effective unless the canal is sufficiently clear of cerumen and exudate to allow contact with inflamed tissue. Patient should lie with affected ear upward for 5 minutes after drops are instilled. When possible, insert a cotton wick; drops placed on the exposed tip of the wick will track down the wick to the infected canal.
   a. Cortisporin otic solution (combination of polymyxin B sulfate, neomycin sulfate, and hydrocortisone), 4 drops in the affected ear 4 times a day for one week.
      or
   b. Domebero otic solution (acetic acid, 2%, in aluminum acetate), 4–6 drops in the affected ear 4 times a day for 1 week.

VII. Complications
A. Severe otitis externa associated with:
1. Swelling of the canal to complete closure.
2. Severe pain.
3. Cellulitis of the canal, auricle, and surrounding tissue.
B. Local allergic reaction to neomycin.
C. Patients with diabetes mellitus may have more severe infections.

VIII. Consultation–Referral
A. Severe otitis externa:
1. Severe pain.
2. Fever.
3. Swelling of external canal sufficient to prevent instillation of drops and requiring a wick.
4. Swelling and tenderness over the mastoid.
B. Cellulitis of ear.
C. Failure to respond to treatment in 1 week.
D. Relapse within a few weeks.

IX. Follow-Up
Return visit if condition persists after 1 week of treatment.

▲ ACUTE PURULENT OTITIS MEDIA: PEDIATRIC AND ADULT

I. Definition
Infection in the middle ear, with accumulation of seropurulent fluid in the middle-ear cavity.

II. Etiology

Eustachian tube dysfunction is of primary importance. The majority of cases are due to bacterial infection. Pneumococcal infection occurs most frequently, but *H. influenzae* is not uncommon, especially in young children. It is not possible clinically to identify those patients with sterile exudate.

III. Clinical Features

A. **Symptoms**

1. Earache.
2. Symptoms of an upper respiratory infection.
3. Fever.
4. Decreased hearing.
5. Sometimes, no symptoms.

B. **Signs**

1. Bulging of any portion of the tympanic membrane with accumulation of exudate in the middle-ear cavity.
2. Disappearance of the malleus (bony landmarks). The short process is often lost first.
3. Perforation of the tympanic membrane, resulting in the presence of exudate in the external canal and distortion of the tympanic membrane. (This must be distinguished from primary otitis externa without otitis media, which is more common in the adult.)
4. Bullae of the tympanic membrane.
5. Decreased or absent movement of the tympanic membrane with insufflation.

Note: Injection or erythema of the tympanic membrane and disappearance or distortion of the light reflex may accompany these signs but alone are not sufficient to diagnose acute purulent otitis media.

IV. Laboratory Studies

None.

V. Differential Diagnosis

A. Erythema of the tympanic membrane associated with an upper respiratory tract infection.

B. Serous otitis media.

C. Otitis externa.

VI. Treatment

A. **Patients under 18 years of age.** Be sure infant is not being fed in the supine position, since this may predispose to otitis media. Parental smoking also increases the incidence of otitis media in young children.

TABLE 5-1

**ORAL PEDIATRIC DOSAGE OF AMOXICILLIN SUSPENSION (125 MG PER 5 ML)
FOR TREATMENT OF ACUTE PURULENT OTITIS MEDIA**

BODY WEIGHT	DOSE	FREQUENCY
6–8 kg (13–18 kg)	100 mg (4 mL)	Every 8 h for 10 days
8–10 kg (18–22 lb)	125 mg (5 mL)	Every 8 h for 10 days

TABLE 5-2

ORAL PEDIATRIC DOSAGE OF AMOXICILLIN SUSPENSION (250 MG PER 5 ML)

BODY WEIGHT	DOSE	FREQUENCY
10–12 kg (22–26 lb)	150 mg (3 mL)	Every 8 h for 10 days
12–15 kg (26–33 lb)	200 mg (4 mL)	Every 8 h for 10 days
Over 15 kg (over 33 lb)	250 mg[a] (5 mL)	Every 8 h for 10 days

[a]Patients weighing over 15 kg (over 33 lbs) who are able to safely swallow capsules may be given amoxicillin capsules, 250 mg 3 times a day for 10 days, or ampicillin, 250 mg 4 times a day for 10 days.

1. Amoxicillin:
   a. Patients weighing 6–10 kg (13–22 lb) (see Table 5-1 for dosage).
   b. Patients weighing over 10 kg (22 lb) (see Table 5-2 for dosage).
2. If patient is allergic to penicillin derivatives, or if there is reason to suspect that the causative organism is an ampicillin- or amoxicillin-resistant strain of *Hemophilus influenzae,* treat with erythromycin and sulfisoxazole combination (Pediazole); see Table 5-3 for dosage.

B. **Patients over 18 years of age**
   1. Amoxicillin capsules, 250 mg 3 times a day for 10 days.
      or
   2. If patient is allergic to penicillin derivatives, treat with 80 mg trimethoprim, 400 mg sulfamethoxazole tablets, two tablets 2 times a day for 10 days.

VII. **Complications**
   A. Chronic serous otitis media (persistent middle ear infusion).
   B. Persistent purulent otitis media.
   C. Mastoiditis.
   D. Chronic otitis media with perforation of the tympanic membrane.

TABLE 5-3

**ORAL DOSAGE OF ERYTHROMYCIN ETHYLSUCCINATE
(200 MG PER 5 ML) AND SULFISOXAZOLE ACETYL (600 MG PER 5 ML)
SUSPENSION COMBINATION (PEDIAZOLE)**

BODY WEIGHT	DOSE	FREQUENCY
6–9 kg (13–20 lb)	2 mL	4 times a day for 10 days
9–12 kg (20–26 lb)	3 mL	4 times a day for 10 days
12–16 kg (26–35 lb)	4 mL	4 times a day for 10 days
16–20 kg (35–44 lb)	5 mL	4 times a day for 10 days
20–24 kg (44–53 lb)	6 mL	4 times a day for 10 days
24–28 kg (53–62 lb)	7 mL	4 times a day for 10 days
28–32 kg (62–70 lb)	8 mL	4 times a day for 10 days
Over 32 kg (over 70 lb)	10 mL	4 times a day for 10 days

    E. Extension into the central nervous system, leading to meningitis or brain abscess.

    F. Cholesteatoma formation associated with chronic otitis media and marginal or pars flaccida perforation.

VIII. Consultation–Referral

    A. Infants under 3 months of age.

    B. Severe pain.

    C. Failure to improve symptomatically in 48 hours.

    D. Signs of meningitis, such as:

        1. Lethargy.

        2. Extreme irritability.

        3. Bulging fontanel.

        4. Stiff neck.

    E. Persistent purulent otitis media, despite adequate course of antibiotics.

    F. More than two episodes of purulent otitis media:

        1. Child—in 1 year.

        2. Adult—over any period of time.

    G. Suspicion of mastoiditis (pain, tenderness, or edema in the postauricular area in older children and adults).

    H. Chronic otitis media with persistent intermittent drainage through perforation of the tympanic membrane.

IX. Follow-Up

Examination in 3 weeks.

▲ SEROUS OTITIS MEDIA: PEDIATRIC AND ADULT

I. Definition

Accumulation of a bacteriologically sterile, nonpurulent effusion in the middle-ear cavity.

II. Etiology

A. Eustachian tube obstruction with subsequent formation of an effusion in the middle ear cavity. The causes of eustachian tube obstruction include:

1. Enlarged adenoids.
2. Upper respiratory tract infection with mucosal edema.
3. Allergic rhinitis with mucosal edema.
4. Cleft palate.
5. Deviated nasal septum.
6. Nasopharyngeal tumor in adults.

B. A complication of purulent otitis media.

C. Possibly, active secretion by the mucosa of the middle-ear cavity in an allergic patient.

III. Clinical Features

A. **Symptoms**

1. Hearing loss.
2. Feeling of fullness in the ear.
3. Snapping sensation when swallowing, yawning, or blowing the nose.
4. Symptoms associated with the disorders listed in **II.A** (e.g., chronic snoring associated with enlarged adenoids).
5. Occasionally, no symptoms, especially if chronic.

B. **Signs**

1. Clear or transparent yellowish fluid (early) or bluish gray fluid (long standing), with or without air bubbles behind the tympanic membrane associated with

   a. Retraction of the tympanic membrane.

   b. Prominence of the malleus, especially the short process, with an abnormally horizontal handle of the malleus drawn inward.

   c. Decreased or absent movement of the tympanic membrane with insufflation. Occasionally, only outward movement with negative pressure is seen.

Note: Injection or erythema of the tympanic membrane and disappearance or distortion of the light reflex, as seen in an upper respiratory tract infection or allergic rhinitis, may accompany these signs but alone are not sufficient to diagnose serous otitis media.

2. Signs associated with the disorders listed in **II.A** (e.g., mouth-breathing associated with enlarged adenoids).

3. Decreased hearing.

IV. Laboratory Studies

None.

V. Differential Diagnosis

A. Acute purulent otitis media.

B. Chronic otitis media.

C. Retraction or erythema, or both, of the tympanic membrane without serous effusion, as seen in an upper respiratory tract infection or allergic rhinitis.

D. Normal retracted appearance of the tympanic membrane of very young infant.

E. Symptoms of eustachian tube obstruction alone, with a normal tympanic membrane.

F. Hearing loss due to other causes.

G. Ménière's disease.

VI. Treatment

A. **Children under 12 years of age**

1. Be sure infant is not being fed in the supine position, which may predispose to otitis media.

2. No therapy. Serous otitis media resolves spontaneously in most patients.

3. Return appointment in 6 weeks. If middle-ear effusion is still present at that time, patient should be referred.

B. **Adults and children over 12 years of age**

1. No therapy if asymptomatic or if symptoms are minimal. Serous otitis media resolves spontaneously in almost all patients in this age group.

2. If patient is symptomatic or if middle ear effusion is still present after 3 weeks, prescribe topical decongestant.

   a. Xylometazoline HCl (Otrivin) 0.1% nasal solution, 2 or 3 drops in each nostril every 8 hours.

   or

   b. Xylometazoline HCl (Otrivin) 0.1% nasal spray, 1 spray followed in 5–10 minutes by a second spray; repeat sequence every 8 hours.

3. If condition is not resolved after 2 weeks of therapy outlined in 2, refer patient.

VII. Complications

A. Chronic serous otitis media (persistent middle ear effusion) with increased risk of

1. Decreased hearing, which can contribute to:

a. Learning difficulties in school.

b. Defective speech development.

2. Adhesive otitis media, with permanent conducive hearing loss.

B. Acute purulent otitis media.

C. Cholesteatoma from chronic severe retraction of pars flaccida.

VIII. Consultation–Referral

A. **Children under 12 years of age**

1. Failure to resolve after 6 weeks.

2. More than two episodes in 1 year.

B. **Adults and children over 12 years of age**

1. Failure to resolve after 2 weeks of therapy outlined in **VI.B.2**

2. More than 2 episodes in 1 year.

IX. Follow-Up

A. See **VI.A** or **B**

B. To avoid complications, always follow patients until resolution occurs.

▲ EPISTAXIS: PEDIATRIC AND ADULT

I. Definition

The spontaneous discharge of blood from the nares.

II. Etiology

A. Spontaneous rupture of a blood vessel in the nose (usually the anterior septum), occurring most frequently in children and in the elderly.

B. Higher incidence in winter, when heating causes drying and cracking of nasal mucosa.

C. Trauma from a direct blow to the nose.

D. Picking of dry, crusted nostrils, particularly in association with an upper respiratory infection.

E. Rarely, hypertension.

F. Rarely, a bleeding disorder.

III. Clinical Features

A. **Symptoms.** Usually, none, other than the awareness of blood dripping down the posterior nasopharynx as well as external bleeding.

B. **Signs**

1. Bleeding from the nares and down the posterior nasopharynx.
2. Localized bleeding point (may or may not be seen in the anterior nasal septum).
3. Usually, normal blood pressure.
4. Usually, no orthostatic fall in blood pressure.
5. Usually, no evidence of bleeding or clotting disorder (e.g., bruises, petechiae).

IV. Laboratory Studies

A. Generally, none.

B. Hematocrit, if history indicates significant bleeding.

V. Differential Diagnosis.

None.

VI. Treatment

A. **Acute bleeding**

1. Keep the patient in an erect sitting position with head tilted forward to prevent blood from going down the posterior nasopharynx.
2. To decrease venous pressure, try to keep children from crying.
3. With thumb and forefinger, apply continuous external compression on both sides of the nose for 15 minutes.

B. **Prevention**

1. Discourage picking of the nose.
2. Advise patient to increase the humidity in the home, especially in sleeping areas, by means of a humidifier or pot of water on a heater.
3. Suggest rubbing petrolatum over the nasal septum twice a day.

VII. Complications.

Anemia, if bleeding is excessive or frequent.

VIII. Consultation–Referral

A. Bleeding not controlled by 15 minutes of compression.

B. Evidence of massive bleeding.

C. Recurrent bleeding within first hour.

D. Second episode within a week.

E. Bleeding from the posterior nasopharynx (usually cannot be controlled by the measures described in **VI.A.**).

IX. Follow-Up

As needed for recurrent episodes.

▲ ALLERGIC RHINITIS: PEDIATRIC AND ADULT

I. Definition

An allergic disease affecting the nasal mucosa and often the conjunctiva. It may be seasonal or perennial (nonseasonal).

II. Etiology

A. Seasonal

1. Pollens that depend on wind for cross-pollination. In the eastern United States, the following are the most common causes (pollination time may vary by several months depending on location):

   a. Trees, April–July.

   b. Grasses, May–July.

   c. Ragweed, August–October.

   d. Combinations of **a**, **b**, and **c**.

B. Perennial

1. House dust. The predominant allergen is found in the feces of house dust mites.

2. Feathers.

3. Mold spores.

4. Animal dander and associated allergens.

5. Cockroaches.

6. Foods. There is disagreement about the role of food in causing isolated allergic rhinitis. Most authorities believe that if foods are causative, other signs of hypersensitivity occur with allergic rhinitis (e.g., urticaria, asthma, gastrointestinal symptoms).

C. Perennial with seasonal exacerbations

D. Aggravating factors

1. Tobacco smoke.

2. Air pollutants.

3. Sudden temperature changes.

III. Clinical Features

A. Symptoms. Onset is usually in childhood and young adulthood, with symptoms decreasing with age. A family history of allergic diseases is common. Symptoms of seasonal allergic rhinitis tend to occur the same time each year and are frequently more severe than those of the perennial form.

1. Sneezing.

2. Nasal itching.

3. Watery rhinorrhea.

4. Nasal stuffiness.

5. Occasionally, other symptoms including:

a. Itching of the eyes, palate, and throat.

b. Snoring and sniffing.

c. Increased tearing and photophobia.

d. Nonproductive cough from irritation of posterior pharyngeal secretions.

e. Fatigue, irritability, anorexia.

B. **Signs**

1. Clear, thin nasal discharge.

2. Pale, edematous nasal mucosa.

3. Enlarged nasal turbinates.

4. "Allergic salute," that is, rubbing of the nose upward and outward (seen especially in children).

5. Mouth-breathing.

6. Conjunctival infection and edema. Occasionally granular, erythematous conjunctivae and swollen eyelids, with extra lines and dark semicircles (allergic "shiners") under the eyes.

7. Allergic facies with perennial allergic rhinitis:

a. Mouth-breathing.

b. Prominent maxilla, high arched palate.

c. Dull expression.

d. Broad midsection of nose, with horizontal crease across lower portion.

IV. **Laboratory Studies**

Wright's or Hansel's stain of smear of nasal secretions may reveal eosinophils, but usually smear is not needed to make a diagnosis.

V. **Differential Diagnosis**

A. **Seasonal**

1. Upper respiratory tract infection.

2. Infectious conjunctivitis.

B. **Perennial**

1. Recurrent upper respiratory tract infections.

2. Vasomotor rhinitis (of unknown cause, noninfectious, nonseasonal, and nonallergic).

3. Deviated nasal septum.

4. Side effect of medications, such as Reserpine and vasoconstricting nose drops.

5. Chronic sinusitis.

VI. Treatment

A. **Identification and avoidance of the offending antigen.** Advise the patient on the following measures *if appropriate* for that individual:

1. **Seasonal**

   a. Avoid areas of heavy concentration of ragweed, trees, or grass during pollinating seasons.

   b. Sleep with bedroom windows closed during the appropriate pollinating season.

   c. Use an air conditioner with an electrostatic precipitating filter to avoid pollen.

2. **Perennial**

   a. Create a dust-free bedroom (patients who must do their own cleaning should use a mouth-and-nose mask):

      (1) Remove everything from the room, including floor coverings, curtains, drapes, and closet contents.

      (2) Clean the room thoroughly—walls, woodwork, ceiling, floor, and closet. Wax the floor.

      (3) Scrub the bed frame and metal springs.

      (4) Cover the mattress, box spring, and pillows with plastic, dustproof covers.

      (5) Make sure the room contains a minimum of furniture, washable rugs, and curtains. Avoid bed pads, heavy rugs, drapes, upholstered furniture, toys, and knickknacks.

      (6) Clean the room at least once a week using a vacuum cleaner, damp cloth, or oil mop. Do not use a broom or duster.

      (7) Keep bedroom windows and door closed. If hot air heating is used, cover vents with coarse muslin and change frequently. Change furnace air filter frequently.

   b. Vacuum, using a water-sealed vacuum cleaner, stuffed furniture and rugs frequently.

   c. Keep pets (dogs, cats) away from the bedroom.

   d. Avoid damp and dusty places (attics, basements, closets, storerooms).

   e. Avoid stuffed toys, if patient is dust-sensitive.

   f. Use an air conditioner with an electrostatic precipitating filter to avoid dust.

B. **Antihistamine.** Use chlorpheniramine (Chlor-Trimeton); see Table 3-4, p. 124, for dosage.

Note: The goal of therapy is to achieve symptomatic relief with a minimum of side effects (e.g., drowsiness, nervousness, dry mouth). Therefore, manipulation of dosage within the prescribed ranges may be necessary. Medication should be taken for several days to weeks during symptomatic periods because antihistamines do not antagonize released histamine but only prevent further release. Intermittent single-dose usage will not be as effective in controlling symptoms. Less sedating antihistamines, such as Seldane and Hismanal, should be used after consultation.

C. Oral decongestants, such as pseudoephedrine, may be used in conjunction with antihistamines.

D. Sympathomimetic nose sprays are discouraged because of the reliance associated with use of decongestant nose sprays for more than several days.

E. Topical corticosteroids—consult physician.

F. Cromolyn sodium—consult physician.

VII. Complications

A. Eustachian tube obstruction causing serous otitis media.

B. Sinus orifice obstruction causing sinusitis.

C. Nasal or sinus polyps from long-standing perennial allergic rhinitis.

D. Dental malocclusion problems from maxillary deformity associated with chronic nasal obstruction.

E. Drowsiness from antihistamine therapy.

VIII. Consultation–Referral

A. Failure to respond to treatment.

B. Consideration for immunotherapy (hyposensitization):

1. Severe or prolonged periods of symptoms not controlled by treatment measures described above.

2. Inability to tolerate antihistamines; symptoms that are more than mild.

3. Patients requiring almost daily medication for perennial allergic rhinitis.

IX. Follow-Up

Return visit in 1 week, and periodically as needed.

▲ PHARYNGITIS (SORE THROAT): PEDIATRIC AND ADULT

I. Definition

Inflammation of the pharynx or tonsils, or both.

II. Etiology

A. Usually nonbacterial (presumed to be viral).

B. Group A beta-hemolytic streptococci. *Streptococcal pharyngitis* is unusual in a child under 3 years of age.

TABLE 5-4

FINDINGS IN PHARYNGITIS SUGGESTIVE OF STREPTOCOCCAL ETIOLOGY

CLINICAL FEATURE	VERY SUGGESTIVE	MODERATELY SUGGESTIVE	QUESTIONABLY SUGGESTIVE	UNUSUAL
Tender enlarged anterior cervical lymph nodes	All ages	—	—	—
Household contact	All ages	—	—	—
Scarletina— form rash	School age Adults	—	—	Infants
Excoriated nares	Infants	—	—	School age Adults
Tonsillar exudate	Adults	School age	Infants	
High fever	—	All ages	—	—
Occurrence during winter and spring	—	All ages	—	—
Acute onset	—	School age Adults	—	Infants
Sore throat	—	School age Adults	—	Infants
Abdominal pain	—	Infants School age	—	Adults
Rhinorrhea	—	Infants	—	School age Adults
Red throat	—	—	All ages	
Hoarseness	—	—	—	All ages
Cough	—	—	—	All ages

Source: Modified from L.A. Wannamaker, *Am. J. Dis. Child.* 124:357, 1972.

C. Much less commonly, *Mycoplasma pneumonia.*

D. Unusual in the United States, *Corynebacterium diptheriae.*

E. Unusual, *Neisseria meningitides* and gonorrhea.

F. Possibly a cause, *Chlamydia trachomatis.*

III. Clinical Features

It is *not* possible to determine the etiology of pharyngitis by clinical features alone. Although Table 5-4 may be helpful, a throat culture is needed to definitely establish if pharyngitis is due to group A beta-hemolytic streptococci.

IV. Laboratory Studies

A. In adults, throat culture for group A beta-hemolytic streptococci is indicated for patients who have two or three of the very suggestive or moderately suggestive findings given in Table 5-4 and do not have a cough. If they have four of these findings, presumptive treatment is indicated. If there is only one, the likelihood of infection is too low to warrant a culture.

B. In pediatrics, culture children with fever and complaint of sore throat or findings of adenopathy or abnormal pharynx or tonsils including inflammation and/or exudate. Some physicians may choose not to culture if fever is accompanied by cough or coryza. Two swabs are used to obtain material from tonsil or pharynx. A rapid strep test is obtained from material on one swab. A positive rapid test indicates treatment and eliminates the need for a culture.If the rapid test is negative, a culture for beta streptococcus is required

C. Throat culture of all *symptomatic* family and close contacts of patient with *Streptococcal pharyngitis.*

D. Throat culture of *all* family and close contacts of patient with *Streptococcal pharyngitis* under the following conditions:

1. The patient or one of the contacts has a history of rheumatic fever.

or

2. There is an outbreak of rheumatic fever or post-streptococcal glomerulonephritis in the community.

E. White blood cell and differential counts and heterophile antibody determination in suspected cases of infectious mononucleosis; see Chapter 16, Infectious Mononucleosis: Pediatric and Adult, pp. 353–355.

V. Differential Diagnosis

A. Infectious mononucleosis.

B. Influenza.

C. Stomatitis (e.g., herpetic).

VI. Treatment

A. **General measures for pharyngitis of any etiology**

1. Acetaminophen (Tylenol) for all ages or aspirin for adults for fever; see pp. 156–157 for adult doses and Table 5-5, p. 156 for pediatric doses of acetaminophen.

2. Warm saline gargle for older children and adults.

3. Increased fluid intake.

B. **Antibiotics for streptococcal pharyngitis.** Ask whether patient is allergic to penicillin.

Note: Tetracycline and sulfonamides should not be used for the treatment of streptococcal pharyngitis.

1. Benzathine penicillin G (Bicillin). (Mixtures containing other penicillin are acceptable; however, the dosage of benzathine penicillin G should *not* be decreased from that listed below.)
   a. Patients weighing less than 25 kg (55 lb): One IM injection of 600,000 units.
   b. Patients weighing more than 25 kg (55 lb): One IM injection of 1,200,000 units.

Note: Patient's reaction should be observed by health care providers for at least 20 minutes after injection.

or

2. **Oral penicillin.** This method of therapy depends on the cooperation of the patient for 10 days. Because many patients do not understand the need for taking medication for the full 10 days, IM benzathine penicillin G is usually the method of choice. If oral penicillin is selected, however, specific counseling outlining the need for the 10 full days of therapy to eradicate the infection and prevent rheumatic fever should be stressed. Dosage is penicillin V, 250 mg 3 times a day for 10 days.

or

3. **If patient is allergic to penicillin**, use
   a. Erythromycin suspension (see Table 3-3, p. 111, for dosage).
   or
   b. If patient is over 25 kg (55 lb), erythromycin tablets (250 mg per tablet) in a dosage of 500 mg (2 tablets) twice a day for 10 days taken 1 hour before meals.

Note: If abdominal discomfort develops, divide dose in half and give 4 times a day.

VII. Complications of Streptococcal Pharyngitis

A. Rheumatic fever.

B. Cervical lymphadenitis, particularly in infants.

C. Otitis media, particularly in children.

D. Peritonsillar abscess in older children and adults.

E. Retropharyngeal abscess in younger children.

F. Sinusitis.

G. Acute glomerulonephritis.

VIII. Consultation–Referral

A. **Cervical adenitis** of 3 cm in diameter or greater.

B. **Peritonsillar abscess.** Consider when the following are present:
   1. Asymmetrical swelling of tonsils, tonsillar fossae, and overlying soft palate. Uvula shifted to opposite side.
   2. Fever persisting 4 days after treatment was started for streptococcal pharyngitis.

3. Trismus, difficulty in swallowing, and feeling of fullness in throat.

4. Extreme enlargement of tonsils.

C. **Prolonged toxic course**

D. **Retropharyngeal abscess.** Consider in infant when the following are present:

1. Difficulty in swallowing.

2. Persistent high fever.

3. Hyperextended head, with difficulty in breathing.

4. Forward bulge in the posterior pharyngeal wall.

E. **Membrane on pharynx** suggesting diphtheria.

IX. Follow-Up

Throat cultures of the patient with streptococcal pharyngitis and family members and close contacts are generally *not* indicated unless:

A. Someone is symptomatic.

B. The patient or a contact has a history of rheumatic fever.

C. There is an outbreak of rheumatic fever or poststreptococcal glomerulonephritis in the community.

Note: If someone has a positive repeat culture for Group A beta-hemolytic streptococci, treat only one more time and do *not* reculture after treatment.

▲ ORAL CANDIDIASIS (THRUSH): PEDIATRIC

I. Definition

Superficial fungal infection of the oral cavity in infants.

II. Etiology

The causative organism is *Candida albicans,* which is usually acquired from the following sources:

A. Mother's vagina during birth.

B. Mother's nipples during breast-feeding.

C. Other infants, by contamination of caretaker's hands or objects shared by babies.

D. Adult with vaginal candidiasis, through contamination of her hands.

E. Patient's own candidal diaper dermatitis.

F. Oral broad-spectrum antibiotic therapy (e.g., ampicillin), as a side effect.

III. Clinical Features

A. **Symptoms**

1. Often none.
2. With extensive involvement, pain during feeding and swallowing.

B. **Signs**

1. White, irregularly shaped plaques appear on the buccal mucosa, lips, palate, and gums. They may produce a confluent white coating on the tongue.
2. Lesions are removable, leaving an inflamed base.
3. The patient may have candidal diaper dermatitis (moist, red, occasionally scaling rash with a sharp border and satellite red papules or pustules.

IV. **Laboratory Studies**

Potassium hydroxide preparation of scrapings of lesions reveals budding yeast with or without hyphae. This study usually is not needed when typical lesions are present.

V. **Differential Diagnosis.**

Milk or food particles remaining in the mouth of the patient.

VI. **Treatment**

Advise parent on the following measures:

A. **Control of source of infection**

1. Wash hands thoroughly between handling of different infants in newborn nursery and before handling any baby.
2. Do not have infants share clothing, pacifiers or nipples.
3. Examine and treat contact with vaginitis or nipple infection.
4. Treat candidal diaper dermatitis (see Chapter 3, Diaper Dermatitis, **VI.D**, p. 98).

B. **Oral antifungal therapy.** Use nyastin (Mycostatin) oral suspension (100,000 units per mL) in a dosage of 2 mL orally 4 times a day for 1 week (1 mL in each side of the mouth, not in back of throat, so that medication is in contact with the lesions for as long as possible). It may help to rub a portion of the dose on the lesions with a cotton swab. This oral antifungal treatment may be continued for another week if there is not marked improvement.

VII. **Complications**

A. Feeding problems due to pain.
B. Candidal diaper dermatitis or perioral dermatitis.
C. Spread of infection to other infants in nursery or home.

VIII. **Consultation–Referral**

A. Feeding problems due to pain.
B. Failure to thrive.

IX. **Follow-Up**

Return visit in 1 week if the infection is not markedly improved.

▲ BACTERIAL SINUSITIS: ADULT

I. Definition

Inflammation of the mucous membrane lining of the paranasal sinuses due to bacterial infection, causing obstruction of normal sinus discharge. In chronic recurrent disease, allergens or irritants such as smoke may initiate symptoms.

II. Etiology

A. Most common

    1. *Hemophilus influenza.*

    2. *Streptococcus pneumonia.*

    3. Various anaerobes.

B. Less common

    1. *Neisseria* species.

    2. Beta-hemolytic streptococci.

    3. *Staphylococcus aureus.*

    4. *Escherichia coli.*

III. Clinical Features

A. Symptoms

    1. Mucopurulent nasal discharge and persistent postnasal drip.

    2. Choking cough at night, often appearing after a recent upper respiratory tract infection.

    3. General malaise.

    4. An ache or pressure behind the eyes.

    5. Toothache-like pain.

    6. Headache (often worse at night and early morning).

B. Signs

    1. Yellow, mucopurulent nasal discharge.

    2. Tenderness over the involved sinus.

    3. Edematous, hyperemic inferior turbinates.

    4. Usually, fever.

    5. Failure of sinus to transilluminate.

IV. Laboratory and Other Studies

A. X-ray (only on physician's orders).

B. Nasopharyngeal cultures correlate poorly with cultures obtained by sinus aspiration and are therefore not indicated.

V. Differential Diagnosis

A. Nonbacterial sinusitis.

B. Undifferentiated upper respiratory tract infection.

C. Persistent rhinitis due to allergy.

VI. Treatment

A. **Nasal congestion and drainage.** Advise patient on the following measures:

1. Keep head raised when lying down.

2. Use a topical decongestant:

a. Xylometazoline HCl (Otrivin) 0.1% nasal solution, 2 or 3 drops in each nostril every 8 hours for a maximum of 2 weeks.

   or

b. Xylometazoline HCl (Otrivin) 0.1% nasal spray, 1 spray followed in 5–10 minutes by a second spray; repeat sequence every 8 hours for a maximum of 2 weeks.

   and/or

3. Start oral therapy:

a. Pseudoephedrine HCl (Sudafed) tablets (60 mg per tablet). 1 tablet 3 or 4 times a day for a maximum of 2 weeks.

   or

b. Phenylpropanolamine HCl (Propadrine) tablets (50 mg per tablet), 1 tablet 3 or 4 times a day for a maximum of 2 weeks.

   or

c. Triprolidine HCl and pseudoephedrine HCl (Actifed) tablets, 1 tablet 3 times a day for a maximum of 2 weeks.

B. **Fever or pain.** Have patient take aspirin (325 mg per tablet), 2 tablets orally every 4–6 hours.

C. **Infection.** Patient can take antibiotics, but prescribe *only* after telephone consultation with physician.

1. Amoxicillin 250 mg tablets for 10 days if not allergic to penicillin.

   or

2. Septra I (double strength) or II (regular strength) twice a day for 2 weeks.

VII. Complications

Complications are infrequent but serious.

A. Abscess.

B. Osteomyelitis.

C. Spread to the central nervous system.

VIII. Consultation–Referral

A. All patients with acute frontal sinusitis.

B. All acutely and severely ill patients.

C. Chronic or recurrent illness.

D. Any indication of involvement of the orbit or central nervous system.

IX. Follow-Up

Have patient call in 2–3 days if there is no improvement.

▲ NONBACTERIAL SINUSITIS: ADULT

I. Definition

Inflammation of the mucous membrane lining the paranasal sinuses due to viral, allergic, vasomotor, or other nonbacterial causes, producing obstruction of normal sinus discharge.

II. Etiology

A. Numerous viruses, pollens, and other allergens.

B. Vasomotor instability secondary to cold or emotional factors, or both.

III. Clinical Features

A. **Symptoms**
1. Clear, nonpurulent nasal discharge.
2. Nocturnal postnasal drip with resultant cough.
3. Pain in the area of the involved sinuses that is usually appreciated as a sensation of pressure or fullness.
4. Minimal or no generalized symptoms, such as malaise or myalgia.
5. Headache.
6. Simulation of a toothache in some cases of maxillary sinusitis.

B. **Signs**
1. Clear nasal discharge.
2. Edema and hyperemia of the nasal mucosa.
3. Tenderness over the involved sinus.
4. No erythema of the area over the involved sinus.
5. No fever.

IV. Laboratory Studies

None.

V. Differential Diagnosis

A. Bacterial sinusitis.

B. Uncomplicated upper respiratory tract infection.

C. Allergic rhinitis.

D. Dental abscess.

VI. Treatment

Advise patient on the following measures:

A. **Nasal congestion.** In sinusitis alone and in sinusitis associated with viral upper respiratory tract infection, the use of decongestants, antihistamines, or both, and topical decongestants is usually sufficient to decrease edema and discomfort. For treatment measures, see Bacterial Sinusiti: Adult, **VI.A**, p. 153.

B. **Pain.** Aspirin (325 mg per tablet), 2 tablets every 4–6 hours as needed.

VII. Complications

Bacterial sinusitis.

VIII. Consultation–Referral

Chronic or recurrent illness.

IX. Follow-Up

Telephone call in 2–3 days if no improvement.

▲ UPPER RESPIRATORY TRACT INFECTION (COMMON COLD): PEDIATRIC AND ADULT

I. Definition

An acute infection of the upper respiratory tract lasting several days.

II. Etiology

Numerous viruses acquired through contact with infected conjunctival or nasal secretions.

III. Clinical Features

A. **Symptoms**

1. General malaise.
2. Nasal stuffiness, nasal discharge, sneezing, cough.
3. Mild sore throat.
4. Watery eyes.
5. Decreased appetite, particularly in infants.

B. **Signs**

1. Erythematous, edematous nasal mucosa, with clear, thin nasal discharge initially. The discharge may become mucoid or purulent as the illness resolves.
2. Mildly erythematous pharynx.
3. Mild conjunctivitis.

4. Sometimes, fever. It is usually of low grade, but may be elevated in infants.

5. Erythematous tympanic membranes in infants.

IV. Laboratory Studies

A. Usually, none.

B. Nasal culture for group A beta-hemolytic streptococci if nasal discharge persists for more than 2 weeks in an infant under 2 years of age and is associated with anorexia, fever, cervical lymphadenopathy, or, especially, excoriation and crusting around the nostrils.

V. Differential Diagnosis

A. Allergic rhinitis.

B. Foreign body, particularly if nasal discharge is unilateral and malodorous, purulent, or bloody.

VI. Treatment

A. **Increased oral fluid intake**

B. **Aspiration of nasal secretions** with rubber suction bulb in infants, particularly before feedings.

C. **Antipyretics and analgesics**

1. **Children.** Acetaminophen (Tylenol) as needed for high fever (see Table 5-5 below for dosage).

2. **Adults**

a. **Acetaminophen** (325 mg per tablet), 1 or 2 tablets as often as every 6 hours as needed.

or

TABLE 5-5

ORAL PEDIATRIC DOSAGE OF ACETAMINOPHEN

	DOSE (10–15 MG/KG/DOSE)		
AGE	DROPS (80MG/0.8 ML)	ELIXIR OF SYRUP (160 MG/5 ML)	FREQUENCY
3 months–1 year	0.8 mL	*or* 2.5 mL	as often as
1–3 years	0.8–1.6 mL	*or* 2.5–5.0 mL	every 4 to 6
3 –6 years	1.6 mL	*or* 5.0 mL	hours
			(5 doses/
Over 6 years*	. . .	*or* 10.0 mL	24 hours)

*Alternative is one-half to one tablet (325 mg per tablet) 3 or 4 times daily.

> b. **Aspirin** (325 mg per tablet), 1 or 2 tablets as often as every 4 hours as needed.

D. **Topical decongestant** for nasal stuffiness or discharge.

1. **Children under 12 years of age.**

Note: The nasal stuffiness and discharge of the common cold are self-limiting, and most patients do not need medication. When symptoms are causing distress or poor feeding and are not controlled by nasal bulb-syringe aspiration in infants, then medication may be helpful.

> a. **Use xylometazoline HCl (Otrivin)** 0.05% nasal solution (see Table 5-6 for dosage).

> b. **For infants less than 6 months of age,** decongestants are not advised. Saline nose drops should be recommended. Commercial preparations may be purchased or saline nose drops may be prepared by distilling 1/4 teaspoon table salt in 8 ounces of warm tap water.

2. **Adults and children over 12 years of age**

> a. Xylometazoline HCl (Otrivin) 0.1% nasal solution, 2 or 3 drops in each nostril every 8 hours as needed. Do not use for more than 3 days.

> *or*

> b. Xylometazoline HCl (Otrivin) 0.1% nasal spray, 1 spray followed by a second spray in 5–10 minutes; repeat sequence every 8 hours as needed. Do not use for more than 3 days.

> *and/or*

> c. Oral decongestant–antihistamine combination, such as triprolidine HCl and pseudoephedrine HCl (Actifed) tablets, 1 tablet 3 times a day.

VII. Complications

A. Serous or purulent otitis media, particularly in infants and young children.

TABLE 5-6

PEDIATRIC DOSAGE OF 0.05% XYLOMETAZOLINE (OTRIVIN) NASAL SOLUTION

AGE	DOSE (IN EACH NOSTRIL)	FREQUENCY
6 months–2 years	2 drops	Every 8 hours while awake as needed*
2–12 years	3 drops	Every 8 hours while awake as needed*

*Do not use for more than 3 days.

   B. Sinusitis.

   C. Lower respiratory tract infection.

VIII. Consultation–Referral

   Only if needed for a complication.

 IX. Follow-Up

   As needed.

6

DISORDERS OF THE LOWER RESPIRATORY SYSTEM

▲ ACUTE LARYNGOTRACHEOBRONCHITIS (VIRAL CROUP): PEDIATRIC

I. Definition

Inflammation of the larynx, often extending to the subglottis, trachea, and bronchi, characterized by hoarseness, barking cough, and inspiratory stridor, usually occurring between ages 6 months and 5 years.

II. Etiology

Predominantly due to myxoviruses (parainfluenza virus types A and B), but may be caused by respiratory syncytial virus, adenoviruses, measles virus and *Mycoplasma pneumoniae.*

III. Clinical Features

A. Symptoms

1. Barking cough.

Patient Care Guidelines for Nurse Practitioners, 4th ed. by Axalla J. Hoole, C. Glenn Pickard, Jr., Ruth M. Ouimette, Jacob A. Lohr, and Robert A. Greenberg. Copyright © 1995 by J. B. Lippincott Company.

2. Inspiratory stridor.
3. Hoarseness.
4. Labored breathing.
5. Symptoms usually occur or become worse at night.
6. Common cold symptoms usually precede onset.

B. **Signs**
   1. Inspiratory stridor.
   2. Barking cough.
   3. Hoarseness.
   4. Labored breathing with respiratory distress.
   5. Low-grade or absent fever.

IV. **Diagnostic Studies**

Chest and lateral neck X-ray films only after consultation, but usually these are not needed.

V. **Differential Diagnosis**

A. Acute epiglottis caused by *Hemophilus influenzae* type B and suggested by the following:
   1. Fever over 101 °F (38.3 °C) rectally.
   2. Sudden onset, with rapid progression.
   3. Severe respiratory distress.
   4. Toxicity, agitation, or prostration.
   5. Drooling, with sore throat or difficulty in swallowing, or both.

Note: Do *not* attempt to look at the epiglottis or upset the patient. This can lead to complete obstruction.

B. Bacterial tracheitis.
C. Congenital laryngeal stridor in infant.
D. Aspirated foreign body.
E. Diphtheria.
F. Angioneurotic edema.

VI. **Treatment**

Advise parent on these measures:

A. Change environmental air to increase humidity.
   1. Let patient breathe outside air when symptoms increase (usually at night).
   2. Place patient in a steam-filled room (e.g., bathroom where hot water had been running).

B. Increase fluid intake.

VII. **Complications**

A. Airway obstruction.

B. Severe tracheobronchitis.

C. Pneumonia.

VIII. Consultation–Referral

A. Signs of epiglotitis. *Refer immediately—this is an emergency.*

B. Respiratory distress.

IX. Follow-Up

Return visit if there is an increase in symptoms.

▲ ACUTE TRACHEOBRONCHITIS: PEDIATRIC

I. Definition

Acute inflammation of the respiratory epithelium of the trachea and bronchi without involvement of the alveoli or supporting lung tissue.

II. Etiology

A. A viral etiology is most common, particularly in young children. Any of the viral respiratory pathogens may be responsible, but the myxoviruses (the parainfluenza viruses and influenza virus types A and B) are most common.

B. *Mycoplasma pneumoniae* is a common cause in school-age children and adolescents.

III. Clinical Features

A. **Symptoms**

1. Cough (persistent, dry, and worse at night).

2. Sometimes, mild tachypnea.

3. Restlessness and irritability associated with cough.

4. Sometimes, preceding or accompanying symptoms of upper respiratory tract infection.

5. Sometimes, systemic symptoms, including myalgia, headache, anorexia and lethargy, particularly with influenza viruses.

B. **Signs**

1. Rhonchi.

2. High-pitched inspiratory or expiratory wheezing that improves with coughing.

3. Fever—usually absent or of low grade; sometimes high, particularly with influenza viruses.

4. Often preceded or accompanied by signs of upper respiratory tract infection.

IV. Diagnostic Studies

Chest X-ray films only after consultation. Usually X-ray not needed.

V. Differential Diagnosis

A. Uncomplicated upper respiratory after consultation. Usually X-ray not needed.

B. Pneumonia.

C. Asthma.

D. Viral croup (laryngotracheobronchitis).

E. Bacterial tracheitis.

F. Aspirated irritants, particularly hydrocarbons.

G. Aspirated foreign body.

H. Tuberculosis and other chronic pulmonary diseases.

I. Congestive heart failure.

J. Environmental irritants including tobacco and marijuana smoking.

VI. Treatment

A. **Prevention.** Influenza virus vaccine (subvirion or split-virus preparations) is strongly recommended for children over 6 months of age with chronic cardiorespiratory diseases or with compromised immune systems.

B. **Therapy**

1. Increase oral fluid intake.

2. Adequate environmental humidity.

3. Soothing preparations, such as lemon juice mixed with sugar.

4. No antibiotics, as most cases are of viral origin.

5. Tuberculin skin test:

a. If there has not been one in a year.

b. If there is a question of exposure to tuberculosis.

c. If symptoms persist.

6. Acetaminophen (Tylenol) for fever (see Table 5-5, p. 156, for dosage).

Note: Aspirin should *not* be used if influenza is suspected, because there is evidence that it may be associated with the development of Reye's syndrome in patients with influenza or chickenpox.

7. Avoid use of cough medications, particularly those which contain cough suppressants, in children.

VII. Complications

A. Usually, none.

B. Rarely, bacterial pneumonia.

VIII. Consultation–Referral

A. Respiratory distress.

B. Evidence of systemic toxicity.

C. More than two episodes in a year.

D. Symptoms lasting more than 3 weeks.

E. Suspicion of aspiration.

IX. **Follow-Up**

A. Clinic visit if no improvement in 7 days.

B. Children with chronic cardiorespiratory disease should be seen again in 2–3 days.

C. Return visit if symptoms of respiratory distress develop.

▲ ACUTE LOWER RESPIRATORY TRACT INFECTION (ACUTE BRONCHITIS): ADULT

I. **Definition**

An infectious inflammatory disease primarily of the bronchi characterized by one or more of these: hyperemia of the bronchial mucosa, increased production of mucous, an inflammatory exudate of mucus and white blood cells. There may be some inflammatory involvement of the alveolar spaces.

Note: Acute lower respiratory tract infections in adults are commonly separated into two categories: "pneumonia" and "bronchitis" depending on whether the inflammation involves the alveolar spaces ("pneumonia") or the bronchi ("bronchitis"). In clinical practice, this precise distinction is rarely possible because many patients who clinically have only "bronchitis" may have X-ray evidence of alveolar involvement (consolidation or infiltrate). In practice, the less seriously ill patients, as described in this guideline, usually have primarily "bronchitis" and are managed as indicated. More seriously ill patients more often have "pneumonia" and may require inpatient evaluation and management.

II. **Etiology**

Viruses are the most common cause. Other common agents are the bacteria *Streptococcus pneumoniae, Hemophilus influenzae,* and *Mycoplasma pneumoniae.* Much less commonly, a wide spectrum of infectious agents can produce acute bronchitis (e.g., *Legionella* and pertussis).

III. **Clinical Features**

A. **Symptoms**

1. Cough is almost always present.

2. The amount and character of sputum produced is of particular importance. Viral bronchitis rarely causes more than 2 tablespoons per day of sputum, which is micropurulent. Bacterial bronchitis is frequently associated with purulent sputum, often more than 2 tablespoons per day.

3. Chest pain, if present, is generally a substernal discomfort aggravated by coughing.

4. Wheezing and slight dyspnea on exertion.

5. There are no frank, shaking chills.

B. **Signs**

1. Temperature is usually less than 101 °F (38.3 °C). No tachypnea at rest.

2. The chest is clear to percussion.

3. Rhonchi or wheezing, or both, are present.

4. Scattered rales may be present.

5. No dullness to percussion or bronchial breath sounds.

IV. **Laboratory and Diagnostic Studies**

A. **Sputum**

1. Sputum is initially clear in viral or mycoplasmal bronchitis, but purulent in bacterial bronchitis.

2. Gram stain and culture of sputum usually are not necessary unless sputum is purulent or pneumonia is suspected.

B. **A chest X-ray** may be taken if the clinical assessment is unclear, but generally is not necessary.

C. **Blood count**

1. A white blood cell count is indicated only if the clinical picture is unclear. Consult with physician.

2. The white blood cell count usually is normal in viral or mycoplasmal disease; the count is rarely elevated, even in bacterial infections.

V. **Differential Diagnosis**

A. Pneumonia.

B. Tuberculosis and other chronic pulmonary diseases.

C. Bronchial asthma.

D. Congestive heart failure.

E. Uncommon causes of bronchitis such as *Legionella,* pertussis, etc.

VI. **Treatment**

A. Bronchitis with production of less than 2 tablespoons of mucoid or mucopurulent sputum per day.

1. Rest.

2. Acetaminophen (Tylenol) for discomfort; see p. 156 for dosage.

3. Vaporizer or humidifier for moisture.

4. Cough suppressants, such as codeine or dextromethorphan hydrobromide, may be used sparingly.

    a. Dextromethorphan hydrobromide, 30 mg orally every 6–8 hours as needed.

    b. Codeine, 15–30 mg orally every 4–6 hours as needed (controlled substance—physician prescription required).

    and/or

  5. Expectorants may be used, although there is debate as to their efficacy. Guaifenesin is available alone or in combination with cough suppressants:

    a. Guaifenesin, 200–400 mg every 4 hours as needed.

  B. Bronchitis with production of more than 2 tablespoons of purulent sputum per day (usually associated with systemic symptoms).

  1. Rest.

  2. Acetaminophen for discomfort (see p. 156 for dosage).

  3. Expectorant (see **A.5**).

  4. Vaporizer or humidifier for moisture; of most value in winter.

  5. Antibiotic:

    a. Erythromycin, 250 mg orally 4 times a day for 10 days.

    or

    b. Amoxicillin, 500 mg orally 4 times a day for 10 days.

    or

    c. Tetracycline, 250 mg orally 4 times a day for 10 days.

    or

    d. Trimethoprim, 160 mg and sulfamethoxazole 800 mg orally 2 times a day for 10 days.

  6. Bronchodilator (if significant wheezing is present)—aminophylline, 200 mg 4 times a day for 10–14 days.

  7. Avoid bronchial irritants.

VII. Complications

Generally, none in simple bronchitis in adults.

VIII. Consultation–Referral

  A. Significant respiratory distress.

  B. Failure to improve in 72 hours.

  C. Elderly patients, particularly those with chronic cardiovascular or pulmonary diseases, who have evidence of worsening cardiovascular status. Patient should contact provider promptly for temperature greater than 39 °C (102 °F), increasing dyspnea or tachypnea, development of pleuritic pain, or if there is no improvement in 72 hours; or if patient is not well in 2 weeks.

▲ INFLUENZA: ADULT

I. Definition
An acute contagious viral illness often occurring in epidemics and characterized by fever, malaise, myalgia, and respiratory symptoms.

II. Etiology
One or another of three myxoviruses having similar properties and categorized as influenza virus types A, B, and C. Influenza A viruses have shown an unusual ability to mutate, resulting in new antigenic strains that frequently produce worldwide epidemics.

III. Clinical Features
A. Symptoms
1. Headache.
2. Malaise, lassitude, and occasionally prostration.
3. Myalgia.
4. Nonproductive cough.

B. Signs
1. Fever, often 39–39.3 °C (102–103 °F).
2. Rhonchi and occasionally scattered rales.

IV. Laboratory Studies
Generally, none.

V. Differential Diagnosis
A. Other viral illnesses.
B. Bacterial pneumonia.
C. Other acute infectious illnesses.

VI. Treatment
A. Supportive therapy
1. Acetaminophen, 325 mg, 2 tablets orally every 4–6 hours for fever and myalgia.
2. Increased fluid intake.
3. Mild cough suppressant, such as Robitussin-DM (guaifenesin and dextromethorphan hydrobromide), 2 teaspoons orally every 6–8 hours as needed.

B. **Amantadine.** In cases of influenza A, amantadine 100 mg orally twice a day for 4–7 days begun within 48 hours of onset of symptoms, is effective in shortening the duration of fever. Because there is no practical way to identify influenza A infection clinically, some practitioners empirically treat epidemic "influenza" with amantadine.

C. Yearly immunization with influenza vaccine.

VII. Consultation–Referral

A. Severely ill patients, particularly the elderly.

B. Respiratory distress or widespread rales or rhonchi on physical examination, or both of these.

C. Pregnant patients.

VIII. Follow-Up

As needed.

▲ BRONCHIAL ASTHMA: PEDIATRIC

I. Definition

A reversible obstructive airway disease characterized clinically by intermittent episodes of cough, dyspnea, and prolonged expiration with wheezing.

II. Etiology

Bronchial asthma is currently felt to be an inflammatory disease characterized by eosinophilic infiltration into the airway. In children, allergy is commonly associated with this inflammation, although non-allergic persons may also have asthma. The bronchi of asthmatics become constricted with a variety of stimuli and are typically more reactive than the bronchi of nonasthmatic persons. Stimuli associated with asthma attacks are listed below:

A. Allergy. Inhalant (house dust mites, animal allergens such as cat dander, molds, and pollen) and rarely food (usually associated with immediate and obvious symptoms after exposure to a given food).

B. Infection. Acute viral upper respiratory tract infection or bacterial sinusitis (but very rarely pneumonia). Viral colds may be the most common triggers of asthma in infants and young children.

C. Nonspecific irritants. Tobacco smoke, air pollution and chemical fumes.

D. Exercise or exertion. May be the only trigger and often occurs in adolescents.

E. Psychogenic factors.

F. Weather changes.

III. Clinical Features

The amount of airway obstruction often determines the severity of signs and symptoms. However, significant airway obstruction may occur without any other symptoms.

A. Symptoms

1. Cough.

2. Wheezing.

3. Dyspnea or chest tightness, anxiety and apprehension.

4. Poor sleep or frequent awakenings associated with cough.

5. May have paroxysmal coughing and vomiting (but other illnesses, including pertussis and parapertussis, may cause such symptoms as well).

B. **Signs**

1. Generalized expiratory wheezing often associated with prolonged expiration. Inspiratory wheezing may also be appreciated as well. Very focal wheezing suggests a focal airway problem (such as an airway abnormality or foreign body aspiration). However, with very severe asthma, chest sounds may be greatly diminished or absent as a result of very diminished airflow.

2. Hyperresonant percussion tone.

3. Tachypnea.

4. Intercostal retractions (usually with more serious exacerbations).

5. Use of accessory muscles of respiration.

6. Increased chest diameter.

7. Cyanosis in a severe attack. Obtain immediate consultation if cyanosis is present.

8. Evidence of upper respiratory tract infection.

9. Presence of allergic rhinitis or sinusitis. Allergic rhinitis may directly worsen asthma and should be treated if found.

10. Fever is only rarely associated with asthma, unless viral infection is triggering asthma and causing the fever.

IV. **Diagnostic Studies**

A. Objective measures of airflow (usually only on children over 5 years of age) can be reliably performed.

1. Peak expiratory flow rate (PEFR).

   a. Measures maximum forced airflow (L/min).

   b. Reflects large airway function only.

   c. Can be used in the office and at home.

   d. Inexpensive.

   e. Can be useful in confirming diagnosis of asthma (via home monitoring or by measuring changes pre- and post-administration of a bronchodilator).

2. Spirometry.

   a. Measures large and small airway function.

   b. Only available in the office.

   c Useful in confirming diagnosis of asthma.

TABLE 6-1
ASSESSMENT OF ASTHMA SEVERITY

	MILD	MODERATE	SEVERE
Exacerbations	1–2/wk	>2/wk	Frequent
Symptoms (between exacerbations)	Rare	1–2/wk	Daily
Nocturnal symptoms	Rare	1–2/month	Frequent
School attendance	Good	Occasional absence	Poor
PEFR	>80% pred.	60–80% pred.	<60% pred.

B. Chest X-Ray.

  1. Rarely needed.

  2. Used to rule out pneumonia (especially with fever).

C. Assessment of severity of asthma: see General Guide, Table 6-1.

V. Differential Diagnosis

A. Acute bronchiolitis.

B. Foreign body.

C. Cystic fibrosis.

D. Cough due to sinusitis or allergic rhinitis.

E. Anatomic abnormality of the airway.

F. *Chlamydia* (infant) or mycoplasmal infection.

VI. Treatment

A. Beta-agonists

  1. Dosage: (if not on as needed schedule)

  a. Metered dose inhaler (albuterol, metaproterenol) 2–4 puffs every 4–6 hours.

  b. Nebulizer

   (1) Albuterol (5 mg/mL): 0.10–0.15 mg/kg in 2 cc normal saline. Maximum dose—5.0 mg.

   (2) Metaproterenol (50 mg/mL): 0.25–0.50 mg/kg in 2 cc normal saline. Maximum dose—15.0 mg.

  c. Oral

   (1) Albuterol: 0.1–0.15 mg/kg every 4–6 hours or as needed, or 4 mg sustained release tablet 2 times a day.

   (2) Metaproterenol: 0.3–0.5 mg/kg q 4–6 hours or as needed.

Side effects: nausea, vomiting, irritability, increased activity, tachycardia, rarely arrhythmias.

B. **Inhaled corticosteroids:** Triamcinolone (100 μg/puff); flunisolide (250 μg/puff); beclomethasone (42 μg/puff).

1. Dosages: 2–4 puffs 2–4 times a day.

2. Side effects:

   a. Known: thrush, hoarseness (minimized by rinsing mouth and using spacer devices).

   b. Possible:

      (1) Mild decrease in growth rate.

      (2) Questionable effect on hypothalamic/pituitary/adrenal axis.

      (3) Clinical experience suggests that side effects are very minimal; studies currently underway.

C. Oral corticosteroids

1. Prednisone or prednisolone 1 mg/kg and decrease as tolerated.

2. Relatively safe for acute exacerbations (used less than 5–10 days).

3. Seek consultation before using for long-term therapy.

4. Side effects with prolonged use extensive: growth delay, adrenal suppression, decreased bone density, immunosuppression. Aseptic necrosis of the femoral head can occur even with short courses of steroids.

D. Steroids and varicella

1. Inhaled corticosteroids are less likely to increase risk of advanced disease and death with varicella but a consultation should be obtained.

2. Brief courses of oral steroids preceding onset of varicella also may increase problems with varicella and consultation is necessary.

3. Risk may be significantly increased with chronic use of oral steroids. Anyone on chronic steroids without a clear history of prior varicella should have varicella titers checked. Post-exposure varicella–zoster immune globulin and/or acyclovir can be used. Seek consultation if these patients acquire varicella.

E. Theophylline

1. Available in immediate release form for dosing every 6 hours or sustained-release form for dosing every 12–24 hours.

2. Liquid and capsule forms available.

3. Blood levels of 5–15 μg/mL required. Levels must be monitored routinely.

4. Side effects include nausea and vomiting, tachycardia, hyperactivity, and, rarely, arrhythmias and seizures.

5. Levels can be affected by other drugs, especially erythromycin.

VII. Treatment of Acute Asthma Attacks in Emergency Room

A. Initial Treatment

1. Nebulized beta-agonist (albuterol or terbutaline) every 20 minutes up to 3 times, and O_2 to keep O_2 saturation >95%. Albuterol dose (0.15 mg/kg/dose up to 5 mg/dose in 6 L oxygen flow).

2. Check peak expiratory flow rate or symptoms after each treatment. Stop if PEFR becomes > 90% of patient's baseline or symptoms abate.

3. Observe for 1 hour. Discharge if symptoms have improved and PEFR is at least >70% of baseline (or predicted if baseline unknown). Use treatment listed below.

4. Nebulized beta-agonist 4 times a day for 24 hours. Have patient call if symptoms return or PEFR becomes <70% of baseline.

5. If cyanosis is present, symptoms are severe, PEFR is <50% predicted, or O_2 saturation <95%—**SEEK IMMEDIATE CONSULTATION.**

B. If incomplete response to initial treatment

1. Repeat beta-agonist as for A.

2. Begin oral prednisone or prednisolone or IV methylprednisolone (2 mg/kg).

3. Observe for 1 hour.

4. If improved (as listed above), discharge with 4 times a day beta-agonist and 1 mg/kg/day of prednisone or prednisolone for 3–10 days.

5. Arrange follow-up by phone in 24 hours and in office by 14 days.

6. If not improved, seek consultation as hospitalization may be necessary.

VIII. Treatment of Acute Attacks at Home

A. Initial Treatment

1. Nebulized or metered dose inhaler beta-agonist (albuterol or terbutaline) every 20 minutes up to 3 treatments. Dose is 2 puffs via metered dose inhaler or 0.15 mg/kg dose of nebulized drug.

2. If cyanosis occurs or PEFR <50% predicted—**GO TO EMERGENCY ROOM IMMEDIATELY.**

3. Give albuterol (or other beta-agonist) every 4 hours. Call if symptoms recur or PEFR <70% of baseline after 1 hour.

4. Maintain all baseline chronic medications.

B. Incomplete response

1. Repeat beta-agonist as in **A**. Call health care provider.

2. Begin home administration of prednisone or prednisolone (1–2 mg/kg/dose first dose then 1 mg/kg/day).

3. If no improvement in one hour, or PEFR falls to <60% of predicted, **GO TO EMERGENCY ROOM or CALL HEALTH CARE PROVIDER.**

4. If improved, arrange telephone follow-up within 24 hours.

C. **Complications of acute asthma**

1. Pneumothorax.

2. Atelectasis.

3. Respiratory failure.

4. Death.

IX. Maintenance Therapy

A. **Asthma treatment strategies.** Asthma is an inflammatory airway disorder in which both symptomatic treatment with bronchodilators and control of inflammation with anti-inflammatory drugs may be necessary. Asthma treatment can vary based on the severity of the disease and particular patient needs. Listed below are general treatment strategies for asthma.

1. Mild asthma: PRN use of beta-agonists and prophylactic use of beta-agonist or cromolyn prior to exercise. beta-agonists as needed can be used via nebulizer, metered dose inhaler, or orally. Oral beta-agonists more likely to cause side effects.

2. Moderate asthma:

   a. Anti-inflammatory treatment

   (1) inhaled corticosteroids (800 to >1000 µg/day as required).

   (2) Oral corticosteroids may be needed on a daily or every other day schedule.

   (3) Obtain consultation if chronic oral corticosteroids are needed.

   (4) Theophylline (not an anti-inflammatory) may be an adjunct to anti-inflammatory drugs. Typically more side effects and blood levels (5–15 mg/mL) must be monitored. Does not decrease underlying airway inflammation.

   b. Bronchodilators:

   (1) Beta-agonists as needed up to 4 times a day (if on a regular schedule of beta-agonist, may still need extra PRN doses).

   (2) May need doses (inhaled or long acting) at bedtime to relieve nighttime symptoms.

4. Ancillary Treatments. If allergic rhinitis or sinusitis is present, concurrent treatment of these diseases can have a marked impact on asthma.

5. Reassess asthma at least every 4–6 months as severity may decrease and treatment plans may be appropriately downgraded.

B. **Patient education.** Patient and family education is essential for successful treatment of asthma.

1. Basic education

   a. Patients need to identify triggers of asthma.

   b. Patients need to understand the reasons specific medications are used as well as the side effects of these medicines.

   c. Patients need to be taught proper use of metered dose inhalers (which should all be used with spacer devices and peak flow meters).

   d. Patients should understand the inflammatory nature of asthma.

2. Specific education

   a. Goals of therapy (to minimize symptoms so that normal activities can be undertaken, including sports and exercise, with a minimum of medicines and side effects).

   b. Specific medication plans: Each patient should have a written plan for everyday (maintenance treatment) and a plan for treatment and evaluation of acute attacks. In allergic individuals, environmental control of allergens is essential. (See Allergic Rhinitis, Chapter 5).

X. **Other Resources**

A. NHLBI Asthma Guidelines—Diagnosis and Treatment of Asthma NIH Publication #3042.

▲ BRONCHIAL ASTHMA: ACUTE ATTACK IN A KNOWN ADULT ASTHMATIC

I. Definition

A clinical syndrome characterized by episodes of wheezing cough and dyspnea due to reversible bronchospasm. Breathing in the intervals between acute attacks is virtually normal.

II. Etiology

An acute attack of bronchial asthma may be of a single, multiple, or unknown cause. Each attack may be associated with one or a combination of the factors listed below. The precipitating factor may not necessarily be the same in each episode.

A. Allergy—inhalant, food.

B. Acute or chronic infection—viral, bacterial, tuberculosis, fungal.

C. Environmental physical factors—humidity, temperature, dust, fumes, odors.

D. Exertion.

E. Psychogenic factors.

III. **Clinical Features**

A. **Symptoms**

1. History of frequent episodes of eczema or atopic dermatitis.

2. Cough.

3. Dyspnea.

4. Wheezing.

B. **Signs**

1. Prolonged expiration with expiratory and, occasionally, inspiratory wheezes. In some cases, with greatly diminished air movement, wheezing may not be found.

2. Tachypnea.

3. Use of accessory muscles of respiration, such as sternomastoid and scalenus.

4. Intercostal retractions.

5. Perspiration.

6. Cyanosis, with severe asthma.

7. Hyperresonant percussion note.

8. Presence of the following, depending on etiology:

    a. Fever.

    b. Rhinorrhea.

    c. Evidence of upper respiratory tract infection or allergy.

IV. **Laboratory and Diagnostic Studies**

A. **Pulmonary function studies.** An objective measure of bronchospasm should be made in all cases.

1. Spirometry. Office spirometry can be used to establish the initial diagnosis of asthma, determine the severity of impairment, evaluate the response to therapy, and evaluate the need for hospitalization. More commonly in office practice, the peak expiratory flow rate is used (see below).

2. Peak expiratory flow rate (PEFR). Simple devices for measuring peak expiratory flow rate are available and can be used to quantitate the severity of the attack and measure responses to therapy. Criteria for severity in normal-sized adults are:

    a. 200 L/min or greater. Mild obstruction. Can usually be treated as outpatient.

    b. 100–200 L/min. Moderate obstruction. Usually should be held in the office for observation of response to therapy.

    c. 60–100 L/min. Severe obstruction. Hospitalization usually required.

B. If infection is suspected, the following should be initiated and a consultation obtained:

  1. Chest x-ray, to demonstrate:

    a. Hyperinflation.

    b. Evidence of pulmonary infection.

    c. Cardiac enlargement and evidence of heart failure, if underlying heart disease is severe.

  2. White blood cell count and differential count:

    a. Eosinophils may be elevated if allergic reaction is an important component of the asthma.

    b. If the white blood cell count is very high, acute infection should be suspected.

  3. Microscopic examination of sputum:

    a. Gram stain of sputum showing polymorphonuclear leukocytes and bacteria should raise suspicion of acute infection.

    b. Wright's stain of sputum will show large numbers of eosinophils if allergic reaction is an important component of the asthma.

  4. Culture of sputum:

    a. *Hemophilus influenzae* and pneumococcus are important pathogens.

    b. "Normal" flora (*Neisseria* and alpha-hemolytic streptococci) may be the cause of an acute attack.

V. Differential Diagnosis

A. Acute bronchitis.

B. Aspirated foreign body.

C. Pneumonia.

D. Allergic reaction to drug, inhalant, or food (anaphylaxis), especially the syndrome of chronic sinusitis, nasal polyps, and asthma that is associated with aspirin ingestion.

E. Congestive heart failure (sometimes called *cardiac asthma*) may closely mimic allergic asthma.

F. Pulmonary emboli.

VI. Treatment

The following regimen is intended for young to middle-aged patients with known asthma and no heart disease. **Warning:** Asthma may deteriorate into status asthmaticus in hours.

A. Ensure adequate hydration of patient by encouraging oral fluid intake.

B. Do not use sedatives.

C. Bronchodilator therapy.

1. Aerosol. Use air compressor-powered nebulizer. Albuterol 5 mg/mL 0.5 mL in 2.5 mL saline administered over 5 min. If not effective may repeat in 20 min.

   or

2. Subcutaneous epinephrine. Initially, inject 0.2–0.3 mL of 1:1000 aqueous epinephrine subcutaneously; reassess in 15–20 minutes and then repeat the dose if the attack persists. Up to 3 injections may be given, with assessment after each injection.

D. Bronchodilator therapy (if **C** is successful):

1. Resume previous maintenance therapy (if patient is not on maintenance therapy, consult physician).

2. Use antibiotics if infection is a significant contributor to the asthmatic exacerbation.

   a. Erythromycin, 250 mg orally 4 times a day for 7 days.

   or

   b. Amoxicillin, 500 mg orally 4 times a day for 7 days (if patient is not allergic to penicillin).

3. Do not use cough suppressants and antihistamines.

E. If **A–C** are not successful, consult physician.

VII. Complications

A. Severe hypoxia.

B. Dehydration.

C. Atelectasis.

D. Pneumonia.

E. Pneumothorax or pneumomediastinum, or both.

F. Respiratory failure.

G. Side effects of bronchodilator drug therapy:

1. Aminophylline or theophylline. Related to excessive plasma levels (e.g., anorexia, nausea, vomiting, nervousness, headache, arrhythmia, convulsions).

2. Terbutaline sulfate. Tachycardia, nervousness, tremors.

VIII. Consultation–Referral

A. All new cases, whether this is the patient's first attack or the first time the patient has been seen.

B. All asthmatics over 60 years of age.

C. All asthmatics with history of heart disease.

D. All patients known to have COPD, if any significant respiratory distress is present.

E. Peak expiratory flow rate >100 L/min.

F. Patients in whom acute therapy A-C fails.

G. Extreme shortness of breath.

H. Side effects of bronchodilator drug therapy (see **VII.G**).

IX. Follow-Up

Patients should be followed regularly every 1–3 months and seen promptly whenever necessary for acute attacks or symptoms or signs of infection, or both.

▲ CHRONIC OBSTRUCTIVE PULMONARY DISEASE (COPD): ADULT

I. Definition

A complex syndrome of decreased pulmonary function made up of three components in various combinations: emphysema characterized by irreversible destruction of the distal airspace; bronchitis characterized by excessive mucus production and inflammation of the bronchi resulting in sputum production; and bronchoconstriction.

II. Etiology

Unknown. Most cases are strongly associated with a history of cigarette smoking. There are usually no symptoms for the first 10–20 years for the smokers who develop COPD. Mild dyspnea after exertion develops first and is followed by cough and sputum production. Serial testing of pulmonary function documents a progressive loss of expiratory volume (FEV). Cessation of smoking does not restore the lost function but does decrease the rate of decline.

III. Clinical Features

A. Symptoms

1. Significant impairment, as detected by spirometry, may be asymptomatic.

2. Shortness of breath, first noticeable with exertion.

3. Chronic cough and sputum production, frequently in the morning.

    4. Often, episodes of wheezing.

B. Signs

    1. Early, no signs on physical examination.

    2. Tachypnea, somewhat labored, with loud breathing.

    3. As the disease progresses, there are increasing signs of hyperinflation and obstruction, depending on the composition of the disease:

        a. Increased anteroposterior diameter of the chest.

        b. Hyperresonant percussion note.

        c. Frequently, rhonchi.

        d. Wheezing.

        e. Distant heart sounds.

        f. Decreased lateral movement of the thorax, with increase in upward vector of the sternum.

        g. Decreased diaphragmatic movement.

        h. Use of the accessory muscles of respiration.

        i. Sometimes, in severe disease, paradoxical inward movement of the lower costal margins.

    4. Signs of right-sided heart failure—peripheral edema, jugular venous distention, hepatomegaly.

IV. Diagnostic and Laboratory Studies

    A. Chest x-ray only after physician consultation. Unsuspected pneumonia is common when there has been worsening of symptoms.

    B. Spirometry (FVC, FEV_1, and FEV_1/FVC).

    C. Sputum culture (occasionally helpful).

    D. Electrocardiogram.

    E. Arterial blood gas determination, after physician consultation.

V. Differential Diagnosis

    A. Allergic asthma.

    B. Acute bronchitis.

    C. Congestive heart failure.

VI. Treatment

    A. Prevention. Complications in patients with known chronic obstructive pulmonary disease may be prevented by:

    1. Yearly immunization with influenza vaccine.

    2. Immunization with pneumonococcal vaccine (Pneumovax).

    3. Cessation of smoking.

    4. Avoidance of foods such as dairy products, spicy food, wine, or other alcohol-containing beverages that in some people may increase bronchospasm and sputum.

5. Avoidance of extremes in temperature.

6. Home humidification of greater than 50% and ingestion of 2–3 L of H_2O per day may help thin their secretions.

B. **Stable chronic disease**

1. Patient should **avoid pulmonary irritants**, especially cigarettes.

2. **Bronchodilator.** Almost all patients with chronic obstructive pulmonary disease have some element of bronchospasm. Use an appropriate bronchodilator, such as

   a. Aminophylline tablets, 200 mg every 6 hours or 4 times a day.

   or

   b. Theophylline tablets, 200 mg every 6 hours or 4 times a day.

Note: Recent evidence suggests considerable variation in the rates of absorption and metabolism of theophylline by patients who do not respond to usual suggested dosages. Rates can best be established by carefully monitoring blood levels of theophylline in these patients. Also, certain long-acting oral preparations may be used to advantage in some patients.

   c. Beta-adrenergic agents by inhaler:

   (1) Metaproterenol 1–3 puffs every 4–6 h.

   (2) Albuterol 2 puffs every 4–6 h.

   (3) Expectorants. There is doubt as to whether these do more good than using a humidifier.

3. **Expectorants.**

   a. Glyceryl guaiacolate, 2 teaspoons by mouth every 4–6 hrs.

   b. Saturated solution of potassium iodide, 15 drops in a glass of water 3 times a day.

   c. Vaporizer.

4. Patient should **avoid sedatives, antihistamines**, and **beta blockers**.

5. Patients with significant bronchitis should follow a routine of **postural drainage** 3 or 4 times a day.

   a. Drink a hot cup of decaffeinated coffee or tea.

   b. Use a vaporizer for 5–10 minutes.

   c. Take an expectorant.

   d. Proceed with postural drainage in four positions, staying in each position for 5 minutes:

   (1) Supine.

   (2) Right side down.

   (3) Left side down.

        (4) Prone, with head down at a 30-degree angle.

  C. Acute attack of bronchitis (manifested by increased symptoms, fever, and change in color and quantity of sputum).

    1. Consult physician.

    2. General therapy as for chronic disease (see B).

    3. Hydration and humidification (extremely important).

    4. Antibiotics (if bacterial infection is suspected based on purulence of expectorated sputum).

      a. Erythromycin, 250 mg orally 4 times a day for 10 days.

      or

      b. Amoxicillin 500 mg orally 3 times a day for 10 days (if patient is not allergic to penicillin).

      c. Trimethoprim 160 mg/sulfamethoxazole 800 mg (Septra, Bactrim) one tablet orally twice a day for 14 days.

    5. Chest X-ray only after physician consultation.

VII. Complications

  A. Pneumonia.

  B. Respiratory failure.

  C. Cor pulmonale.

  D. Side effects of bronchodilator or drug therapy: see Bronchial Asthma: Acute Attack in a Known Adult Asthmatic, **VII.G.**

VIII. Consultation–Referral

  A. All new cases of suspected COPD.

  B. Pneumonia.

  C. Coexisting acute or chronic bronchitis if the patient has any significant change in respiratory function or a temperature greater than 38.3 °C (101 °F).

  D. Failure to improve within 48 hours.

  E. Suspected respiratory failure, manifested by severe dyspnea or any confusion or clouding of consciousness, or both.

  F. Side effects of bronchodilator drug therapy; see Bronchial Asthma: Acute Attack in a Known Adult Asthmatic, **VII.G.**

IX. Follow-Up

  A. Acute attack. Telephone call if there is no improvement in 3 days, or immediately if condition worsens.

  B. Stable chronic disease

    1. In 3 months for review.

    2. Repeat spirometry every year.

    3. Development of symptoms or signs of respiratory infection or increased shortness of breath, or both. Emphasize to patient the importance of promptly consulting the nurse practitioner or physician.

▲ ACUTE BRONCHIOLITIS: PEDIATRIC

I. Definition

A generalized inflammation of the bronchioles, characterized by signs of expiratory obstruction, occurring usually as an epidemic disease in winter and early spring in children under 3 years of age.

II. Etiology

A. Epidemic forms are usually caused by respiratory syncytial virus.

B. Sporadic cases are usually viral in origin, but bacteria, allergy, and *Mycoplasma pneumoniae* (particularly in adolescents) may be responsible.

III. Clinical Features

A. **Symptoms**

1. Onset as an upper respiratory tract infection.

2. Paroxysmal coughing.

3. Expiratory wheezing.

4. Dyspnea.

5. Difficulty sleeping and eating.

B. **Signs**

1. Rapid respirations.

2. Symmetric expiratory wheezing or grunting, or both.

3. Air-trapping causing liver to be pushed down, hyperresonant percussion note, and prolonged expiratory phase.

4. Increased heart rate.

5. Sometimes, fever (usually of low-grade).

6. Sometimes, rales.

IV. Diagnostic Studies

Chest X-ray only after consultation. Usually, X-ray is not needed.

V. Differential Diagnosis

A. Pneumonia.

B. Asthma.

C. Tracheobronchitis.

D. Pertussis.

E. Aspirated foreign body, especially with unilateral signs.

VI. Treatment

A. Maintain adequate fluid intake.

B. Therapeutic trial of B_2 adrenergic agonist aerosol may be considered after physician consultation.

C. Antibiotics are indicated only for complications such as acute otitis media.

VII. Complications

A. Hypoxia.

B. Progressive exhaustion followed by respiratory failure.

C. Dehydration from loss of water through lungs combined with poor fluid intake (usually with the accompanying upper respiratory disease.

D. Superimposed bacterial infection, including acute otitis media associated with the accompanying upper respiratory disease.

VIII. Consultation–Referral

A. Respiratory distress.

B. Children under 3 months of age.

C. Children with congenital heart disease.

D. More than 2 episodes. Refer to evaluation of possible underlying causes.

IX. Follow-Up

A. Phone contact in 24 hours.

B. Return visit if there is no improvement in 48 hours.

▲ PNEUMONIA: PEDIATRIC

I. Definition

Inflammation of the lung involving the alveoli or interstitial tissues, or both.

II. Etiology

A. A viral etiology is most common, particularly in preschool children. Respiratory syncytial virus and parainfluenza virus type 3 are particularly common causes in children under 3 years of age.

B. *Mycoplasma pneumoniae* probably accounts for at least half of the cases of pneumonia seen in school-age children, adolescents, and young adults. It is usually characterized by insidious onset and mild, but protracted, disease.

C. Bacterial pneumonia other than *Mycoplasma pneumoniae* is less common than viral pneumonia and is usually due to pneumococcus, *Hemophilus influenzae,* or, rarely, *Staphylococcus aureus.* Marked toxicity and consolidation or pleural fluid are usually present.

III. Clinical Features

A. Symptoms

1. Upper respiratory tract infection that precedes or accompanies the pneumonia.
2. Cough.
3. Fever.
4. Rapid or labored breathing, or both.
5. Lethargy.
6. Anorexia.
7. Abdominal pain and distention.
8. Vomiting.

B. **Signs**
1. Rapid breathing.
2. Labored breathing.
   a. Grunting on expiration.
   b. Flaring of nostrils.
   c. Intercostal and subcostal retractions.
3. Fine, crackling rales.
4. Evidence of consolidation or pleural effusion, or both:
   a. Decreased breath sounds.
   b. Dullness to percussion.
5. Sometimes, marked fever, lethargy, and anorexia.

IV. **Diagnostic Studies.**
Chest X-ray only after consultation. X-ray is not needed in mild cases.

V. **Differential Diagnosis**
A. Bronchiolitis and tracheobronchitis.
B. Aspirated foreign body.
C. Tuberculosis.

VI. **Treatment**
A. Increased fluid intake.
B. Rest, as needed.
C. Acetaminophen (Tylenol) for fever (see Table 5-5, p. 156 for dosage).
D. Antibiotics for bacterial, mycoplasmal, or chlamydia disease, after consultation.
E. Avoid cough medications, particularly those which contain cough suppressants, in children.

VII. **Complications**
A. Empyema.
B. Atelectasis.
C. Bronchiectasis.

    D. Pneumothorax.

    E. Dehydration.

VIII. Consultation–Referral

    A. All cases of pneumonia.

    B. Failure to improve in 48 hours.

    C. Failure to resolve in 3 weeks.

IX. Follow-Up

    A. Telephone call, home visit, or clinic visit every day until patient is afebrile and has no respiratory distress.

    B. Return visit in 3 weeks.

    C. Repeat chest X-ray for severe disease or persisting symptoms and signs. Consult physician for review of initial X-ray film for decision on the necessity for and timing of follow-up films.

7

▼

DISORDERS OF THE CARDIOVASCULAR SYSTEM

▲

▲ ANGINA PECTORIS: ADULT

I. Definition

Pain, usually in the substernal region of the chest, occasionally in the epigastrium, neck, back, or arms, caused by an imbalance between the work required of the myocardium and the oxygen supply to the myocardium.

II. Etiology

Usually, atherosclerosis of the coronary arteries. Risk factors for developing atherosclerosis include: family history of atherosclerosis, hypertension, cigarette smoking, hyperlipidemia, male gender, obesity, diabetes mellitus, and sedentary lifestyle.

III. Clinical Features

A. **Symptoms.** Diagnosis is based primarily on the history of characteristic pain.

1. Location. Pain usually located in the substernal region of the chest, but occasionally is present in the epigastrium, neck, back, or arms.

2. Onset. Pain usually occurs with an increase in the workload on the heart and is relieved by a decrease in the workload. Classi-

Patient Care Guidelines for Nurse Practitioners, 4th ed. by Axalla J. Hoole, C. Glenn Pickard, Jr., Ruth M. Ouimette, Jacob A. Lohr, and Robert A. Greenberg. Copyright © 1995 by J. B. Lippincott Company.

cally, this relation is demonstrated by pain occurring with work and relieved by rest (usually within 3–5 minutes and less than 15 minutes). Pain, however, may occur at rest. Rest angina suggests more serious disease and requires immediate attention.

3. Description. The pain is usually described as squeezing or pressurelike, sometimes as expanding, and seldom as sticking sharp or burning.

4. Radiation of pain. Pain often radiates to the neck, shoulder, or arms (the left arm more often than the right).

5. Accompanying symptoms. Sometimes there is a slight shortness of breath, mild diaphoresis, or slight nausea, or a combination of these. The pain is not pleuritic.

B. **Signs.** There should be no signs in uncomplicated angina. Nonetheless, one should carefully examine the heart and lungs for signs of congestive heart failure (CHF) which may be caused by the ischemic event (see Congestive Heart Failure, p. 186).

IV. Diagnostic Studies

(With new onset angina, a consultation with the physician is necessary.)

A. Electrocardiogram. The ECG may show characteristic abnormalities, particularly during an attack of pain. The ECG, however, is normal in 50%–70% of patients.

B. Other studies, such as an exercise ECG, should be ordered only after consultation.

C. Hematocrit, thyroid function tests.

V. Differential Diagnosis

A. Acute myocardial infarction.

B. Musculoskeletal pain (e.g., costochondritis).

C. Esophagitis, esophageal spasm, and other gastrointestinal causes of chest pain.

D. Pleurisy and other pulmonary causes of chest pain.

E. Malingering.

F. Cervical spine root compression.

VI. Treatment

Angina pectoris can be divided into two broad categories, stable angina and unstable angina, which are treated quite differently.

A. **Stable angina** is previously diagnosed angina that recurs with approximately the same amount of exertion with the same frequency and intensity of pain, and is relieved after approximately the same period of rest (less than 15 minutes) and/or the same number of nitroglycerin tablets.

1. General measures:

a. Reduction or elimination of risk factors.

  b. Reduction of workload on the heart:

    (1) Reduction of exertion by the patient.

    (2) Reduction of workload by control of other diseases that tend to increase the workload.

        (a) Control of hypertension (see Uncomplicated Essential Hypertension, pp. 194).

        (b) Correction of anemia.

        (c) Treatment of anxiety.

        (d) Weight loss.

  c. Improvement of cardiac performance without changing workload. Treatment leading to compensation of CHF (see Congestive Heart Failure, **VI**, p. 191).

  2. Specific therapy

  a. Nitroglycerin, 1 tablet (0.3–0.4 mg) sublingually every 3–5 minutes until pain is relieved or headache results. Not to exceed a total of 3 tablets.

  b. Long-acting nitrates. Consult physician for choice of agent and regimen.

  c. Beta blockers. Consult physician for choice of agent and regimen.

  d. Calcium channel blockers. Consult physician for choice of agent and regimen.

 B. **Unstable angina** consists of angina de novo (the first attack or attacks of angina) or a worsening of previously stable angina and is characterized by more severe or persistent pain, pain on less exertion, or pain at rest. These patients should be referred and hospitalization considered.

VII. Complications

 A. Myocardial infarction.

 B. Congestive heart failure.

VIII. Consultation–Referral

 A. Unstable angina, including angina de novo.

 B. Development of congestive heart failure.

 C. Angina not relieved after 3 nitroglycerin tablets.

 D. Angina persisting more than 15 minutes.

IX. Follow-Up and Maintenance of Stable Angina

 A. Frequency of assessment. Frequency can vary considerably, depending on the severity of the disease and the presence or absence of other conditions, such as hypertension and CHF. For angina uncomplicated by other problems, a visit every 2–4 months should be adequate. Any time angina becomes unstable (see **VI.B**), the patient should be advised to seek care.

B. Content of assessment

1. Assessment of basic disease process

a. Subjective evaluation:

(1) Stability of angina.

(2) Symptoms of CHF.

b. Objective evaluation:

(1) Assessment of heart and lungs, particularly for signs of CHF.

(2) Resting ECG every 2 or 3 years.

2. Assessment of chronic medical regimen

a. Sublingual nitroglycerin. For drug and dosage, see **VI.A.2.**

(1) Subjective.

(a) Frequency and number of tablets required for relief of angina.

(b) Activity of medication. (Tablets should be replaced every 6 months as nitroglycerin deteriorates rapidly.)

(c) Occurrence of headache after only one tablet suggests need for lower dose.

b. Long-acting nitrates.

(1) Drug and usual dosage. Isosorbide 20–40 mg orally every 6 hours while awake.

(2) Assessment of side effects.

(a) Subjective (review at each visit).

[1] Headaches. Usually decrease or disappear with dosage reduction or passage of time.

[2] Dizziness on arising from sitting or lying.

(b) Objective. Check for postural drop in blood pressure.

c. Beta blockers. Many agents are available. Consult physician for choice of agent and regimen.

(1) Assessment of side effects of beta blockers.

(a) Subjective.

[1] Fatigue.

[2] Depression or sleep disturbance.

[3] Bronchospasm or worsening of asthma or chronic obstructive pulmonary disease (COPD).

[4] Onset or worsening of CHF (see below).

(b) Objective:

[1] Pulse rate less than 60/min.

[2] Wheezing.

[3] Signs of CHF (see below).

d. Calcium channel blocking agents. Many agents are available. Consult physician for drug and regimen.

(1) Assessment related to possible side effects of calcium channel blockers.

(a) Subjective:

[1] Onset or worsening of CHF (see below).

[2] Syncope or near syncope due to atrioventricular block.

(b) Objective:

[1] Pulse rate less than 60/min.

[2] Signs of CHF (see below).

▲ CONGESTIVE HEART FAILURE (CHF): ADULT

I. Definition

A complicated state of altered cardiac function in which there is inadequate cardiac output to meet the oxygen demand of metabolizing tissues, leading to excessive retention of salt and water.

II. Etiology

Any process that damages the heart. In the United States, the most common causes are arteriosclerotic heart disease and hypertensive heart disease. In addition, one must look for secondary factors that may aggravate or precipitate CHF. These include increased physical activity, inadequate control of hypertension, increased sodium intake, failure to take medications properly, anemia, renal failure, thyrotoxicosis, cardiac arrhythmia, intercurrent illness such as pneumonia, and emotional stress.

III. Clinical Features

A. Heart failure itself

1. Symptoms

a. Dyspnea on exertion which may progress to dyspnea at rest.

b. Orthopnea.

c. Paroxysmal nocturnal dyspnea.

d. Ankle swelling.

e. Nocturia.

f. Dry hacking cough or wheezing, particularly at night.

g. Chronic fatigue.

2. Signs

a. Tachycardia.

    b. Weight gain, reflecting fluid retention.

    c. Neck vein distention.

    d. Rales, particularly over the base of the lungs.

    e. S_3 gallop rhythm.

    f. Bilateral dependent edema.

    g. Hepatomegaly with severe, usually chronic, heart failure.

    h. Rarely, ascites.

    i. Rarely, plural effusion.

B. Secondary factors that aggravate or precipitate CHF

    1. Symptoms

      a. Palpitation.

      b. Symptoms of intercurrent illness such as cough with sputum production.

      c. Symptoms of thyrotoxicosis such as decreased heat tolerance, increased sweating, etc.

      d. Anxiety.

    2. Signs.

      a. Arrhythmia.

      b. Signs of hyperthyroidism such as sweating, tremor, tachycardia, etc.

      c. Signs of intercurrent illness such as evidence of pulmonary consolidation, etc.

IV. Laboratory and Diagnostic Studies

    A. Chest X-ray may be indicated to confirm diagnosis and to better assess the magnitude of the problem.

    B. An ECG may be helpful in determining the cause of failure; it is not helpful in establishing a diagnosis of failure or in monitoring response to therapy.

    C. Serum NA^+, K^+, HCO_3^-, CL^-, and creatinine levels are useful as a baseline and should be measured before treatment is instituted.

    D. Hematocrit or hemoglobin should be measured, because anemia may contribute to the pathogenesis of CHF.

    E. Thyroid function studies.

V. Differential Diagnosis

    A. Other causes of dyspnea, such as chronic lung disease and asthma.

    B. Other causes of edema, such as renal disease, liver disease, and local venous problems.

    C. Recurrent pulmonary emboli.

    D. Other causes of wheezing, such as asthma. In the elderly, particularly with chronic obstructive pulmonary disease (COPD), establishing cause of wheezing may be difficult.

VI. Treatment

The general goal of therapy is to rid the body of excess salt and water by a combination of measures designed to improve cardiac function and to increase renal excretion of salt and water.

Note: Physician should be consulted before any treatment is begun.

A. **Initial therapy**

1. Low sodium diet. Generally, few patients can restrict their sodium intake below 85 mEq per day without major alterations in their style of living and eating. However, in refractory cases, further restriction should be attempted.

2. Measures to improve myocardial function:

   a. Reduction of systemic blood pressure to normal levels if it is elevated. Consult physician for regimen.

   b. Correction of anemia, if present.

   c. Use of digitalis preparations, such as Digoxin. Consult physician for initial dosage regimen and establishment of maintenance therapy (see **IX.C.1**).

   d. Measure to decrease peripheral resistance (afterload reduction) and to produce central vasodilation (preload reduction). (See **IX.C.2.**)

      (1) Long acting nitrates (e.g. Isosorbide). Consult physician for initial dosage and for long term maintenance regimen.

      (2) Angiotensin connecting enzyme (ACE) inhibitors. (e.g., Captopril, Enalapril, and others). Consult physician for initial dosage and for long term maintenance regimen.

3. Measures to increase renal excretion of sodium and water:

   (a) Oral diuretics if the patient is not acutely ill.

      (1) Hydrochlorothiazide, 25–50 mg every morning.

         or

      (2) Furosemide, 20–40 mg every morning.

   (b) I.V. diuretics should not be used without physician consultation.

B. **Maintenance therapy (see IX).**

VII. Complications

A. Worsening CHF.

B. Arrhythmias.

C. Hepatomegaly, ascites, profound peripheral edema.

D. Pulmonary embolism.

E. Digitalis toxicity (see **IX.C.1**).

F. Side effects of medications (see **IX.C**).

VIII. Consultation–Referral

A. All new patients should initially have a physician consultation.

B. All patients should be followed by the nurse practitioner with close physician consultation until their condition is stable on a maintenance regimen. The nurse practitioner may then follow and alter the regimen as needed on the basis of the follow-up and maintenance guidelines (**IX**), but should consult frequently with a physician.

C. Worsening CHF. In previously compensated patients who develop worsening CHF, consider these possible causes:

   1. Failure to adhere to low-sodium diet.

   2. Failure to comply with medical regimen.

   3. Progression or development of ischemic heart disease, even in the absence of pain.

   4. Failure to control blood pressure in hypertensive patients.

   5. Development of renal failure.

   6. Development of anemia.

D. Arrhythmia.

E. Suspected drug toxicity.

IX. Follow-Up and Maintenance

A. Frequency of assessment

   1. Initial follow-up in 24 hours to determine if patient has improved.

   2. Then every 1–2 weeks until patient is symptom-free and dry weight is achieved.

   3. Then every month for 3 months.

   4. Then every 3 months, indefinitely.

B. Content of assessment (related to basic diseases)

   1. Subjective symptoms:

      a. Dyspnea on exertion.

      b. Orthopnea.

      c. Paroxysmal nocturnal dyspnea.

   2. Objective evaluation:

      a. Neck veins. Look for distention.

      b. Chest examination. Listen for rales.

      c. Cardiac examination. Listen for gallop rhythm or arrhythmia.

      d. Abdomen. Look for hepatomegaly.

    e. Extremities. Check for edema.

    f. Weight. Patient should be weighed at every visit (change in body weight is one of the most sensitive measurements of fluid balance).

  3. Laboratory tests:

    a. Blood urea nitrogen (BUN), serum creatinine, Na^+, K^+, HCO_3^-, and CL^- initially; then, BUN and K^+ at 2 weeks and 8 weeks; and then BUN and K^+ every 6 months if patient is stable.

    b. Hematocrit or hemoglobin, every year.

C. Long-term treatment

  1. Digitalis (Dosage or drug should not be altered without physician consultation.)

    a. Digoxin is the most commonly used preparation. Maintenance dose is digoxin, 0.125–0.375 mg orally every day.

    b. Assessment of digitalis toxicity.

      (1) Subjective symptoms (assess at each visit):

        (a) Nausea, vomiting, anorexia.

        (b) "Yellow vision," blurred vision

        (c) Palpitations.

        (d) CNS symptoms (headache, disorientation, fatigue, malaise).

      (2) Objective signs (assess at each visit):

        (a) Bradycardia of 60 beats or less.

        (b) Arrhythmias, commonly premature ventricular contractions.

  2. **Diuretics** (dosage or drug should not be altered without physician consultation).

    a. Drugs and usual maintenance dosage

      (1) Hydrochlorothiazide, 50 mg orally every day or

      (2) Furosemide, 20–40 mg orally every day (occasional patient may require much larger dosage).

    b. Assessment related to possible side effects of diuretics

      (1) Subjective symptoms (review at each visit):

        (a) Hypokalemia. Lethargy, muscle cramps.

        (b) Gout. Acute joint pain.

        (c) Diabetes. Polyuria, polydipsia, weight loss.

      (2) Objective evaluation of orthostatic hypotension—obtain supine and standing blood pressure at each visit.

      (3) Laboratory tests:

(a) BUN, serum creatinine, Na+, K+, HHCO$_3^-$, CL$^-$ initially; then BUN and K+ at 2 weeks and 8 weeks; and then BUN and K+ every 6 months if patient is stable.

(b) Uric acid, at 3 months and then annually.

(c) Urinalysis for glucose; check if polyuria, polydipsia, or polyphagia develops.

3. Long-acting nitrates (see Angina Pectoris: Adult, pp. 185–189).

4. ACE inhibitors.

a. Many agents are now available, such as captopril, enalapril, lisinopril, etc. Maintenance dosage should be established with physician consultation and any changes in regimen implemented only after consultation.

b. Side effects related to ACE inhibitors.

(1) Symptoms (review at each visit):

(a) Dizziness on arising.

(b) Cough.

(c) Angioedema.

(2) Signs:

(a) Check for postural drop in blood pressure.

(b) Presence of angioedema, usually of face or lips.

▲ UNCOMPLICATED ESSENTIAL HYPERTENSION: ADULT

I. Definition

Persistent elevation of the arterial blood pressure greater than 150/95 mm Hg but less than 200/110 (present on weekly determinations over 1–2 weeks) without demonstrable cause and with no associated symptoms or signs of end-organ involvement.

II. Etiology

Unknown.

III. Clinical Features

A. Symptoms

1. Usually, the patient is asymptomatic.

2. Hypertension of this magnitude can rarely be shown to be associated with the symptoms that the general population associates with high blood pressure. These symptoms— dizziness, stuffiness, lightheadedness, and headaches have not been found to be predictably present when blood pressure is elevated.

3. In uncomplicated hypertension, symptoms of target organ involvement are not present:

    a. Symptoms of angina pectoris.

    b. Symptoms of congestive heart failure.

    c. Symptoms of cerebral ischemia or stroke syndrome.

    d. Severe headaches, nausea and vomiting.

    e. Alterations in level of consciousness.

B. Signs

1. Elevation of arterial blood pressure greater than 150/95 mm Hg, but less than 200/110 (present on weekly determinations over 1–3 weeks).

2. Sometimes, narrowing, copper-wiring, or arteriovenous nicking of the arterioles of the optic fundi. Usually there are no hemorrhages or exudates, and there is no papilledema.

3. Chest clear to percussion and auscultation.

4. The heart is usually normal, although it may show minimal to moderate left ventricular hypertrophy. No gallop rhythm is present.

5. No bruit over abdomen or flank or in back.

6. No edema.

7. Intact neurologic system.

8. No signs of Cushing's syndrome, hyperthyroidism, or pheochromocytoma.

IV. Laboratory and Diagnostic Studies

  A. Before treatment

    1. Blood urea nitrogen or serum creatinine.

    2. Serum Na^+, K^+, HCO_3^-, and CL^-. levels.

    3. ECG.

    4. Chest X-ray.

    5. Urinalysis.

    6. Studies to detect causes of secondary hypertension are deferred until the patient has been seen by the physician, or after consultation with the physician.

  B. After treatment. See **VI.C.**

V. Differential Diagnosis

  A. Headaches and dizziness from other causes.

  B. Secondary hypertension:

    1. Systolic hypertension

      a. Arteriosclerotic vascular disease.

      b. Hyperthyroidism.

      c. Anxiety.

2. Diastolic hypertension
   a. Renal disease.
   b. Coarctation of aorta.
   c. Pheochromocytoma.
   d. Cushing's syndrome.

VI. Treatment

The goal of treatment is the achievement and maintenance of a reasonable blood pressure (less than 150/95) and the prevention of complications of either the disease or the treatment regimens.

A. **Initial therapy**. If the patient meets the criteria as outlined for uncomplicated benign essential hypertension, proceed with the following: ·

1. Salt restricted diet. Salt intake should approximate 85 mEq (2 gm) sodium daily, but may be altered as necessary, depending on such factors as the patient's socioeconomic status, habits of living and eating, and ability to comprehend.

2. Weight reduction.

3. Drugs.

   With the introduction of new agents including beta blockers, calcium channel blockers, ACE inhibitors and newer central sympatholytics, the choice of therapy has become very complicated. This is particularly true when cost of therapy is considered because the newer agents are more expensive than the older agents. For this reason, the use of thiazides as initial therapy should be considered as well as the use of reserpine as a sympatholytic agent. We have therefore continued to include these drugs in our recommendations.

   Because of the wide spread use of the newer agents, however, we have included others. That will enable nurse practitioners to follow patients who have had their regimen on these agents established.

   a. Thiazide diuretic
      (1) Hydrochlorothiazide:
          (a) Initial dosage is 25 mg orally every day.
          (b) Dosage may be increased in 4–6 weeks to 50 mg orally every day. Higher doses are seldom effective and should not be used.

          or

      (2) Chlorthalidone:
          (a) Initial dosage is 50 mg orally every day. Higher doses are seldom effective and should not be used.

   Note: Thiazide diuretics cause renal potassium loss. If a patient is on digitalis, supplemental potassium should be given after renal function is established. If patient is not on digitalis and serum potassium stays above 3.0 mEq per liter, potassium need not be given. Because many patients do not need supplemental potassium and are maintained on only one drug, we do not advocate using a formulation that combines thiazide with triamterene, a weak diuretic that decreases potassium loss. These combination drugs are expensive and necessitate two drugs when one is usually sufficient.

B. **Sympatholytic therapy.** If thiazide therapy is not effective in bringing the blood pressure to normal levels, begin sympatholytic therapy while maintaining the previously established dose of thiazide diuretic.

A wide variety of drugs is available for sympatholytic therapy. For nurse practitioner practice, we still recommend that reserpine be the drug of first choice (see orders below) because it is effective, inexpensive, produces few side effects, and is safe. It should always be given with a thiazide diuretic. Several thiazide-reserpine combination tablets are available and can be recommended because administration of a single once-a-day tablet often improves compliance.

A wide range of additional agents is currently available. We do not feel these agents should be initially prescribed by the nurse practitioner without physician consultation, because of the number of side effects and complications of therapy. Once maintenance dosage is established, however, we feel nurse practitioners can safely monitor patients, and we have included orders for following patients on beta blockers, calcium channel blockers, ACE inhibitors, and clonidine.

1. Reserpine. Begin with reserpine 0.125 mg orally every day. May increase to 0.25 mg orally every day, if needed, in 6 weeks. Higher doses are not recommended.

2. Beta blockers. Consult physician for drug and dose.

C. **Other therapies.** Many patients will respond to other drugs. In general these are more effective when used with a diuretic.

1. Calcium channel blockers. Consult physician for drug and dose.

2. ACE inhibitors. Consult M.D. for drug and dose.

3. Clonidine. Consult physician for dose.

D. **Follow-up and maintenance—general.**

1. Frequency of assessment

   a. Every 1–2 weeks until normal blood pressure is achieved.

   b. Then every month for 3 months.

   c. Then every 6 months, indefinitely.

2. Content of assessment (related to hypertension)

    a. Subjective symptoms:

        (1) Headaches.

        (2) Dizziness.

        (3) Angina.

        (4) Congestive heart failure.

        (5) Cerebral ischemia or stroke syndrome.

        (6) Nausea, vomiting.

        (7) Alterations of level of consciousness.

    b. Objective evaluation:

        (1) Blood pressure—Measure supine and standing at each visit.

        (2) Appropriate examination related to symptoms.

        (3) Routine examination of heart, lungs, and nervous system every 6 months.

3. Assessment related to thiazide

    a. Subjective symptoms (review at each visit):

        (1) Hypokalemia. Lethargy, muscle cramps.

        (2) Gout. Acute joint pain.

        (3) Diabetes. Polyuria, polydipsia, weight loss.

    b. Objective evaluation:

        (1) Orthostatic hypotension. Obtain supine and standing blood pressure at each visit.

        (2) Serum potassium level. Measure initially; repeat after diuretic dose is established; and repeat every 6 months thereafter.

        (3) Serum uric acid level. Check any time joint pain develops. Check at end of the first 3 months of therapy, and then annually.

        (4) Blood sugar level. Check routinely at end of the first 3 months of therapy and then annually, 2 hours after eating. Check if polydipsia, polyuria, or polyphagia develops.

4. Assessment related to resperine

    a. Subjective symptoms:

        (1) Nasal stuffiness.

        (2) Depression.

        (3) Epigastric pain.

        (4) Impotence.

    b. Objective evaluation— obtain an hematocrit and a stool for occult blood prior to consultation if patient has epigastric pain or symptoms such as melena suggesting gastrointestinal bleeding.

5. Assessment related to clonidine.

a. Subjective symptoms:

(1) Dry mouth.

(2) Drowsiness.

(3) Dizziness.

b. Objective symptoms: Postural hypotension.

6. Assessment related to maintenance of patients on beta blockers (see Angina Pectoris, pp. 185–189).

7. Assessment related to maintenance of patients on calcium channel blockers (see Angina Pectoris, pp. 185–189).

8. Assessment related to maintenance of patients on ACE inhibitors (see CHF).

VII. Complications

A. Angina pectoris.

B. Congestive heart failure.

C. Transient cerebral ischemia or other stroke syndrome.

D. Secondary renal disease.

E. Complications of therapy.

F. Poor response to therapy.

VIII. Consultation–Referral

A. Any patient who does not achieve blood pressure of 150/95 or less while on therapy, or any patient exhibiting signs of complications of hypertension.

B. Any patient who has complications related to the treatment regimen.

IX. Follow-Up (see VI.C).

See (**VI.C**).

▲ CHRONIC OCCLUSIVE ARTERIAL DISEASE OF THE EXTREMITIES: ADULT

I. Definition

A chronic decrease in blood flow to one or more extremities, leading to partial or complete occlusion of one or more of the peripheral blood vessels, almost always in the lower extremities.

II. Etiology

Usually, atherosclerosis (see Angina Pectoris for risk factors for atherosclerosis). Congenital lesions, trauma, and other mechanisms may be causative. The condition frequently is associated with diabetes.

III. Clinical Features

A. **Symptoms.** The location of symptoms, depending on the site of occlusion, is the buttocks, thigh, calf, or, rarely, the arm.

   1. Intermittent claudication (cramping pain in the muscles on exercise that is relieved by rest).

   2. Occasionally, nocturnal muscle cramps.

   3. Feeling of coldness in involved extremity.

B. **Signs.**

   1. The involved extremity may demonstrate any or all of these:

     a. Decreased pulses.

     b. Coolness.

     c. Loss of hair.

     d. Shiny, atrophic skin.

   2. Ischemic necrosis (gangrene) in advanced disease.

   3. Bruits may be heard over the involved vessel, particularly the femoral arteries and abdominal aorta.

IV. Laboratory Studies

A. 2 hour P.C. blood sugar determination to screen for diabetes mellitus.

B. Lipid panel.

C. Arterial Doppler flow study.

V. Differential Diagnosis

A. Raynaud's disease

B. Raynaud's phenomenon

C. Scleroderma

D. Problems with venous stasis; see Stasis Ulcer of the Lower Extremity: Adult, pp. 201–202).

VI. Treatment

A. The patient should be instructed in methods of skin care using lanolin, lamb's wool between toes, and properly fitting shoes.

B. The patient should be cautioned about the dangers of excessive heat or cold.

C. Vasodilating drugs are of no proven benefit and need not be prescribed. Consult with physician for patients who are already on previously prescribed vasodilators.

D. The patient should eliminate or reduce risk factors for atherosclerosis. (See Angina Pectoris: Adult, pp. 185–189.)

E. Trental, which apparently acts by allowing blood cells to flow more freely, has been shown to increase walking distance but not to change ultimate outcome. Dose 400 mg twice a day to promote symptomatic improvement. Consult physician before starting Trental.

VII. Complications

A. Gangrene, ulceration.

B. Impaired nail and hair growth.

VIII. Consultation–Referral

A. All patients should be discussed with the physician or referred within 2 weeks for evaluation regarding further diagnostic studies and consideration for revascularization.

B. Any patient with acute onset of symptoms should be referred that day.

C. Patients with gangrene or skin ulcers should be referred.

IX. Follow-Up

A. All patients should be seen every 3–6 months to follow their circulatory status; physician should be consulted if there is progression of the disease.

B. All patients should be instructed to return if symptoms increase or if skin abrasions, lacerations or other breaks in skin surface, inflammation, or infection occur.

▲ STASIS ULCER OF THE LOWER EXTREMITY: ADULT

I. Definition

A chronic ulcerative lesion of the lower extremity caused by poor circulation due to venous stasis.

II. Etiology

Chronic impairment of venous return secondary to varicose veins, a previous episode of thrombophlebitis, or congestive heart failure.

III. Clinical Features

A. Symptoms

1. Pain at the ulcer site.

2. History of varicose veins or thrombophlebitis.

3. History of congestive heart failure.

B. Signs

1. A chronic ulcer of the lower extremity with minimal surrounding inflammation or infection.

2. Associated varicose veins.

3. Usually, pitting edema of the involved leg.

    4. Frequently, brawny edema.

    5. Negative Homans' sign.

    6. Intact peripheral pulses in the involved extremity.

IV. Laboratory Studies

None.

V. Differential Diagnosis

    A. Chronic lymphedema.

    B. Arterial occlusive lesion (see Chronic Occlusive Arterial Disease of the Extremities: Adult, pp. 199–201).

VI. Treatment

    A. Rest and elevation of the involved leg.

    B. Muscular activity of elevated leg by such measures as using a footboard during bed rest.

    C. Initial vigorous cleansing of the ulcer by the nurse practitioner followed by twice daily cleansing of the ulcer by the patient at home, using povidone-iodine (Betadine) and water, or hydrogen peroxide. Apply dry dressing after cleansing. A povidone-iodine soak may be necessary before beginning cleansing.

    D. Application of Unna's paste boot if measures A–C do not result in healing in 3 weeks, particularly if the patient is unable or unwilling to follow the regimen.

    E. For ongoing treatment after the ulcer heals, use support stockings or compression stockings.

VII. Complications

    A. Severe extension of ulcer.

    B. Cellulitis.

VIII. Consultation–Referral

    A. Surrounding inflammation or infection.

    B. Positive Homans' sign.

    C. Failure to heal within 1 month.

IX. Follow-Up

Return visit every 5–7 days until ulcer is healed or consultation is required.

8
▼

DISORDERS OF THE GASTROINTESTINAL SYSTEM

▲

▲ AEROPHAGIA (GASEOUS DISTENTION SYNDROME): ADULT

I. Definition

A syndrome characterized by gaseous distention of the abdomen, which is usually worse after meals and relieved in part by eructation or passage of flatus.

II. Etiology

Most of the offending gas is due to air-swallowing. Most of these patients suffer from tension-anxiety states.

III. Clinical Features

A. Symptoms
  1. Abdominal distention.
  2. Mild, nonlocalized abdominal discomfort.
  3. Eructation and passage of flatus, often with partial relief.
  4. Often, worsening of symptoms just after meals.
  5. No nausea or vomiting.

Patient Care Guidelines for Nurse Practitioners, 4th ed. by Axalla J. Hoole, C. Glenn Pickard, Jr., Ruth M. Ouimette, Jacob A. Lohr, and Robert A. Greenberg. Copyright © 1995 by J. B. Lippincott Company.

    6. No change in bowel habits or character.

    7. No melena.

  B. Signs

    1. No weight loss.

    2. No fever.

    3. Minimal, nonlocalized abdominal tenderness.

    4. Slight to moderate abdominal distention with hyperresonance to percussion.

    5. No fluid wave or shifting dullness.

    6. No masses or visceromegaly.

    7. Normal to slightly hyperactive bowel sounds.

    8. Negative rectal examination.

IV. Laboratory Studies

  A. Negative stool guaiac test.

  B. Normal hematocrit.

V. Differential Diagnosis

  A. Intestinal obstruction of any etiology such as adhesions, carcinoma of colon, etc.

  B. Ascites.

  C. Drugs—such as anticholinergics, antidepressants—causing decreased intestinal motility.

VI. Treatment

  A. Reassurance and explanation of the nature of the problem.

  B. Prescribe a non-gas producing diet.

  C. Simethicone (Mylicon), 80 mg, 1 or 2 tablets chewed with each meal.

  D. Reconsider medicines causing decreased intestinal motility and discontinue or change if possible.

VII. Complications

  None.

VIII. Consultation–Referral

  Symptoms persisting more than 4–6 weeks.

IX. Follow-Up

  Return visit if there is no improvement in 2–3 weeks.

▲ CONSTIPATION: PEDIATRIC

  I. Definition

  Difficulty in passing stools, commonly associated with excessive firmness of stools and a decrease in frequency of defecation.

II. Etiology

A. Acute constipation (a change of a few days to several months duration from a pattern that was within normal limits).

  1. Pain on defecation with secondary retention of stools

    a. Anal fissure.

    b. Anal irritation from diaper dermatitis.

    c. Rarely, perianal abscess.

  2. Functional causes

    a. Acute illnesses, especially if associated with decreased appetite and activity (e.g., upper respiratory tract infection in an infant).

    b. Uncomfortable circumstances for defecation (e.g., outdoor toilet in cold weather, unfamiliar location of toilet facilities, school where permission is required).

    c. Emotional upset.

    d. Disruption of usual daily routine.

  3. Hard stools

    a. Drying of stools retained because of the conditions cited in 1 and 2.

    b. Recent change to a constipating diet (e.g., excessive milk products or chocolate and not enough fruits or vegetables or other foods with significant residue).

    c. Thickening of formula (i.e., reflux treatment).

B. Chronic constipation

  1. Psychogenic stool-holding.

  2. Chronic neuromuscular disease (i.e., cerebral palsy, spina bifida occulta).

  3. Aganglionic megacolon (Hirschsprung's disease).

  4. Hypothyroidism (acquired or congenital).

III. Clinical Features

A. Symptoms

  1. Acute

    a. Pain on defecation if stool is hard, or anal fissure or irritation is present, or both.

    b. Straining on defecation.

    c. Firm stools.

    d. History of blood-tinged stool if anal fissure is present.

    e. Decrease in frequency of defecation from usual pattern.

    f. No vomiting.

    g. Abdominal pain.

2. **Chronic**

   a. Psychogenic stool-holding:

     (1) Onset in infancy or early childhood (often begins at toilet training).

     (2) Huge bowel movements at long intervals.

     (3) Encopresis (also enuresis).

     (4) Evidence of behavior problems.

     (5) Chronic diarrhea (overflow).

   b. Chronic neuromuscular disease: abdominal distention, poor attainment of motor milestones.

   c. Aganglionic megacolon:

     (1) Congenital anomaly.

     (2) No spontaneous passage of formed stool.

     (3) No encopresis or overflow diarrhea unless obstruction overcome by instrumentation (suppository, thermometer).

     (4) Abdominal distention, anorexia, vomiting may be presenting symptoms in neonate.

     (5) Failure to thrive, abdominal distention may be presenting signs in older infant or child.

B. **Signs**

  1. Acute constipation

   a. Physical examination is usually normal.

   b. Anal fissure, marked diaper dermatitis, or perianal abscess may be present.

   c. Mild abdominal distention with palpable firm stool is apparent on abdominal and rectal examination.

  2. Chronic constipation

   a. Psychogenic stool-holding:

     (1) Rectum is large and filled with soft or hard stool.

     (2) Mild abdominal distention may be present.

     (3) Stool often palpable on abdominal examination.

     (4) Remainder of physical examination usually is normal.

   b. Aganglionic megacolon:

     (1) Very tight anal canal with no obvious rectal vault.

     (2) Abdominal distention with palpable stool masses may be present.

     (3) Growth may be poor.

C. Neuromuscular disease

  1. Hypotonia and hyperreflexia.

2. Mental retardation.

3. Failure to thrive.

4. Palpable stool on abdominal exam and rectal exam, having tuft of hair on back, deep sacral pit.

D. Hypothyroidism

   1. Apathy.

   2. Cold intolerance.

   3. Hypotonia.

   4. Short stature, chubby.

IV. Laboratory Studies

None.

V. Differential Diagnosis

A. Normal patient. Parents may not appreciate or accept the wide variation of patterns of defecation that are within normal limits.

B. Intestinal obstruction. Abdominal pain and vomiting usually are present.

VI. Treatment

A. **Acute constipation**

   1. Treat underlying cause:

      a. Diaper dermatitis (see Chapter 3, Diaper Dermatitis).

      b. Anal fissure:

         (1) Warm sitz baths.

         (2) Gentle cleansing with soap and water.

         (3) Anusol HC 1–2 a day.

         (4) Stool softener (milk of magnesia) 1 cc/kg/day.

      c. Reassure parent if constipation is associated with an acute self-limiting illness.

      d. Encourage parents to help child avoid or cope with environmental or emotional circumstances that promoted constipation.

   2. Fecal impaction:

      a. Fleet enema.

         (1) <2 years—pediatric preparation.

         (2) >2 years—adult preparation.

B. Chronic constipation

   1. Senokot liquid or tablets for 5 days.

   2. Stool softener— milk of magnesia or mineral oil 1–2 cc/kg/day.

VII. Complications

A. **Acute constipation**

1. Fecal impaction.
2. Overresponse of parents, whose excessive, abnormal concern with and manipulation of child's bowel function can lead to behavior problems, encopresis, stool-holding, and parent–child interaction problems.

B. Chronic constipation

1. Fecal impaction.
2. Secondary behavior and psychosocial problems.
3. Failure to thrive and colitis (due to aganglionic megacolon).

VIII. Consultation–Referral

A. Chronic constipation.

B. Recurrent fecal impaction.

C. Failure to respond to treatment.

▲ CONSTIPATION: ADULT

I. Definition

Properly defined as excessive *hardness* of stool without regard to frequency of bowel movements. Normal frequency of bowel movements can vary greatly, from two or three movements daily to one every 3–5 days; however, a decrease in frequency from the patient's usual routine may be significant. In simple constipation there is no intrinsic bowel disease.

II. Etiology

A. Decreased fluid intake.

B. Bed rest.

C. General debility or chronic illness.

D. Chronic laxative abuse.

E. Side effect of many medicines including antidepressants, anticholinergics, calcium channel blockers, opiates.

F. Hypothyroidism.

III. Clinical Features

A. Symptoms

1. Increased hardness of stool or difficulty in moving bowels.
2. Decreased frequency of bowel movement; this is not important if stools are soft and not difficult to pass, unless the decrease in frequency has been a recent change.
3. Sometimes, abdominal distention.
4. *No abdominal pain* in simple constipation.
5. No nausea or vomiting.

6. No history of blood in stools.

B. Signs

1. No *abdominal tenderness* on palpation.
2. No rectal mass.
3. Normal bowel sounds (absence of bowel sounds does *not* occur in simple constipation).
4. No hyperactive rushes or tinkles.
5. Fecal impaction may occur, particularly in bedridden, debilitated, or elderly patients.
6. Sometimes, palpable fecal material. Feces feel firm, but may be indented. No other intra-abdominal mass may be molded.

IV. Laboratory and Other Studies

A. Stool specimen, if obtained, is negative for occult blood.

B. X-ray or other studies are not indicated for simple constipation.

V. Differential Diagnosis

A. Constipation from obstructive lesions of the bowel.

B. Hypothyroidism.

C. Neurotic preoccupation with bowel function (rather than true constipation).

VI. Treatment

A. Check for the presence of fecal impaction in elderly or debilitated patients. (Remember that fecal impaction often presents as diarrhea.) Disimpact by digital manipulation if needed.

B. Increase fluid intake to at least six 8-oz glasses per 24 hours.

C. Drink warm water or coffee early in the morning to initiate bowel movement.

D. Increase intake of fruits, bulky vegetables, or cereals.

E. Prescribe a regular exercise program.

F. If measures **A–D** do not work, the patient can try the following medications (starting with the milder agents, listed first):

1. Psyllium hydrophilic mucilloid (Metamucil), 2 tablespoons in glass of water 2 times a day and at least 6–8 glasses of fluid every 24 hours.
2. Glycerine suppository, per rectum.
3. Milk of magnesia, 15–30 mL before bed with sufficient fluids (contraindicated in patients with chronic renal disease).
4. Dioctyl sodium sulfosuccinate (Colace), 100 mg twice a day.

G. Schedule a regular time for defecation.

H. Rarely, an adult Fleet enema is necessary for relief of severe constipation in chronically ill patients.

      1. Saline solution, 1–2 L rectally.

      2. Adult Fleet enema.

VII. Complications

  A. Hemorrhoids.

  B. Rectal fissures.

  C. Fecal impaction.

VIII. Consultation–Referral

  A. Any suspicion of an acute abdominal condition.

  B. Abdominal pain or tenderness.

  C. Nausea or vomiting associated with failure to move bowels.

  D. Hyperactive bowel sounds, or rushes or tinkles.

  E. Absence of bowel sounds.

  F. Occult blood in stool.

  G. Failure to respond to conservative treatment in 3-6 weeks (as outlined in **VI**).

IX. Follow-Up

Patients should be followed until "normal" bowel function resumes, that is, passage of soft stool without difficulty, because failure to improve may indicate more serious underlying illness.

▲ ACUTE DIARRHEA: ADULT

I. Definition

Frequent loose or watery stools persisting 3–5 days that are not bloody, purulent, or greasy in character.

II. Etiology

  A. Infectious (usually, acute viral, rarely bacterial, infections).

  B. Psychophysiologic disturbances (often related to stress).

  C. Dietary indiscretion, particularly simple sweets.

  D. Laxatives.

III. Clinical Features

  A. Symptoms

      1. Frequent loose or watery stools.

      2. Sometimes, mild crampy abdominal pain just prior to bowel movement.

      3. Absence of gross blood.

      4. Epidemiology: Knowledge of similar cases occurring in the community is very helpful in making a diagnosis of viral gastroenteritis.

5. No rectal pain with defecation.

B. **Signs**

1. Low-grade or no fever.
2. Abdomen may show slight diffuse tenderness. No localized tenderness. No rebound or referred rebound tenderness.
3. Hyperactive bowel sounds.
4. No high-pitched rushes or tinkles.

IV. **Laboratory and Other Studies**

A. Stool guaiac test is negative.
B. Methylene blue stain of fecal specimen for white blood cells. Presence of significant numbers of white blood cells suggests bacterial etiology.
C. Studies such as barium enema should be done only after consultation.
D. Stool culture or testing of stool for ova and parasites initially is not necessary.

V. **Differential Diagnosis**

A. Inflammatory causes of diarrhea.
1. Bacterial causes such as *Salmonella, Shigella,* enteropathogenic *Campylobacter,* or staphylococcal or clostridial toxin.
2. Regional enteritis.
3. Ulcerative colitis.
4. Diverticulitis.
5. Certain bowel cancers.
B. Steatorrhea. Malabsorption syndrome.

VI. **Treatment**

A. **Symptomatic management**
1. Diphenoxylate HCl and atropine sulfate (Lomotil), 1 or 2 tablets 4 times a day until diarrhea stops, not to exceed 8 tablets in 24 hours.

or

2. Loperamide (Imodium) 4 mg (2 capsules) orally followed by 2 mg (1 capsule) orally after each loose stool, not to exceed 16 mg (8 capsules) in 24 hours.
B. **Clear liquid diet** of tea, carbonated beverages, or soups to maintain hydration until improvement.

VII. **Complications**

A. With simple diarrhea—generally, none.
B. With severe diarrhea—dehydration, electrolyte imbalance, vascular collapse, or shock.

VIII. Consultation–Referral

A. Bloody stools.

B. Absence of bowel sounds.

C. Positive methylene blue stain for fecal leukocytes.

D. Abdominal tenderness or rebound tenderness.

E. High fever or toxicity.

F. Dehydration.

G. Weight loss greater than 5% of body weight.

H. Diarrhea persisting 10–14 days.

IX. Follow-Up

Return visit if no improvement within 48 hours.

▲ FUNCTIONAL BOWEL DISEASE (IRRITABLE COLON SYNDROME): ADULT

I. Definition

A syndrome characterized by frequent passage (up to 4–6 movements per day) of small amounts of loose, watery stool associated with mild lower abdominal discomfort and a frequent sensation of a need for further defecation recurring in tense, anxious patients, particularly at times of stress. Occurs in the absence of any GI pathology. It is in the final analysis a diagnosis of exclusion.

II. Etiology

In some manner, tension and anxiety in susceptible patients produce increased intestinal motility and decreased transit time, leading to frequent loose, watery stool. The bowel itself is not inflamed and appears normal on examination. The disturbance is in bowel function.

III. Clinical Features

A. Symptoms

1. Frequent passage (up to 4–6 movements per day) of loose, watery stool.

2. Mild lower abdominal discomfort, often preceding and relieved by defecation.

3. No nausea or vomiting.

4. No history of blood in stools.

5. Stools often contain mucus.

B. Signs

1. No weight loss.

2. No fever.

3. Minimal lower abdominal tenderness.

4. No rebound or referred rebound tenderness.

5. Normal to slightly hyperactive bowel sounds.

6. No masses or visceromegaly.

IV. Laboratory Studies

A. Stool guaiac test is negative.

B. Hematocrit reading is normal.

V. Differential Diagnosis

A. Inflammatory bowel diseases (e.g., ulcerative colitis and regional enteritis).

B. Infectious causes of diarrhea.

C. Parasitic infestations.

D. Tumors of the large bowel.

VI. Treatment

A. Reassurance as to the nature of the problem.

B. Reduction of stress in life situation.

C. Mild tranquilizer, after physician consultation.

D. Antidiarrheal agents, such as paregoric or Lomotil, are not indicated.

E. Dicyclomine hydrochloride (Bentyl) 10 mg PD, 4 times a day.

VII. Complications

None.

VIII. Consultation–Referral

Failure to improve in 4–6 weeks.

IX. Follow-Up

Return visit if no improvement in 3–4 days.

▲ ACUTE GASTROENTERITIS: PEDIATRIC

I. Definition

An acute inflammation of the gastrointestinal tract characterized by passage of stools that are more liquid than normal, usually with an increase from the patient's normal frequency. The disorder is often preceded by or associated with vomiting and/or fever.

II. Etiology

A. Often of unknown cause. Many cases are due to viral infections (Rotavirus most often identified but also reovirus, adenovirus, Norwalk, etc.).

B. Occasionally due to the following:

    1. Bacterial infection

        a. *Shigella* (relatively common in some areas, especially summer).

        b. *Salmonella* (summer).

        c. *Campylobacter* (well water).

        d. *Yersinia.*

        e. Certain *Escherichia coli.*

    2. Side effect of oral antibiotics (mild to severe colitis).

    3. Food poisoning

        a. *Salmonella.*

        b. Staphylococcal enterotoxin (not an actual infection).

    4. Parasitic infestation.

        a. *Giardia Lamblia* (also, cryptospritum, *Dientamoeba fragilis, Hastocystidrominus,* etc.).

III. Clinical Features

  A. **Symptoms**

    1. Increased liquid content of stools with no specific color change.

    2. Increased frequency of stools.

    3. Vomiting.

    4. Abdominal pain.

    5. Sometimes, coexisting respiratory tract infection or otitis media.

    6. Sometimes, flecks of blood in stool as diarrhea continues.

    7. With dehydration— listlessness and lethargy.

    8. Sometimes, family history of similar illness.

  B. **Signs**

    1. Fever may be low grade or marked.

    2. Abdominal distention (usually mild).

    3. Abdominal tenderness (usually generalized, but may be more prominent in any area).

    4. Increased bowel sounds.

    5. With dehydration—sunken eyes, dry mucous membranes, decreased skin turgor, weight loss, lethargy, apathy, no or decreased urine output (not all symptoms may be present at the same time).

IV. Laboratory Studies

  A. Usually, none are necessary.

  B. Stool culture for bacteria should be done if any of these apply:

    1. Blood-tinged mucus in stool.

2. Fever over 102 °F rectally or 101 °F(38.3 °C) orally.

3. Family or closed population outbreak.

4. Diarrhea persisting over several days.

5. History of possible exposure to a bacterial pathogen.

V. Differential Diagnosis

A. Normal patient. Parents may not appreciate or accept the wide variation of patterns of defecation that are within normal limits.

B. Intussusception. This usually occurs in a patient aged 3–24 months who has a sudden onset of severe, paroxysmal abdominal pain and vomiting. It may be followed within 8-12 hours by loose stools containing blood and mucus. May be accompanied by mental status change.

C. Appendicitis. Rarely, a pelvic appendix can cause diarrhea if appendicitis develops.

D. Toddler's diarrhea (irritable bowel syndrome of infancy).

VI. Treatment

A. **General management**

1. Explain to parents that there is no specific therapy to stop symptoms immediately but that attention to diet and fluid management (see **3** below) is needed. Discourage use of antidiarrheal and antiemetic medications.

2. Search for early signs of dehydration:

   a. Instruct parents to record nature and amount of fluid intake, occurrence of vomiting, the number and character of stools, and frequency and amount of urination.

   b. Weigh the patient carefully at the initial visit and each follow-up visit to determine the state of fluid balance. Infants should be weighed naked, and older children, with the same, minimal clothing at each visit.

   c. Examine for sunken eyes, dry mucous membranes, and decreased skin turgor, lethargy, irritability, tachycardia, skin capillary refill.

3. Dietary management of mild diarrhea and vomiting may be varied, depending on age (older children are less likely to progress to dehydration) and rapidity of improvement. Advise patients on these guidelines:

   a. Infants (<12 months)

      (1) If breast-feeding, continue and supplement with a prepared electrolyte solution.

      (2) If bottle feeding, discontinue for 4–6 hours and replace with a prepared electrolyte solution.

      (3) Encourage more frequent feedings of small volumes;

the total volume for a 24 hour period should exceed the usual 24-hour volumn.

(4) Instruct parents to give small specific amounts of fluid every 15 minutes to start.

(5) If diarrhea is improved, may start diluted formula fluids in 12–24 hours in addition to clear liquids (there is no difference in amount of increased diarrhea with regard to lactose vs. lactose-free formulas). Increase diet to full strength formula in the next 24 hours as tolerated.

(6) When infant is taking solids, start easily ingested foods such as mashed potatoes, dry toast, rice cereal, crackers, or bananas as soon as infant will accept them.

(7) Increase to regular diet by end of day 3.

(8) Using these guidelines, the infant will (1) stay hydrated, (2) stay nourished, (3) will not have hyper osmotic fluids contributing to diarrhea once acute episode is over.

(9) Fatty foods should be withheld until foods in 7 are well tolerated.

(10) Most acute viral diarrheal illness lasts 5–7 days regardless of management.

(11) If a return to milk exacerbates the diarrhea, consult a physician.

b. Older children. Basically the same as for the infant, only they will not take fluids such as Pedialyte, etc.

B. Bacterial gastroenteritis.

1. Rehydration/maintenance are the same.

2. Contact physician about the need for antimicrobial therapy (e.g., antibiotic therapy for *Shigella*).

C. **Side effects of oral antibiotics**

1. Diarrhea is usually mild and the antibiotic may be continued unless diarrhea increases.

2. If diarrhea increases, consult physician about substituting an alternative antibiotic and consideration of enterocolitis due to clostridium difficile toxin or staphylococcus investigation.

VII. Complications

A. Dehydration.

B. Hypovolemic shock (severe dehydration).

C. Inability to tolerate milk during recovery period (uncommon).

VIII. Consultation–Referral

A. Vomiting and/or diarrhea in a child less than 3 months of age.

B. Dehydration >5% (estimated).

C. Severe abdominal pain.

D. Moderate amount of blood in stools (more than just flecks).

E. Failure to improve with treatment within 48 hours.

F. Inability of a young infant to tolerate return of milk formula to diet >1 week.

G. Bacterial infections or food poisoning.

H. Chronic diarrhea.

IX. Follow-Up

A. <12 months—daily weight checks until improved.

B. >12-36 months—weight check in 24 hours and 40 hours, then if improved, phone follow-up/additional visits as needed until symptoms resolved.

C. >36 months—return visit in 24 hours, phone follow-up daily (with additional visits as needed) until symptoms resolved.

▲ HIATAL HERNIA WITH ESOPHAGITIS: ADULT

I. Definition

Herniation of the stomach through the diaphragm. Hiatal hernia is generally asymptomatic unless associated with esophagitis due to reflux of acid into the esophagus. Reflux may occur in some patients due to faiiure of the gastroesophageal sphincter without a hiatal hernia.

II. Etiology

Unknown. Certain factors known to contribute to reflux and esophagitis include:

A. Obesity.

B. Pregnancy.

C. Nicotine.

D. Caffeine.

E. Alcohol.

III. Clinical Features

A. **Symptoms**

1. Burning substernal pain that is worse when bending over or lying down, particularly after meals. Pain often relieved by antacids.

2. Regurgitation of acid into posterior pharynx, particularly when lying down.

3. Dull substernal pain from esophageal spasm.

B. **Signs.** Physical examination is usually normal, but patient may have minimal tenderness on palpation of the epigastrium.

IV. Laboratory Studies

A. Hematocrit or hemoglobin is normal.

B. Stool guaiac test is negative.

V. Differential Diagnosis

A. Strictures due to chronic esophagitis.

B. Pains of myocardial infarction or other nasogastrointestinal problems.

C. Peptic ulcer.

D. Esophagitis of other causes, such as alcohol or certain medication.

VI. Treatment

Advise patient to:

A. Eat small amounts frequently.

B. Avoid food 4 hours before bedtime or lying down.

C. Take antacids, 2 tablespoons (30 cc; 1 oz) 1 hour after meals and just before bedtime.

or

Alginic acid antacid tabs (Gaviscon)—2–4 tablets chewed and swallowed 1 hour before meals and at bedtime.

D. Elevate head of bed on 6- to 8-inch blocks.

E. Reduce weight (if overweight).

F. Avoid tight clothing around the abdomen and chest.

G. Anticholinergics, theophylline, beta adrenergic agents, diazepam, meperidine, nicotine, and calcium channel blocking agents all may exacerbate reflux and should be reevaluated and discontinued if possible.

H. Medications: If symptoms are not improved by **A-G** above, may initiate therapy with H_2 blockers as below:

1. Tagamet 400 mg orally twice a day. May increase to 800 mg orally twice a day.

2. Zantac 150 mg orally twice a day. May increase to 300 mg orally twice a day. If no improvement, may add Reglan 5–10 mg orally 1/2 hour before eating.

VII. Complications

A. Gastrointestinal bleeding.

B. Anemia.

C. Aspiration.

D. Stricture formation.

VIII. Consultation–referral

A. Gastrointestinal bleeding.

B. Persistent symptoms.

C. Severe anemia.

D. Weight loss.

E. Dysphagia.

F. Vomiting.

IX. **Follow-Up**

A. Weekly, until patient is asymptomatic; then whenever necessary for recurrence of symptoms.

B. Barium swallow and upper gastrointestinal X-ray series, if symptoms change (after consultation with physician).

▲ UNCOMPLICATED ACID PEPTIC DISEASE: ADULT

I. **Definition**

Ulceration of duodenal mucosa producing pain but *not* bleeding or obstruction.

II. **Etiology**

The etiology is unknown, but peptic ulceration can be related to the following factors:

A. **Neuropsychiatric disorders**

1. Stress.

2. Personality trait.

B. **Endocrine disorders.** These conditions are related to increased hydrochloric acid production:

1. Hyperparathyroidism.

2. Zollinger–Ellison syndrome.

C. Recurrent ulcers are often associated with *Helicobacter pylori.*

D. **Drugs**

1. Aspirin.

2. Nonsteroidal antiinflammatory agents such as indomethacin, phenylbutazone, ibuprofen, piroxicam, naproxen, sulindac, tolmetin, meclofenamate.

3. Reserpine.

4. Corticosteroids such as prednisone.

5. Cigarette smoking.

6. Alcohol.

E. **Other diseases**

1. Cirrhosis.

2. Pancreatitis.

3. Pulmonary disease.

 4. Arthritis.

III. Clinical Features

A. Symptoms

 1. Epigastric pain usually 1–2 hours after meals (sooner, if gastric ulcer is present).
 2. Pain relief with food and antacids.
 3. Occurrence of pain at night but not just before breakfast.
 4. Intermittent nausea, vomiting, and belching.
 5. No history of hematemesis or melena.

B. Signs

 1. Abdominal examination may be normal.
 2. Direct epigastric tenderness without rebound or referred rebound tenderness.
 3. Normal stool with *no* melena on rectal examination.

IV. Laboratory and Other Studies

 A. Hematocrit.
 B. Negative test for occult blood in stool.

V. Differential Diagnosis

 A. Functional disease.
 B. Hiatal hernia.
 C. Coronary insufficiency.
 D. Gastric ulcer.
 E. Less frequently, mild pancreatitis and biliary colic.

VI. Treatment

 A. Diet. Small frequent feedings. Fats, milk and cream are not necessary and only increase the risk of atherosclerosis. Avoid caffeine, strong spices, alcohol and cigarettes.
 B. Antacids. 2 tablespoons (30 cc; 1 oz) 1 hour and 3 hours after meals and at bedtime.
 C. Cimetidine (Tagamet) or ranitidine (Zantac) 150 mg orally twice a day.
 D. Anticholinergics. Rarely used; consult physician.

VII. Complications

 A. Gastrointestinal bleeding.
 B. Perforation of the stomach or duodenum and development of peritonitis.
 C. Intractable pain.
 D. Obstruction.

VIII. Consultation–Referral

A. Failure of diet or medicines to relieve symptoms in 4–6 weeks.

B. Gastrointestinal bleeding manifested by melena, occult blood in stool, or a drop of more than 4% in the hematocrit reading, even in the absence of recognized bleeding.

C. Progressive weight loss.

D. Signs and symptoms of an acute abdominal condition, including rigidity and rebound or referred rebound tenderness.

E. All gastric ulcers.

F. All recurrent ulcers.

IX. Follow-Up

A. Every 2 weeks for 4 weeks after acute onset of symptoms of pain (without gastrointestinal bleeding) to check for:

1. Response of pain to diet adjustment and medicines.

2. Evidence of gastrointestinal bleeding (history of hematemesis or melena or positive test for occult blood in stool).

B. Check for side effects of antacids, such as diarrhea and constipation. Watch for development of congestive heart failure in elderly patients if Maalox, Gelusil, or other antacids with high sodium content are used (Riopan has a low sodium content).

C. Check for side effects of H_2 blockers, such as confusion.

D. An upper endoscopy series generally is not necessary in the clinical follow-up of a duodenal ulcer that becomes asymptomatic.

E. After 6–8 weeks of effective therapy (relief of symptoms), H_2 blockers may be reduced to a single dose at bedtime; after another 6–8 weeks of effective therapy, their use may be stopped. Recurrence of ulcer symptoms suggests infection with *H. pylori,* and the physician should be consulted.

▲ HEMORRHOIDS (PILES): ADULT

I. Definition

Varices of the hemorrhoidal veins, which drain the area of the anus, are called hemorrhoids. Internal hemorrhoidal veins and internal hemorrhoids occur on the mucosal side of the mucocutaneous junction; external hemorrhoidal veins and external hemorrhoids occur on the skin side.

II. Etiology

The principal cause of hemorrhoids is loss of support of the connective tissue of the anus and dilation of the submucous veins, resulting in the formation of varicosities of the hemorrhoidal veins. Often, such factors as position, straining at stool, and occupation are thought to contribute to the pathogenesis of hemorrhoids.

III. Clinical Features

A. Acute external hemorrhoids

1. **Symptoms.** Constant mild to moderate pain, itching, and irritation aggravated by defecation and sitting.

2. **Signs**

   a. Bluish, firm (thrombosed) varix protruding around the anus and covered with skin. May occupy only a small portion of area around anus or may surround it entirely.

   b. Bleeding occurs from an external hemorrhoid if the varix ruptures.

B. Chronic external hemorrhoids.
May appear as painless swellings around anus, which appear when patient strains at stool, then disappear. The stretching of skin over repeated acute episodes of thrombosis may leave a redundancy of tissue, or an "appendage," after the acute state has resolved. These "appendages" are easily seen and palpated and are called tags.

C. Acute internal hemorrhoids

1. **Symptoms**

   a. If not prolapsed through anus, painless bleeding may be only symptom. Bleeding from internal hemorrhoids is bright red blood, usually occurring at the end of defecation. The blood may actually drip into the toilet bowl.

   b. With prolapse and thrombosis, patient may have severe pain.

2. **Signs**

   a. Normally not visible externally; usually not palpable unless thrombosed.

   b. Through an anoscope, appear as soft, red-to-purple varices just proximal to the mucocutaneous junction.

   c. When prolapse occurs, hemorrhoids protrude through anus and resemble an external thrombosed varix.

   d. May have chronic mucous discharges from rectum.

Note: A patient with hemorrhoids usually has a combination of both external and internal types. Internal hemorrhoids are responsible for painless bleeding; either can cause painful swelling.

D. Chronic internal hemorrhoids

1. **Symptoms**

   a. Painless bleeding; see III.C.1.

   b. Occasional prolapse occurs with straining or long standing and is easily reduced. Generally there is little pain.

IV. Differential Diagnosis

A. Prolapse of internal hemorrhoids must be differentiated from thrombosis of external hemorrhoids. A hemorrhoid visible outside the anus and covered with rectal mucosa is an internal hemorrhoid. One covered with skin is external.

B. Condyloma acuminatum (venereal wart).

C. Condyloma latum (a lesion of secondary lues).

D. Other causes of rectal bleeding: carcinoma, polyps, inflammatory bowel disease, anal fissures.

V. Laboratory Studies

Generally, none, unless severe bleeding occurs; then a hematocrit is indicated.

VI. Treatment

A. Chronic external hemorrhoids. No treatment is necessary.

B. Acute thrombosed external hemorrhoids

1. **Early.** Surgical consultation for clot extraction or complete excision.

2. **After 24–48 hours.** Conservative treatment (advise patient on the following measures):

   a. Stay off feet; prone position is preferred as much as possible.

   b. Sitz bath for 20 minutes 3 times a day.

   c. Liquid diet during acute phase.

   d. Avoidance of constipation via high fiber diet and stool softener if needed to prevent recurrences.

C. Chronic internal hemorrhoids

1. **Protrusion.** Reinsert into rectum.

2. **Bleeding.** Decrease straining at stool by using stool softener, such as Colace, 100 mg twice daily. If diarrhea is present, use antidiarrheal agent (see Acute Diarrhea: Adult, **VI.A,** p. 211).

3. May use rectal suppositories, such as Preparation H or Anusole, which are astringents.

D. Acute thrombosis of internal hemorrhoid with prolapse requires physician consultation.

VII. Complications

A. Bleeding and subsequent anemia.

B. Necrosis or thrombosis with ulceration.

VIII. Consultation–Referral

A. Acute thrombosed internal hemorrhoid if severe, or if there is prolapse of internal hemorrhoid.

    B. Chronic bleeding that has caused anemia.

    C. If conservative treatment is ineffective.

IX. Follow-Up

As needed for recurrence of symptoms.

9

DISORDERS OF THE GENITOURINARY SYSTEM

▲ CYSTITIS: ADULT FEMALE

I. Definition

A condition characterized by inflammation of the bladder, marked by dysuria and frequency, and not accompanied by systemic complaints. It is frequently seen in females at the onset of or change in sexual activity. Dysuria and frequency, without fever or flank pain, may be associated with a number of problems (see **Differential Diagnosis**). Previously a culture of 100,000 colonies per high-powered field was thought necessary to prove bacterial infection; however, counts as low as 1,000 colonies per high-powered field of pathogenic bacteria occur in symptomatic females with urinary tract infection limited to bladder and urethra.

II. Etiology

A. Bacteria are identified in 60–70% of patients with symptoms of cystitis, of these, *Escherichia coli* is the most frequently encountered in the ambulatory population. *Staphylococcus saprophyticus* a gram positive organism, has been identified in a small number of

Patient Care Guidelines for Nurse Practitioners, 4th ed. by Axalla J. Hoole, C. Glenn Pickard, Jr., Ruth M. Ouimette, Jacob A. Lohr, and Robert A. Greenberg. Copyright © 1995 by J. B. Lippincott Company.

patients. The bacteria originate in the gastrointestinal tract. Women with urinary tract infection may have increased adherence of pathogenic bacteria to vaginal vestibule prior to infection. Entrance to the bladder is through the urethra; sexual activity may milk bacteria into the bladder.

B. Occasionally nonbacterial pathogens such as *Chlamydia* are identified in symptomatic females with >5 WBCs/HPF, but no bacteria.

III. Clinical Features

A. Symptoms

1. Dysuria, frequency, urgency.
2. Occasionally, gross hematuria.
3. Occasionally, low back or lower abdominal pain. No flank or costovertebral pain.
4. No shaking chills.
5. Usually, no gastrointestinal complaints.
6. No vaginal or urethral discharge.

B. Signs

1. No fever, or temperature less than 37.8 °C (100 °F).
2. Only slight lower abdominal tenderness.
3. No peritoneal signs.
4. Normal bowel sounds.
5. No costovertebral angle tenderness.
6. In the elderly there may be few urinary tract symptoms; only failure to thrive.

IV. Laboratory Studies

Urine for examination must be collected carefully (see Urinary Tract Infection: Pediatric, **IV.A.1**, p. 232). A clean-catch urine specimen is particularly important for females because of the possibility of vaginal contamination. If epithelial cells appear in a clean-catch urine specimen, the specimen has been contaminated.

A. Urinalysis. White and red blood cells and bacteria may be present.

1. In a spun sediment greater than 10 white blood cells per high-power field has only a 50% correlation with cultures of 100,000 colony-forming units, but 4 WBCs/HPF has a good correlation with lower counts (10^{2-4}) of colony-forming units.
2. The presence of any bacteria in an unspun urine specimen has a high correlation with significant cultures.

B. Urine culture. A colony count >1000 of a single urinary tract pathogen per milliliter may indicate an infection. If bacteria or significant WBCs or both are present and symptoms clearly indicate cystitis that is not a relapse (see **V.A.1**), cultures need not be done.

If there is a problem of relapse or a complicated history, cultures should be obtained.

V. Differential Diagnosis

A. Recurrent attack of cystitis. Patient may symptomatically appear to have cystitis, but if attacks are recurrent an effort should be made to differentiate between relapse and reinfection.

1. **Relapse**

   a. Usually occurs within a few weeks after previous infection.

   b. Bacteria obtained from culture are the same as that from the previous episode.

   c. Bacteria obtained from urine may be antibody coated, which indicates parenchymal invasion and usually suggests kidney involvement.

   d. Suggests pyelonephritis, anatomic abnormality, or nephrolithiasis that provides a focus for infection that has been inadequately treated.

   e. May require a long course of antibiotics.

2. **Reinfection**

   a. Occurs sporadically, with no relation to previous infection.

   b. Bacteria obtained from urine are not the same as that found during previous infection.

   c. Bacteria are not antibody coated.

   d. Suggests infection limited to bladder from reentry of bacteria from below.

   e. Responds rapidly to a wide variety of antibiotics. Recent studies suggest that a single dose or short course of one of a wide variety of antibiotics may be sufficient.

B. Acute pyelonephritis. Patient is sick. Although dysuria and frequency may be present, these symptoms are overshadowed by systemic complaints of high fever and flank pain. Patient has occasional shaking chills. Occasionally pyelonephritis may cause only lower-tract complaints.

C. Vaginitis. Complaints are predominantly vaginal, with accompanying dysuria and frequency.

D. Urethritis. Dysuria is the chief complaint; a discharge, which may be purulent, is present (an unusual finding in females).

E. Acute abdominal disorder. Severe abdominal pain and rebound tenderness, which are not found in cystitis, are present.

F. Cervicitis.

G. Salpingitis.

VI. Treatment

A. Relapse or pyelonephritis should be referred to physician.

B. Initial occurrence or obvious reinfection:

1. Recent studies indicate that a single dose of either sulfisoxazole, sulfamethoxazole and trimethoprim (Septra, Bactrim), or amoxicillin is effective in treating cystitis. However, a short course of 3 days of therapy is associated with fewer relapses. Three-day therapy is recommended rather than single dose. This maneuver also may separate patients with lower-tract infection from those with upper-tract disease; those who have recurrent symptoms after three-day therapy may have upper-tract disease and need to be more closely evaluated. Use three-day treatment if:

   a. Symptoms last fewer than 3 days.

   b. Vaginitis or overt upper-tract infection is not present.

   c. No complicating factors exist such as diabetes, urinary-tract stones, anatomic abnormalities, pregnancy, or recurrent infection.

   d. Patient can be relied upon for follow-up visits.

2. Antibiotics. Treatment may be instituted with any of these:

   a. Ampicillin, 500 mg every 6 hours for 3 days.

   b. Trimethoprim, 80 mg and sulfamethoxazole, 400 mg; or double-strength trimethoprim, 160 mg and sulfamethoxazole, 800 mg (Bactrim, Septra) tablets. Give two regular strength or one DS (double strength) twice a day for three days.

   For patients with symptoms of cystitis for whom single-dose therapy is not indicated, one of these may be used:

   c. Sulfisoxazole (Gantrisin), 1 gm orally 4 times a day for 10 days.

   or

   d. If patient is allergic to sulfonamides, use trimethoprim, 100 mg twice a day for 10 days.

   or

   e. Tetracycline, 250 mg 4 times a day for 10 days

   f. Fluoroquinolones such as ciprofloxacin or norfloxacin should not be used for routine treatment of cystitis, but reserved for complicated infections.

C. **Urinary infections in pregnancy**

1. **Cystitis uncomplicated.** Treatment is the same as outlined, but there is higher incidence of recurrence and the following precautions should be taken during pregnancy:

   a. Ampicillin may be used at all stages of pregnancy.

   b. Cephalexin (Keflex), 250 mg 4 times a day for 10 days, may be used in patients who are allergic to ampicillin.

    c. Nitrofurantoin macrocrystals (Macrodantin), 100 mg 4 times a day for 10 days, may be used in patients allergic to ampicillin, but not after 36 weeks into gestation or if any renal impairment is expected.

    d. Sulfisoxazole (Gantrisin) may be used up to 30 weeks in gestation.

    e. Septra (or Bactrim) and tetracycline should not be used.

    f. Recurrence of cystitis requires consultation.

  2. Pyelonephritis of pregnancy. Patients with symptoms of pyelonephritis require immediate consultation and often need hospitalization for parenteral antibiotics.

VII. Complications

  A. Chronic infection.

  B. Pyelonephritis.

VIII. Consultation–Referral

  A. Failure to improve in 3 or 4 days.

  B. Recurrent cystitis:

    1. Reinfection within 2 weeks.

    2. More than three episodes in one year.

  C. Growth of original pathogen on follow-up urine culture.

  D. All males with cystitis.

  E. Patient with diabetes or known kidney stones.

IX. Follow-Up

Urine cultures are expensive. If patient is asymptomatic, urine cultures need not be obtained routinely after antibiotic therapy has been completed.

▲ ACUTE PYELONEPHRITIS: ADULT

I. Definition

An infectious disease involving the collecting system and the renal parenchyma of the kidney.

II. Etiology

Bacterial infection, usually with a gram-negative organism; *Escherichia coli* is the most common.

III. Clinical Features

  A. Symptoms

    1. Usually, flank pain.

    2. Often, frank, shaking chills.

    3. Often, nausea or vomiting, or both.

   4. Dysuria, frequency, urgency. (These are primarily symptoms of cystitis, but they may be present in pyelonephritis.)

   5. No vaginal or urethral discharge.

B. **Signs**

   1. Usually, fever of 38.5 °C (101 °F)

   2. Tenderness on percussion over costovertebral angle.

   3. Negative abdominal examination except for tenderness to deep palpation in the involved flank area.

   4. Patient generally has systemic illness and appears very sick.

IV. **Laboratory Studies**

   (Use clean-catch urine specimens.)

   A. **Urinalysis** shows white blood cells (frequently in clumps), white cell casts, proteinuria, and red blood cells.

   B. **Urine culture** shows a colony count greater than 100,000 of the urinary tract pathogen.

V. **Differential Diagnosis**

   A. Cystitis.

   B. Prostatitis.

   C. Other causes of flank pain. (The general public commonly and erroneously considers any back pain as tantamount to kidney infection.)

VI. **Treatment**

   These measures are for an initial occurrence of acute pyelonephritis in an otherwise healthy patient; all patients require at least a consultation and any complicated patient requires a referral for possible admission. If patient is feeling well enough to care for himself or herself, can take oral medicines, and is not dehydrated, therapy can be instituted at home. Hospitalization may be required for systemically ill or septic patients or those with complicating diseases such as diabetes.

   A. **Antibiotics.** Amoxicillin, 500 mg orally 3 times a day for 10 days.

   B. The patient must be followed closely. If vomiting becomes a problem, intramuscular medications are necessary.

   C. Antibiotics may need to be changed on the basis of clinical response and results of sensitivity testing of the organism.

VII. **Complications**

   Chronic pyelonephritis.

VIII. **Consultant–Referral**

   A. Severely ill or toxic patient; patient requiring intramuscular medication because of nausea, vomiting.

   B. Diabetic patient.

C. Elderly or debilitated patient.

D. Any recurrence.

E. Positive culture obtained in follow-up (see **IX.B** and **C**).

IX. **Follow-Up**

A. The patient should be in telephone contact in 24 hours and then every day or every other day until asymptomatic.

B. A repeat urine culture is carried out 1 week after cessation of treatment.

C. A second repeat culture in about 6 months is desirable.

▲ URINARY TRACT INFECTION: PEDIATRIC

I. **Definition**

A bacterial infection of the kidneys, collecting system of the kidneys, or bladder, or a combination of these.

II. **Etiology**

A. Approximately 80% of cases are due to *Escherichia coli.*

B. The remainder are usually due to *Klebsiella, Proteus mirabilia, Enterobacter, Staphylococcus epidermidis, enterococci,* or *Pseudomonas.*

III. **Clinical Features**

A. **Epidemiology**

1. **Newborn infants.** Significant bacteriuria is more common in males than females and has an overall frequency of about 1%. It is often associated with bacteremia.

2. **Preschool children.** Symptomatic urinary tract infection is relatively common in this age group. Urinary tract infection in general is 10–20 times more common in females than males.

3. **School-age children.** Symptomatic urinary tract infection is less frequent than in the preschool period, but at least one episode of significant asymptomatic bacteriuria will occur in at least 5–6% of females between 6 and 17 years of age. The prevalence of asymptomatic bacteriuria is 30 times greater in females. Asymptomatic bacteriuria is associated with increased risk of symptomatic infection in the future.

B. **Symptoms**

1. Urinary tract symptoms may be present:

a. Urgency, frequency, dysuria.

b. Enuresis in a child who had achieved control.

c. Flank pain.

d. Suprapubic pain.

   e. Foul-smelling or cloudy urine.

   f. Occasionally, hematuria in acute cystitis.

2. Various combinations of other symptoms, with or without urinary tract symptoms, may be present:

   a. Gastrointestinal symptoms, such as anorexia, nausea, and vomiting.

   b. Abdominal pain.

   c. Lethargy, irritability.

   d. Unexplained fever.

C. **Signs**

1. Often, normal physical examination.

2. Suprapubic tenderness.

3. Costovertebral angle percussion tenderness.

4. Fever, alone or with other signs and symptoms.

5. Failure to thrive.

IV. Laboratory Studies

The diagnosis of a urinary tract infection is based on the finding of significant growth of bacteria from a urine culture.

A. **Urine culture**

1. **Collection of specimen** (trained personnel should assist in collecting specimen).

   a. Urine specimen should be collected in a sterile container after the urethral meatus and surrounding area have been thoroughly sponged with an ordinary liquid soap solution and rinsed with water-soaked sponges. Four soaped sponges followed by four rinse sponges should be used for females and wiping direction should be from front to back. One soaped sponge and one rinse sponge are sufficient for males after the foreskin of uncircumcised males is retracted (the foreskin should not be forcibly retracted).

   b. After infancy, a clean-voided *midstream* urine specimen should be collected.

   c. Specimen should be cultured immediately after it is collected. If there is any delay, store specimen in refrigerator.

   d. Drug sensitivity studies for potential urinary pathogens should be requested.

2. **Minimal diagnostic criteria**

   a. Two consecutive clean-voided specimens revealing 100,000 or more of the same, single urinary pathogen per milliliter of urine are diagnostic.

   b. If only one specimen for culture can be obtained before

symptoms require therapy, urinalysis should reveal abundant bacteria in order to make a preliminary diagnosis of urinary tract infection.

c. Lower colony counts (10,000–100,000 organisms per milliliter) may represent infection, especially in patients with recurrent or chronic urinary infections, in patients on suppressive but inadequate antibiotic therapy, and in patients who are emptying their bladders frequently. When the count is between 10,000 and 100,000 organisms per milliliter, culture should be repeated.

d. A colony count of fewer than 10,000 organisms per milliliter usually indicates contamination.

e. Cultures producing colony counts of 100,000 or more per milliliter of mixed organisms should be repeated, as they suggest contamination in a patient who has not had urinary tract instrumentation.

B. **Urinalysis** on a clean-voided specimen (examine urine as soon as possible).

1. More than 20 bacteria per high-power field in the sediment of a centrifuged specimen usually indicate the presence of 100,000 or more organisms per milliliter.

2. Pyuria *alone* is *not* a reliable guide to the presence of an infection:

a. Pus cells may be contaminants from the vagina and vulva.

b. Pyuria is absent in up to 50% of patients with significant bacteriuria.

c. Pyuria may persist for several days after an infection has been successfully treated.

d. There are other diseases that cause sterile pyuria.

3. Urine should be examined for other elements—casts, red blood cells, protein, specific gravity.

V. **Differential Diagnosis**

A. Vulvovaginitis.

B. Urethritis.

C. Prostatitis (in postpubertal male).

D. Nonbacterial cystitis (e.g., hemorrhage cystitis associated with adenovirus type 11).

VI. **Treatment**

Consultation is required *before* instituting treatment for a urinary tract infection (see **VIII**). Treatment, after consultation, will usually consist of:

A. **Antibiotic.** Usually, an oral sulfonamide is prescribed (see Table 9-1) for dosage of sulfisoxazole (Gantrisin) suspension. Be certain

TABLE 9-1

ORAL DOSAGE OF SULFISOXAZOLE (GANTRISIN) SUSPENSION (500 MG PER 5 ML)

BODY WEIGHT	INITIAL DOSE GIVEN IN CLINIC	SUBSEQUENT DOSES	FREQUENCY
5–7 kg (11-15 lb)	500mg (5 mL)	250 mg (2.5 mL)	
7–9 kg (15–20 lb)	600 mg (6 mL)	300 mg (3 mL)	
9–12 kg (20–26 lb)	800 mg (8 mL)	400 mg (4 mL)	
12–15 kg (26–33 lb)	1000 mg (10 mL)	500 mg (5 mL)	4 times a day
15–18 kg (33–40 lb)	1200 mg (12 mL)	600 mg (6 mL)	for 10 days
18–22 kg (40–48 lb)	1500 mg (15 mL)	750 mg (7.5 mL)	
22–25 kg (48–55 lb)	1800 mg (18 mL)	900 mg (9 mL)	
Over 25 kg* (over 55 lb)	2000 mg (20 mL)	1000 mg (10 mL)	

*Patients weighing over 25 kg (55 lb) who are able to swallow tablets safely may be given sulfisoxazole (Gantrisin) tablets (500 mg per tablet), 1000 mg (2 tablets) four times a day for 10 days.

the patient is not allergic to the drug. Other commonly used antibiotics include amoxicillin, nitrofurantoin, and trimethoprim sulfamethoxazole.

B. Ample fluid intake and frequent voiding.

VII. Complications

A. Failure to control infection because organism is resistant to antibiotic prescribed.

B. Marked systemic toxicity (high fever, vomiting), with possible bacteremia associated with pyelonephritis. Patient may not be able to tolerate oral therapy.

C. Recurrent infection. In school-age girls, 80% of patients will have at least one recurrence of significant bacteriuria, which may or may not be symptomatic.

D. Rarely, chronic infection, with progressive renal damage. Patients at risk are usually discovered when radiologic study of the urinary tract is performed.

VIII. Consultation–Referral

A consultation is required before instituting treatment for a urinary tract infection.

A. If patient is asymptomatic or only mildly symptomatic, consultation may be requested after the results of the urine cultures are known.

B. If patient is moderately or markedly symptomatic, consultation should be requested after the results of urinalysis are known.

C. A consultation is again required at the follow-up visit 2 or 3 days after treatment has been started under the following circumstances:

1. Patient is still symptomatic.

2. Original urine cultures were not diagnostic of urinary tract infection.

3. Antibiotic sensitivity studies reveal resistance to prescribed drug.

IX. **Follow-Up**

A. After 2 or 3 days of therapy:

1. Assessment of clinical status.

2. Review original culture results.

B. If medication is changed at the first follow-up visit, a return visit is again needed in 2 or 3 days for clinical assessment.

C. One week after completing a course of antibiotic therapy:

1. Assessment of clinical status.

2. Urinalysis on clean-voided specimen.

3. Urine culture and antibiotic sensitivity testing.

D. *If no further infections occur,* the following schedule of visits for clinical assessment, urinalysis, and urine culture is required:

1. After 1 month.

2. Then every 6 months for 1 year.

3. Then routine health maintenance visits.

E. Consultation should be requested 6–8 weeks after treatment has been completed for an intravenous pyelogram and a voiding cystourethrogram.

▲ PRIMARY GONOCOCCAL INFECTION: ADULT

I. **Definition**

Gonococcal infection of the genitourinary tract, oropharynx, or anorectum. Urethral infections may be accompanied by asymptomatic pharyngeal or rectal infection in those who have orogenital contact. Occasionally pharyngitis or proctitis may be the presenting complaint. The occurrence of one sexually transmitted disease is a trigger for inquiring about other STDs and risks for disease.

II. **Etiology**

A. *Neisseria gonorrhoeae.*

B. Antibiotic resistant *Neisseria gonorrhoeae.*

C. Coexistent chlamydial infection in up to 45% of patients.

III. Clinical Features

A. **Males.** Primary infection may be urethral, pharyngeal, or anorectal.
1. Occasionally, asymptomatic.
2. Urethritis (most frequent acute presentation) begins acutely only a few days after exposure.
   a. Dysuria and frequency.
   b. Purulent discharge.
3. Pharyngitis from orogenital contact.
4. Anorectal infection:
   a. Anorectal burning.
   b. Mucopurulent discharge.
   c. Painful bowel movements.

B. **Females.** Primary infection may be urethral, endocervical, pharyngeal, or anorectal.
1. Occasionally, asymptomatic.
2. Urethritis (dysuria, frequency).
3. Salpingitis:
   a. Bilateral lower abdominal pain.
   b. Adnexal tenderness.
   c. Tenderness with manipulation of cervix.
   d. Elevated temperature and chills in some cases.
   e. Occasionally, females with gonococcal infections will develop pain in the right upper quadrant.
4. Pharyngitis from orogenital contact.
5. Anorectal infection (see **A.4**).

IV. Laboratory Studies

A. Gram stain of urethral discharge in both male and female.
B. VDRL test for syphilis.
C. Culture in cases unproved by gram stain. Culture area under suspicion—pharynx, anus, urethra, endocervix. (For urethral culture, insert small swab or wire several centimeters into meatus.) Endocervix is best site for screening in females. In patients with urethritis and history of orogenital exposure, consider culture of pharynx and rectum to detect asymptomatic disease. Gonococcal infections in these areas have a high failure rate to amoxicillin, ampicillin, or spectinomycin.
D. *Chlamydia* culture.
E. See Chapter 16, The Asymptomatic HIV-Infected Adult, pp.363–365.

V. Differential Diagnosis

A. Nongonococcal urethritis.

B. Urinary tract infection.

C. Acute abdominal disorder in females with salpingitis.

D. Nongonococcal prostatitis.

VI. Prevention

A. Counsel patients (male or female) on use of condoms and discuss high-risk lifestyles.

B. Counsel concerning early treatment of recurrence or reinfection.

C. Counsel on necessity of contact information in order to prevent further spread of disease.

D. Recommend abstinence from sexual activity for at least 48 hours.

VII. Treatment

A. **Patients for treatment**

1. Patients with urethral discharge containing gram-negative intracellular and extracellular diplococci.

2. Patients with known recent exposure to gonorrhea.

3. Patients with positive cultures.

B. **Drugs for uncomplicated urethral, endocervical, or rectal infections.*** Because of increasing incidence of antibiotic resistant Neisseria gonorrhea and coexistence of chlamydia, each of these should be covered by initial therapy:

1. Therapy of choice:

Ceftriaxone 250 mg IM once

plus

Doxycycline 100 mg orally 2 times a day for 7 days.

2. Alternative regimens.

For patients who cannot take ceftriaxone, the preferred alternative is spectinomycin 2 g IM in a single dose plus doxycycline. There are a number of other regimens for which experience is less extensive.

a. Tetracycline 500 mg 4 times a day may be substituted for doxycycline but has the disadvantage of being taken 4 times a day.

b. For patients who cannot take tetracycline, erythromycin base

---

*Based on recommendations of the Center for Disease Control, Atlanta, GA. MMWR Sept. 1, 1989, Vol. 38, No. S-8, pp. 22–23.

or stearate 500 mg 4 times a day for 7 days or erythromycin ethylsuccinate 800 mg 4 times a day for 7 days may be substituted. Tetracycline or doxycycline alone is no longer considered adequate therapy for gonococcal infection.

C. **Instructions to patient**
   1. Avoid sexual activity for 2 days.
   2. Ask sexual contacts to come to clinic for diagnosis and treatment.
   3. Advise about safe sexual behavior and risks involved.

VIII. **Complications**
   A. **Associated complications**
      1. Urethral stricture.
      2. Rectal stricture.
      3. Sterility (infrequent).
   B. **Infections beyond site of primary infection**
      1. Monarticular septic arthritis.
      2. Disseminated gonococcal infection manifested primarily as skin lesions.
      3. Gonococcal endocarditis.
   C. **The reappearance of urethral discharge** after several days absence.

IX. **Consultation–Referral**
   A. Pharyngitis.
   B. Proctitis.
   C. Acute abdominal disorder or salpingitis.
   D. Tender, swollen adnexa.
   E. Fever above 100 °F (37.8 °C).
   F. Arthritis.
   G. Disseminated gonococcal infection with skin lesions.
   H. Endocarditis
   I. Recurrence or positive follow-up culture.
   J. Suspicion of penicillinase-producing N. gonorrhea.

X. **Follow-Up.**
   Reculture in 1–2 months to find treatment failures and infections.
   A. **Males.** Urethral culture.
   B. **Females.** Cervical and anal cultures.

XI. **Contact and Reporting**
   A. Contact and treat all sexual partners.
   B. Report primary case to the health department in the patient's county of residence.

▲ NONSPECIFIC URETHRITIS (NONGONOCOCCAL URETHRITIS): ADULT MALE

I. Definition

Infection of the urethra not caused by *Neisseria gonorrhoeae.*

II. Etiology

Chlamydia is felt to be the cause in at least half the cases. In the remainder, the cause has not been identified.

III. Clinical Features

A. Symptoms

1. In contrast to gonococcal infections, may have had 1–2 weeks of symptoms.

2. Dysuria.

3. Increased urinary frequency.

B. **Signs.** Urethral discharge, which is usually not as copious as in gonorrhea and may initially be present only on arising in the morning. The discharge may be milky in appearance and not purulent; however, this condition may mimic gonorrhea, presenting with extreme dysuria and purulent discharge.

IV. Laboratory Studies

A. Gram stain does not reveal gram-negative diplococci.

B. Culture for *Neisseric gonorrhoeae* should be obtained.

V. Differential Diagnosis

This syndrome must be differentiated from gonococcal urethritis. Although there are some clinical differences, the diagnosis must be established by laboratory findings. There also may be a mixed infection of gonococcus and *Chlamydia.* In this case discharge may initially disappear following treatment with penicillin, only to reappear in several days, often in a less purulent form. The second infection, postgonococcal urethritis (PGU), is from *Chlamydia* not affected by penicillin.

VI. Treatment

If gram stain does not reveal gram-negative intracellular diplococci, treat with:

A. Tetracycline, 500 mg 4 times a day for 7 days, or

B. Doxycycline, 0.1 gram orally, 2 times a day for 7 days.

C. If culture grows *Neisseria gonorrhoeae,* add ceftriaxone 250 mg IM.

VII. Complications

A. Usually there are no complications.

B. In a small percentage of patients with a gram stain on which no gram-negative intracellular diplococci are found, the culture will be positive.

VIII. Consultation–Referral

Failure of urethritis to respond to tetracycline.

IX. Follow-Up

A. Return visit if symptoms do not improve.

B. Return visit if culture is positive for *N. gonorrhoeae,* for follow-up culture for *N. gonorrhoeae,* subsequent and treatment if necessary.

▲ ACUTE BACTERIAL PROSTATITIS: ADULT

I. Definition

Acute bacterial infection of the prostate gland.

II. Etiology

Usually, *Escherichia coli* or other gram-negative bacteria that frequently cause infections of genitourinary tract.

III. Clinical Features

A. **Symptoms**

   1. **Local:**

      a. Pain in the lower back and perineum, which may be referred into the inguinal area and testes.

      b. Symptoms of urinary obstruction or cystitis, or both.

      c. Tenesmus.

   2. **Systemic:**

      a. Fever.

      b. Nausea.

      c. Malaise.

      d. Painful sexual intercourse or loss of libido.

B. **Signs**

   1. Extremely tender, enlarged prostate. Do not massage.

   2. Sometimes, temperature above 38.5 °C (101 °F).

   3. Sometimes, penile discharge that is usually milky white, but may be purulent.

IV. Laboratory Studies

A. Urinalysis usually shows both white and red blood cells.

B. Urine culture may be positive.

C. Gram stain of spun sediment may reveal bacteria.

V. Differential Diagnosis

A. Low back pain from muscle strain or chronic prostatitis.

B. Febrile syndromes (e.g., "flu" syndrome) associated with backache.

VI. Treatment

A. **Antibiotic.** Begin treatment when diagnosis is made—do not wait for results of culture:

1. Ampicillin, 500 mg orally 4 times a day for 10 days.
2. TMS/SMX 1 double strength twice a day or 2 regular twice a day for 2 weeks.

B. **General**

1. Analgesic for pain.
2. Sitz bath for 30 minutes 3 times a day.

VII. Complications

A. Chronic bacterial prostatitis.
B. Urinary retention.

VIII. Consultation–Referral

A. No improvement in 2 days.
B. Recurrence.
C. Temperature above 100° F (37.8 °C).
D. Patient with diabetes mellitus.
E. Tenderness or swelling of epididymis or testicle.
F. Urinary retention.

IX. Follow-Up

Reculture in 3 weeks if initial culture was positive.

▲ CHRONIC PROSTATITIS: ADULT

I. Definition

A condition of chronic infection or inflammation and congestion of the prostate, or both; may be bacterial or nonbacterial.

II. Etiology

A. **Bacterial.** The gram-negative bacteria commonly associated with genitourinary infection. Rarely, gram-positive organisms, such as *Staphylococcus saprophyticus.*

B. **Nonbacterial.** Cultures may be negative because of an antibacterial agent in prostatic fluid, Mycoplasma or *Chlamydia* may be the responsible organism, or the architecture of the prostate makes recovering bacteria from the infected site difficult.

III. Clinical Features

A. **Symptoms**

1. Early morning penile discharge.
2. Vague urinary discomfort, frequently at the termination of micturition.

3. Dull ache in the perineum, often radiating into the groin or testicles.

4. Diminution of libido.

5. Low back pain.

6. No fever.

B. **Signs.** The prostate is slightly tender and slightly enlarged; it may be asymmetrical or boggy. Normal landmarks are preserved. There should be no nodules and massage may cause the described pain.

IV. Laboratory Studies

The ideal material for study is prostatic fluid. If this material cannot be obtained, a urine specimen voided after prostatic massage is satisfactory. This sample may be compared with a urine specimen collected before massage.

A. **Bacterial**

1. Prostatic fluid contains greater than 10 white blood cells per high-power field, and gram stain of fluid shows bacteria.

2. Urine obtained after prostatic massage should contain more white blood cells and bacteria than in premassage urine.

3. Culture of prostatic fluid or urine voided after prostatic massage should produce gram-negative bacteria, or, rarely, gram-positive organism, such as *Staphylococcus saprophyticus*.

B. **Nonbacterial**

1. Urine or prostatic fluid contains more than 10 white blood cells per high-power field but no bacteria.

2. Culture of urine or prostatic fluid does not produce bacteria.

V. Differential Diagnosis

A. Acute bacterial prostatitis.

B. Other causes of low back pain.

C. Diseases of the anus, fissure, hemorrhoids.

D. Prostatodynia, a painful disease of prostate not associated with infection or WBCs.

VI. Treatment

A. **Bacterial.** Chronic bacterial prostatitis does not respond to many drugs because of poor diffusion of the drug into prostatic fluid and duration of therapy is not well established. Some practices may decide to treat for up to six weeks.

1. **Antibiotics**

   a. Doxycycline, 100 mg twice a day for 2 weeks.

   or

   b. Trimethoprim and sulfamethoxazole combination, 2 tablets twice a day for 4 weeks.

    c. Erythromycin, 250 mg 4 times a day for 2 weeks, is used for gram-positive organisms; because of high levels possible in the prostate, may have some action against gram-negative bacteria.

    d. A fluoroquindone such as ciprofloxacin may be used after consultation if the bacteria is not sensitive to **a** or **b**.

  2. **General measures**

    a. Sitz bath, 2 or 3 times a day for 15–20 minutes if pain is significant.

    b. Explain to patient that increased sexual activity may help reduce prostatic congestion.

    c. Analgesic for pain.

    d. Stool softeners.

 B. Nonbacterial

  1. **General treatment.** See VI.A.2.

  2. Prostatic massage may relieve pain from congestion.

VII. Complications

  A. Obstruction of urinary outflow.

  B. Chronic pain in the back and groin.

VIII. Consultation–Referral

  A. **Bacterial.** Failure of infection to resolve after 2 week antibiotic course.

  B. **Nonbacterial.** failure of symptoms to resolve after prostatic massage.

  C. **Recurrence of any symptoms.**

IX. Follow-Up

  A. **Bacterial.** Return in 3 weeks for repeat evaluation and urinalysis.

  B. **Nonbacterial.** Return if symptoms persist.

◢ BENIGN PROSTATIC HYPERTROPHY: ADULT

I. Definition

Hyperplasia of the periurethral glands and fibromuscular stroma, with overall enlargement of the gland and compression of the true prostatic tissue.

II. Etiology

The cause of benign prostatic hypertrophy (BPH) is unknown, but normal testes seem to be necessary for BPH to occur. The disorder occurs with aging of the male, with symptoms and obstruction developing in 20% of males over 50–60 years of age and progressing to 50% of males over 80.

III. Clinical Features

A. Symptoms

1. Difficulty in starting micturition.
2. Difficulty in stopping urine flow.
3. Small urinary stream.
4. Small amounts voided frequently.
5. Nocturia.

Note: Nocturia is an important finding and suggests that there have been changes in the bladder wall sufficient to cause post-void residual and frequently indicates the need for surgery.

B. Signs

1. Diffuse enlargement of the prostate gland is present. Size does not correlate with the degree of obstruction.
2. No nodules are present. Normal landmarks are preserved.
3. Bladder may be palpable or percussible above the symphysis pubis if obstruction is present.

IV. Laboratory Studies

A. Blood urea nitrogen and creatinine levels.

B. Urinalysis, including microscopic examination.

C. Urine culture (clean-catch urine specimen).

D. PSA is not recommended as a screening test for cancer because of the large number of false positives.

V. Differential Diagnosis

A. Other causes of obstruction to urinary flow, particularly urethral structure.

B. Carcinoma of the prostate.

C. Inflammation of the prostate.

D. Other causes of nocturia, such as diabetes and congestive heart failure.

Note: In diabetes and congestive heart failure, patients pass large volumes of urine. In benign prostatic hypertrophy, there is frequent, difficult voiding of small amounts of urine.

VI. Treatment

A. Patients with known BPH should be instructed about common medicines that might worsen obstruction. Some of these are over-the-counter decongestants such as pseudoephedrine that have adrenergic properties and antidepressants, antipsychotics, and antispasmodics which have anticholinergic effects.

B. There is currently no widespread medical therapy for BPH. However, recent evidence suggests that finasteride, a 5-alpha reductase inhibitor that blocks the conversion of testosterone to dihydroxytesterone may reduce prostatic size and improve the symptoms of prostatism. When symptoms of obstruction occur, consult about medical therapy or referral to an urologist for surgical therapy. Because of the prevalence of this problem in elderly males, one must be aware of the potential complications of an enlarged prostate.

VII. Complications

A. Increasing obstruction.

B. Secondary infection.

C. Renal failure.

D. Congestive heart failure.

Note: In patients with compromised cardiac function, the inability to pass sufficient urine can lead to fluid retention and congestive heart failure.

VIII. Consultation–Referral

A. Significant symptoms of obstruction or a palpable or percussible bladder, or both.

B. Nocturia of 2–3 times a night.

C. Acute or symptomatic infection of the prostate, or both.

D. Laboratory evidence of decreased renal function.

E. Recurrent urinary tract infection.

IX. Follow-Up

Obtain voiding-related history at least once a year, or every visit if visits occur less frequently than once a year. Also, do rectal examination annually.

▲ VULVOVAGINITIS: PEDIATRIC

I. Definition

Inflammation of the vulva and vagina, commonly presenting with discharge, pruritus, and erythema.

II. Etiology*

A. **Nonspecific origin.** This type of vulvovaginitis is usually associated with poor hygiene, and no specific microorganism is incriminated. Culture reveals mixed flora of colonic bacteria (the most common cause in prepubertal females). Inflammation may be

---

*For any complaints related to the genital area the examiner should explore the possibility of sexual abuse.

aggravated by tight undergarments, especially pantyhose or leotards.

B. **Irritant**

1. Bubble bath (relatively common).

2. Foreign body in vagina (often wads of toilet paper not palpable on rectal examination). Bloody, purulent discharge may ensue.

C. **Bacteria**

1. Group A beta-hemolytic streptococci (occasionally associated with scarlet fever).

2. Gonococcus, causing vaginitis in prepubertal females and endocervicitis in older females. In prepubertal patients, gonococcal infection strongly indicates sexual abuse.

3. Other organisms, including *Staphylococcus aureus* (labial abscess or impetigo causing vulvitis) and *Gardnerella vaginalis* (more common in older females).

D. **Parasites**

1. Pinworms, which move from the anus into the vagina, where they cause mechanical irritation and scratching.

2. *Trichomonas vaginallis* common *after* puberty; prepubertal suggests sexual abuse.

E. **Fungus.** Vulvovaginitis due to *Candida albicans* is common *after* puberty, but occasionally is seen in very young infants, where spread is by hands from vaginitis in an adult.

F. **Virus**

1. Herpesvirus hominis type 2 usually causes infection in the postpubertal period; see Chapter 3, Herpes Simplex: Pediatric and Adult.

2. Vulvovaginitis may be associated with measles or varicella.

III. **Clinical Features**

A. **Symptoms**

1. Pruritus.

2. Vaginal discharge.

3. Dysuria.

4. Enuresis.

5. Pain with walking or sitting.

6. In a younger child, awkward motions, keeping thighs together while moving, or scratching.

B. **Signs**

1. Vaginal discharge is usually purulent, and occasionally blood-tinged if a foreign body is present.

2. Excoriations may be present.

3. Erythema of vulva may be present.

4. If hygiene is poor, one may see either bits of stool in the perineal area or pasty, white material between the labial grooves.

5. A foreign body, if hard, may be felt on compression of the vagina during rectal examination.

IV. Laboratory Studies

A. **Smear of vaginal discharge**

1. Obtain a fresh specimen with a cotton swab or dropper after cleansing the vulva.

2. Wet preparation with saline is used to identify *Trichomonas vaginalis* organisms.

3. Wet preparation with potassium hydroxide is used to detect *Candida* budding yeast with or without hyphae.

4. Gram stain results are sometimes difficult to interpret because of the larger variety of organisms found in the normal prepubertal vagina. Gram stain is also unreliable for diagnosing gonococcal infection because of the similar appearance of some nonpathogenic organisms.

B. **Culture of vulval and vaginal secretions.**

1. Obtain vaginal specimen by inserting a moist sterile cotton swab after culturing and cleansing the vulva.

2. Order routine bacterial culture.

3. Order gonococcal culture.

Note: The normal prepuberal vagina has a great variety of bacteria, including *Escherichia coli, Klebsiella,* enterococci, alpha streptococci, *Staphylococcus epidermidis, Proteus,* diphtheroids, *Lactobacillus,* and *Pseudomonas.*

V. Differential Diagnosis

A. Discharge seen normally in first two weeks of life (white, nonpurulent, nonodorous, and nonirritating).

B. Discharge seen normally in pubertal and immediate prepubertal period (asymptomatic and white or mucoid).

VI. Treatment

Treatment is specific, depending on etiology:

A. **Patient should discontinue bubble bath.**

B. **Treat for pinworms** if they are seen by a reliable observer (see Chapter 15, Pinworms: Pediatric and Adult, **VI,** p. 348), but **consult also** because of the possibility of trapped vaginal pinworms.

C. **Treat for specific pathogenic bacteria** after review of culture results and clinical evidence with consultant.

D. See guidelines in Chapter 14 for **candidal vaginitis** and **trichomonal vaginitis** in postpubertal patients. Because *Tri-*

chomona vaginalis may be transmitted venereally, counsel patient appropriately.

E. Use the following measures for **nonspecific vulvovaginitis** and as **general treatment** for all patients:

1. **Perineal hygiene.** Instruct patient in the following hygiene practices:

   a. Bathe the perineum gently but carefully with warm water and nonperfumed, nonmedicated soap twice a day and after defecation.

   b. Remove smegma from between interlabial grooves.

   c. Blot dry—do not rub with a towel.

   d. Then air-dry, with perineum exposed to warm, dry air.

   e. Wear loose, clean, absorbent (cotton) underpants, and change them frequently. Do not wear pantyhose or leotards.

   f. After defecation, wipe from front to back, with hand coming from behind.

   g. Educate child about perineal hygiene if she is old enough. Have mother observe child practicing.

2. **Sitz baths.** Patient should take a daily sitz bath with an acidifying solution (2 tablespoons of vinegar per quart of warm water) to make the vulval and vaginal mucosa less favorable for bacterial growth and to provide symptomatic relief.

C. **Cold compresses.** If the vulva is very edematous and tender, patient can apply cold compresses of tap water to aluminum acetate (Burow's) solution for 20 minutes 4 times a day.

VII. Complications

Irritation of the perineum, with development of dermatitis and secondary bacterial skin infection.

VIII. Consultation–Referral

A. Clinical or laboratory evidence of a bacterial pathogen. Review bacterial culture results with the physician if the organisms are not listed as nonpathogenic in **IV.B. Note.**

B. Pinworm infestation and vulvovaginitis.

C. Suspicion of a foreign body.

D. Failure to respond to treatment within 1 week. These patients will probably need vaginoscopy to rule out a foreign body.

E. *Trichomonas vaginalis* in prepubertal child.

F. Any case in which sexual molestation is a possibility.

IX. Follow-Up

Return visit in 1 week or sooner if results of culture indicate a need for additional therapy.

⚠ ENURESIS: PEDIATRIC

I. Definition

An involuntary passage of urine during the day or night. Nocturnal enuresis occurs in about 10–16% of 5 year olds; by 8 years of age the incidence drops to half that figure, by 10 years of age to approximately 5%, and by 15 years of age to 1%.

II. Etiology

A. **Unknown cause.** This is the most common category. Numerous etiological theories have been advanced; however, there is no unanimous agreement among authorities. These theories include:

1. Psychologic factors, emotional problems.

2. Limited bladder capacity.

3. Delayed neurologic maturation; failure of arousal; sphincteric incompetence.

4. Profound sleep state.

B. **Variation of normal.** Under 5 years of age, enuresis can be considered normal unless there are signs and symptoms suggesting a specific cause. While most children will have bowel control by 3 to 5 years of age, it often takes longer to learn control of the bladder. Most will achieve nighttime dryness by five years of age.

C. Urinary tract infection.

D. Obstructive lesions of the urinary tract.

E. Primary neurologic disorder.

F. Disorders associated with decreased urine-concentrating ability, and increased volume, causing enuresis.

G. Child abuse.

H. Allergies.

I. Pinworms.

J. Antidiuretic hormone insufficiency.

III. Clinical Features

A. **Symptoms**

1. The passage of urine may occur from rarely to several times daily, day or night. In children who have achieved good control, there may be periodic lapses at night for several years.

2. Boys are affected somewhat more frequently than girls.

3. There is a familial tendency.

B. **Signs.** Results of a complete physical examination are usually normal; however, particular attention should be paid to:

1. Evidence of psychologic and behavior problems.

    2. Lumbosacral skin abnormalities.

    3. Abnormalities of the genitalia, including the urethral meatus.

    4. Poor rectal sphincter tone.

    5. Decreased perineal sensation to pinprick.

IV. Laboratory Studies

    A. Urinalysis and measurement of specific gravity (ideally on a first morning specimen to assess concentrating ability).

    B. Urine culture: see Urinary Tract Infection: Pediatric, **IV.A**, p. 232, for technique and interpretation.

V. Differential Diagnosis

None.

VI. Treatment

    A. **General counseling**

        1. If child is under 5 years of age, reassure that enuresis is normal at that age unless symptoms or signs suggest a specific cause.

        2. Advise parents not to ridicule or punish for enuresis, as it is not voluntary. Secondary psychologic problems can result if enuresis is managed inappropriately by the family.

        3. Reassure that even if nothing is done, enuresis is most often a self-limiting condition if no specific underlying cause can be found.

    B. **Therapy for children over 5 years of age** (after examination and laboratory studies reveal no specific cause)

        1. Have patient keep a diary of wet and dry days and nights for 1 month.

        2. If daytime enuresis occurs, consult physician.

        3. If only nocturnal enuresis occurs, suggest the following measures (the efficacy of these suggestions has not been proved, but each has the support of some clinicians):

            a. Limit fluid intake after evening meal and have child urinate before going to bed.

            b. Suggest that before the parents go to bed, they awaken the child to urinate.

            c. Encourage the child to become involved in the therapeutic process:

                (1) Have the patient keep a diary of wet and dry nights.

                (2) Have parents give praise and small rewards for dry nights.

                (3) Suggest that the patient retain urine for progressively longer periods during the day.

      d. Schedule return visit in 1 month.

      e. If enuresis has not decreased, consult the physician.

      f. If enuresis has decreased, give praise and continue to see the patient periodically on the basis of degree of improvement and need for counseling.

   4. Punishment or ridicule by family should be strictly prohibited.

   5. Moisture sensors may be an appropriate initial therapeutic modality.

VII. Complications

Secondary psychologic problems because of:

  A. Punitive or ridiculing family attitude.

  B. Inability of child to participate in certain social activities, such as camp and overnight visits.

VIII. Consultation–Referral

  A. Daytime enuresis.

  B. Evidence suggesting specific organic cause.

  C. Severe psychologic problems.

  D. Failure to improve after treatment.

  E. Consideration of desmopsiam (DDAVP).

IX. Follow-Up

See **IV.B.3.d–f.**

▲ URINARY INCONTINENCE: ADULT

I. Definition

Involuntary passage of urine that is a social or hygienic problem for the patient.

II. Etiology

Urination occurs when pressure within the bladder overcomes resistance of the sphincter. Bladder and sphincter tone is maintained by a complex neurologic system that extends from cortical centers through the spinal column to the bladder detrusor muscles. Sphincter competence is further supported by estrogen effects on the urethral mucosa and by the vesico-urethral angle.

  A. Instability of the detrusor muscle (spastic bladder). Bladder contractions overcome normal sphincter tone. May cause more than 70% of incontinence in the elderly.

  B. Overflow incontinence (incontinence at very high bladder volumes). Associated with bladder outlet obstruction, decreased bladder tone, and decreased bladder sensation.

  C. Stress incontinence. (Decreased sphincter competence.) Besides neuromuscular structures, sphincter competence is maintained by estrogen effects on the urethral mucosa and maintenance of vesico-urethral angle.

D. Functional incontinence related to other medical conditions, fecal impaction, urinary infection, medications, or altered mental status.

E. Factors that may worsen incontinence from one of the above causes, are diuretics, physical restraints, sedatives, or antipsychotics, (which may decrease attention) or muscle relaxants.

III. Clinical Features

A. **Symptoms.** Workup should include a detailed history of the pattern (onset, duration, amount of urine lost, and times of incontinence), of incontinence, as well as precipitants, past history of urologic and neurologic disease, and medications.

   1. Patients with detrusor instability may have a sensation of bladder fullness or urgency with little warning before passage of urine.

   2. Overflow incontinence is manifested by frequent loss of small amounts of urine.

   3. Stress incontinence may be precipitated by coughing, laughing, or later, by simply rising from a chair.

   4. Functional incontinence may occur in the setting of a progressive dementing illness, sedating medication, or in association with diminished communication or motor function after a CVA.

B. **Physical examination**

   1. Neurologic examination including mental status.

   2. Abdominal and pelvic examination for evidence of a distended bladder, cystocele, or atrophic vaginitis (secondary to estrogen deficiency).

   3. Test for perineal sensation including anal sphincter tone.

   4. Rectal examination to rule out fecal impaction or prostatic disease.

   5. Assessment of functional ability to carry out a complete urinary maneuver.

   6. Other assessments may be indicated by deterioration in general condition.

C. **General considerations**

   1. A palpable or percussible bladder suggests overflow incontinence.

   2. The absence of signs of overflow suggests detrusor instability.

   3. Stress incontinence particularly in older women may occur. May not be the only problem, but may accompany detrusor instability.

IV. Laboratory Studies

A. Urinalysis for evidence of infection; blood glucose, BUN, calcium.

B. Catheterization for post-void residual urine.

C. The above tests are sufficient for initial evaluation. Some patients may need further tests following consultation, particularly patients found to have obstruction, overflow or stress incontinence. These patients may benefit from studies which include an IVP, cytoscopy, or urodynamic measurements.

V. Conditions Associated With Incontinence

A. Fecal impaction.

B. Urinary tract infection.

C. Medication effect (diuretics, sedatives).

D. Atrophic vaginitis.

E. A variety of neurologic diseases, including spinal cord lesions. The simultaneous occurrence of urinary and fecal incontinence is suspicious for a spinal cord lesion.

VI. Treatment

The above conditions should be treated. If incontinence remains, consultation is required. Many, perhaps most of the remaining cases of urinary incontinence in the elderly can be successfully treated, especially if intervention is begun soon after symptoms appear. Treatment is specific to type of incontinence found. Plans of care should be developed after physician consultation and must anticipate multiple trials of therapy. Diapering or permanent indwelling catheters represent failures of medical treatment.

VII. Complications

A. Social isolation of the patient and frustration for the family.

B. Skin breakdown.

VIII. Consultation–Referral

All cases of new-onset urinary incontinence require physician consultation once fecal impaction and urinary infection have been ruled out and a careful medication review has been performed.

IX. Follow-Up

Therapy of urinary incontinence may require therapeutic trials or a number of medications or behavioral interventions. Frequent follow-up is necessary after every intervention, and supportive contact with family is helpful.

10

▼

DISORDERS OF THE MUSCULOSKELETAL SYSTEM

▲

▲ MINOR ANKLE SPRAIN: PEDIATRIC AND ADULT

I. Definition
An injury to the ankle resulting in stretching of the ligament. In a mild sprain, there is no significant tear of the ligament.

II. Etiology
Sprain is most often due to inversion-plantar flexion injury ("I turned my ankle").

III. Clinical Features
A. Symptoms
   1. Pain over the lateral aspect of the ankle.
   2. Patient did *not* hear or feel a "pop" or "snap" at the time of injury (these suggest a ligamental tear or fracture).

B. Signs
   1. *No* ecchymoses.
   2. Minimal or *no* swelling.
   3. Minimal, somewhat diffuse tenderness over the medial or lateral malleolus.

Patient Care Guidelines for Nurse Practitioners, 4th ed. by Axalla J. Hoole, C. Glenn Pickard, Jr., Ruth M. Ouimette, Jacob A. Lohr, and Robert A. Greenberg. Copyright © 1995 by J. B. Lippincott Company.

4. *No* focal area of exquisite tenderness.

IV. Diagnostic Studies

With mild injury, X-ray films are not indicated.

V. Differential Diagnosis

A. Ligamental tears.

B. Fractures.

VI. Treatment

A. Tell patient to keep weight off the ankle, with either bed rest or use of crutches. Keep ankle elevated when at rest.

B. Wrap ankle with Ace bandage.

C. An ice pack may be applied to the ankle for the first 24 hours to prevent swelling. Follow with heat to the ankle if necessary to reduce swelling.

D. Ibuprofen, 800 mg every 8 hours for analgesic and anti-inflammatory effects for adults.

or

E. Acetaminophen (325 mg per tablet), 2 tablets orally 4 times a day. For pediatric dosage, see Table 5.5, p. 156.

VII. Complications

None with minor sprain.

VIII. Consultation–Referral

All sprains associated with ecchymoses, focal or moderate to severe tenderness, more than minimal swelling, or instability of a joint. These findings indicate a possible fracture or severe ligamental tear.

IX. Follow-Up

Return visit in 24 hours; if the sprain is not significantly improved, refer for X-ray study and consultation.

▲ MINOR STRAINS AND SPRAINS*: PEDIATRIC AND ADULT

I. Definition

Minor injury to a joint where the nature of the trauma was mild, resulting in minimal stretching of the involved ligaments and contusion of the surrounding soft tissues.

II. Etiology

Strains and sprains usually result from a fall, a blow from another per-

---

*Excluding ankle sprains. For these, see Minor Ankle Sprains: Pediatric and Adult, p. 254.

son, or an automobile accident. In cases to be managed by the nurse practitioner, the history of the nature of the injury should suggest only minor trauma; for example, falling on the ground, a child's receiving a blow from another child, or a minor automobile accident. Although minor trauma does not ensure that the injury is not severe, it is an important point to notice. All cases involving major trauma, such as severe automobile accidents, should *not* be managed by the nurse practitioner. Child abuse and neglect may present as minor strain or sprain.

III. **Clinical Features**

    A. **Symptoms**

        1. Mild pain around the site of the injury.

        2. Minimal or no loss of function of the involved area.

    B. **Signs**

        1. No ecchymoses.

        2. No instability.

        3. No focal tenderness over the involved ligaments or bones.

        4. No crepitations.

        5. *Minimal* or *no* swelling of the involved area.

IV. **Diagnostic Studies**

    X-ray films are not indicated in minor injuries.

V. **Differential Diagnosis**

    A. Severe sprain with or without fracture, suggested by these symptoms:

        1. Severe pain.

        2. Loss of function.

        3. Ecchymoses.

        4. Point tenderness.

        5. Instability.

        6. Crepitations.

        7. Moderate or severe swelling.

    B. Fractures.

VI. **Treatment**

    A. Immobilization of joint for 24–36 hours. Elevate joint when at rest.

    B. Ice pack for 24 hours.

    C. Local heat after first 24 hours, if needed.

    D. Ibuprofen (Motrin) 800 mg q 6 h for analgesic and antiinflammatory effects for adults.

        or

    E. In case of intolerance to NSAIDs in adults, Acetaminophen (325 mg per tablet), 2 orally 4 times a day. For pediatric dosage, see p. 156.

VII. Complications

None.

VIII. Consultation–Referral

All injuries associated with

A. Signs and symptoms found in V.A.

B. Cases where child abuse or neglect is suspected.

IX. Follow-Up

A return visit is mandatory if there is *no* improvement in 24 hours or incomplete resolution in 1 week.

▲ MUSCULOSKELETAL CHEST PAIN: ADULT

I. Definition

Pain in the chest arising from (1) the bony structures of the rib cage and associated upper limb girdle, (2) the skeletal muscle related to the chest and upper limb, or (3) a combination of these.

II. Etiology

The pain frequently is related to unusual muscular exertion involving the upper limb or chest, or both. Trauma may be implicated. In many cases, the cause is unknown.

III. Clinical Features

A. **Symptoms**

1. The pain is usually aggravated by activity that produces either movement of the chest cage or upper extremity or pressure on the chest, or both, and is relieved by rest or release of pressure.

2. The pain is *not produced by general exertion,* such as walking up a flight of stairs, or other exertion not requiring movement of the chest or arm.

3. The pain often occurs late in the day after the patient has indulged in strenuous exertion involving the chest or arm.

4. The pain is frequently described as sharp, momentary, and stabbing.

B. **Signs**

1. Pain is often reproduced by either movement of the arm or chest or pressure on the chest cage or muscles involved, or both.

2. The chest is clear on auscultation.

3. Cardiac examination is normal and patient is hemodynamically stable.

IV. Diagnostic Studies

A. Seldom indicated.

B. Electrocardiography may be done in older patients for reassurance. One should not rely on the electrocardiogram to rule out ischemic heart disease as a cause of chest pain, however.

V. Differential Diagnosis

A. Angina pectoris.

B. Myocardial infarction.

C. Pleuritic chest pain.

D. Esophagitis and other gastrointestinal causes of chest pain.

E. Cervical spine disease (disc disease and osteophytosis produce nerve root compression).

VI. Treatment

A. Reassure patient as to the origin of the pain.

B. Advise patient on these measures:

   1. Heat to the involved area.

   2. Rest.

   3. Acetaminophen (325 mg per tablet), 2 tablets orally every 4–6 hours; or Ibuprofen (Motrin) 800 mg orally 3 times a day.

VII. Complications

These are primarily psychologic, relating to the patient's concern that the pain is cardiac in origin.

VIII. Consultation–Referral

A. Unclear diagnosis.

B. Unusual patient anxiety, even if the diagnosis seems readily apparent.

IX. Follow-Up

As needed to reassure both the patient and the nurse practitioner.

▲ LUMBOSACRAL STRAIN: ADULT

I. Definition

A painful condition involving the lower back. It is usually recurrent, with acute exacerbations often related to physical stress (80% of adults will develop back pain at some time).

II. Etiology

Pain arises from strain of the ligaments and musculature of the lumbosacral area, and not from the vertebrae, articular cartilage or nerve roots.

III. Clinical Features

A. Symptoms

1. Usually mild to moderately severe pain located across the lumbosacral area, generally worsened by movement, such as getting out of bed, rising from a sitting position, or bending over.
2. No radicular pain.
3. No radiation of pain to legs, groin, or testes.
4. No costovertebral angle pain.
5. No dysuria, frequency, or other genitourinary symptoms.
6. No bladder or bowel incontinence.

B. **Signs**

1. No fever.
2. Pain and muscle spasm on palpation over lumbosacral area may be present.
3. No pain in flanks on percussion.
4. Straight leg-raising should not produce pain that radiates down the leg.
5. Normal neurologic examination of lower extremities, including sensory and motor function and reflexes.
6. Intact pulses in lower extremities.

IV. **Diagnostic Studies**

None.

V. **Differential Diagnosis**

A. Lumbosacral disc disease.
B. Genitourinary infections: cystitis rarely causes back pain and pain with pyelonephritis is usually in the flanks, even with prostatitis which can cause midback pain. There should be other discriminating symptoms.
C. Vascular occlusion at the level of the aortic bifurcation.
D. Cancer with bony metastases (cancer of the prostate often presents in this manner).
E. Gynecologic disorders (e.g., endometriosis and fibromyomas).
F. Compression fracture in the elderly.

VI. **Treatment**

Advise patient on these measures:

A. Education about back care.
B. For moderately severe pain, bed rest for 2–3 days may be useful. For minimal pain, restriction of activity, particularly lifting.
C. Bed board.
D. Local heat.
E. Back flexion exercises.
F. Ibuprofen (Motrin), 800 mg orally 3 times a day.

or

   G. In case of intolerance to NSAIDs, acetaminophen (325 mg tablets), 2 orally 4 times a day.

VII. Complications

Prolonged disability that is probably due to a combination of physical, psychologic, social, and economic factors.

VIII. Consultation–Referral

   A. Severe, disabling pain.

   B. Prolonged pain (lasting more than 2 weeks).

   C. Recurrent pain (more than three attacks).

   D. Neurologic deficit (motor or sensory).

   E. Bladder or bowel incontinence, which may indicate involvement of autonomic nerves.

IX. Follow-Up

If there is no improvement within a week.

▲ NONSPECIFIC MUSCULOSKELETAL PAIN: ADULT

I. Definition

Vague aching of the muscles, bones, joints, or ligaments (alone or in any combination), usually poorly localized to areas such as the arm and shoulder, the hip and leg, and the anterior chest and arm.

II. Etiology

   A. Trauma or straining of the involved area by excessive use is often implicated.

   B. Frequently, no cause can be ascertained.

   C. Nonspecific musculoskeletal pain is often associated with tension–anxiety states.

III. Clinical Features

   A. Symptoms

      1. A vague aching of the muscles, bones, joints, or ligaments, usually poorly localized to areas such as the arm and shoulder, the hip and leg, and the anterior chest and arm.

      2. *No* generalized myalgia.

      3. *No* localized musculoskeletal pain, as in bursitis or arthritis.

      4. *No* neurologic symptoms, such as sensory loss or localized weakness.

      5. Sometimes, history of trauma to or excessive or unusual use of the involved area.

   B. Signs

1. No fever.
2. No objective inflammation, that is, no redness, swelling, heat, or warmth of any part of the painful area.
3. No demonstrable sensory or motor deficit.
4. Sometimes, vague, poorly localized tenderness to palpation of the involved muscles, joints, ligaments, or bones.

IV. Diagnostic Studies

None.

V. Differential Diagnosis

A. Specific localized inflammatory conditions affecting the musculoskeletal system (e.g., arthritis, bursitis, tendinitis, and gout).

B. Generalized myalgia accompanying systemic illnesses (e.g., influenza, Rocky Mountain spotted fever, and pneumonia).

C. Specific localized symptoms related to known trauma (e.g., sprained ankle).

VI. Treatment

Advise patient on these measures:

A. Rest of the involved area.

B. Heat by means of a hot water bottle, heating pad, warm soaks, hot showers, etc.

C. Ibuprofen (Motrin), 800 mg orally 3 times a day.

or

D. In case of intolerance to NSAIDs, acetaminophen (325 mg tablets), 2 orally 4 times a day.

VII. Complications

Prolonged disability.

VIII. Consultation–Referral

A. Severe, disabling pain.

B. Course prolonged more than 2 weeks.

C. Recurrent pain (more than three attacks).

D. Symptoms suggesting systemic illness.

IX. Follow-Up

As needed.

▲ DEGENERATIVE JOINT DISEASE (OSTEOARTHRITIS): ADULT

I. Definition

A disorder usually restricted to elderly people and characterized by degeneration of articular cartilage and hypertrophy of bone, usually in weight-bearing joints and in the distal interphalangeal joints of the fingers.

II. Etiology

Degenerative joint disease is associated with aging and trauma, but no specific cause has been found.

III. Clinical Features

A. **Symptoms**

1. Joint pain and stiffness are present. The pain characteristically improves with rest and worsens with exercise, while the stiffness improves with exercise.

2. Pain is usually mild and rarely progresses to the point of invalidism, although it may become difficult to move the affected fingers easily and with precision.

3. Cervical lesions may lead to neck pain and may cause radicular neuropathy, with pain and weakness in the arm or the shoulder girdle. In rare instances central osteophytes may compress descending tracts and effect the lower extremities.

B. **Signs**

1. The joints most commonly affected are the knees, hips, lumbar vertebrae (weight-bearing joints), cervical vertebrae, and distal interphalangeal joints of the fingers.

2. Affected joints are not hot or erythematous, but may be mildly tender.

3. Classically, interphalangeal involvement leads to Heberden's nodes—firm, knotty, enlargements of the distal interphalangeal joints—which may be present alone without other joint involvement.

4. Larger joints and vertebrae usually appear grossly normal.

IV. Laboratory and Other Studies

A. An X-ray film of the involved joint is useful if the diagnosis is in question (Heberden's nodes do not require X-ray).

B. Determination of the sedimentation rate also may be helpful to establish the presence of an inflammatory process. Should be normal in degenerative joint disease.

V. Differential Diagnosis

A. **Polyarthritis**

1. Acute rheumatoid arthritis is usually easily differentiated because the affected joints are inflamed, there may be constitutional signs and symptoms, the sedimentation rate is elevated, and it occurs less frequently in elderly people.

2. Chronic rheumatoid arthritis affects the proximal interphalangeal and the metacarpo-phalangeal joints.

3. In addition to bone involvement, there is swelling of synovial tissue and edema around the joints in both acute and chronic rheumatoid arthritis.

B. **Monarticular arthritis**

1. Gout (see Chapter 12, Gout and Hyperuricemia: Adult, pp. 288–292).

2. Traumatic arthritis. Generally, the joints are swollen and tender, and there is a history of trauma.

3. Infection. Inflammatory arthritis is frequently associated with gonococcal infection occurring in a much younger age group.

Note: Osteoarthritis may be present along with an inflammatory arthritis. If the degree of pain and inflammation seems incompatible with osteoarthritis, one should seek another cause.

VI. Treatment

Advise patient on these measures:

A. Rest of the involved joints.

B. Physical therapy of the joints.

C. Acetaminophen (325 mg) for pain, 2 tablets orally every 4–6 hours, or ibuprofen (Motrin), 800 mg orally 3 times a day.

D. Heat to the involved joints.

E. Weight loss and elimination of trauma.

F. In some cases, a neck or back support.

VII. Complications

A. Generally, osteoarthritis is not severe or crippling and usually results in no systemic complaints.

B. Cervical vertebral lesions occasionally lead to radicular neurologic problems.

VIII. Consultation–Referral

A. Inflammatory arthritis.

B. Neurologic involvement.

IX. Follow-Up

A. These patients may be seen as needed for exacerbation of pain or dysfunction.

B. Special visits generally are not necessary; the osteoarthritis may be evaluated during visits for other problems or for health maintenance.

▲ OSTEOPOROSIS: ADULT

I. Definition

A heterogeneous group of diseases resulting in a reduction in bone mass per unit volume below the level required for adequate mechanical support. The ratio of mineral to matrix material remains normal. This reduction may ultimately lead to fractures, most frequently in hip, spine, and wrist.

II. Etiology

Multiple known causes for osteoporosis include corticosteroid therapy, chronic heparin therapy, prolonged immobilization, thyrotoxicosis, Cushing's disease, malabsorption, renal tubular acidosis. Most cases, however, are of unclear etiology. The risk of osteoporosis increases with age, female sex, white race, and menopause, especially secondary to surgical removal of the ovaries before menopause. Thin women are also at greater risk than obese women.

III. Clinical Features

A. **Symptoms**
   1. Most patients are asymptomatic as they undergo slow reduction in their bone density.
   2. Back pain related to vertebral compression fractures is the most common symptomatic presentation.
   3. Fracture of the hip may be the first indication of significant bone disease.

B. **Physical examination**
   1. May have no physical signs.
   2. Kyphosis.
   3. Loss of height.

IV. Laboratory and Diagnostic Studies

A. X-rays may show decreased bone density, but this may be evident only after >40 % of bony mass is lost.

B. Bone densitometry may detect early bone loss, but its precise role is unclear.

C. Complete blood count, calcium, and alkaline phosphatase should be obtained, but will be normal in idiopathic osteoporosis.

V. Differential Diagnosis

A. Vitamin D deficiency.

B. Metastatic carcinoma.

C. Multiple myeloma.

D. Cortisol excess, either intrinsic (Cushing's disease) or from use of exogenous steroids.

E. Osteoarthritis may cause back pain, but has a very different clinical course and X-ray picture.

VI. Treatment

A. **Prevention.** Primary prevention of bone loss seems to be more effective in preventing symptoms than treatment after pain or fractures have occurred.

1. Women who have undergone premature surgical oophorectomy should receive estrogen replacement. Patients with carcinoma of the breast in a first degree relative are at risk for carcinoma and consultation is necessary.

2. Estrogen replacement in women at the time of physiologic menopause is indicated particularly in women at risk for fractures (white race, thin body habitus, family history of fractures).

3. Maintenance of an adequate calcium intake (greater than 1.0 gram elemental calcium per day) may have some protective effect, and is unlikely to do harm. This addition may be in the form of increased intake of dairy products or use of over-the-counter calcium supplements. Such dietary supplementation, when administered, should begin well before menopause. After menopause, some authors recommend 1.5 grams of elemental calcium per day. The utility of supplemental vitamin D in patients with adequate natural intake is controversial.

4. Maintenance of moderate physical activity with aging may preserve bony mass.

Note: Use of conjugated estrogens has been linked with later development of endometrial cancer. When this class of medications is administered to a patient with a uterus, the patient should be informed of the risks. Conjugated estrogen 0.625 mg should be given for the first 25 days each month and 5 mg of medroxy progesterone for the last 10 days of estrogen therapy. This combination will cause withdrawal bleeding which some patients may find troublesome. The monthly endometrial shedding putatively decreases the risk of endometrial cancer. Continuous therapy using lower dose progestogens are being used, but the relationship of continuous therapy to endometrial cancer is uncertain.

VII. Complications

A. Fracture of the femoral neck with mild or minimal trauma.

B. Other fractures, including vertebral compression fractures.

C. Breakthrough bleeding.

VIII. Consultation–Referral

A. Consultation for all patients with symptomatic back pain related to compression fractures.

B. Bleeding before the 12th day of progestogen therapy.

IX. Follow-Up

A. Preventive interventions should be addressed at health care maintenance visits.

B. Follow-up for symptomatic patients should be individualized.

11

DISORDERS OF THE NERVOUS SYSTEM

▲ Dizziness: Adults Less Than Sixty Years Old

I. Definition

A vague sensation of unsteadiness or lightheadedness, or both, occurring episodically in adults less than 60 years old. This is a common complaint in all ages, but in the young adult most often is inconsequential and must be differentiated from the problems below.

II. Etiology

Most often seen in association with tension-anxiety states.

III. Clinical Features

  A. Symptoms

    1. A vague sensation of unsteadiness, as though one might fall in one direction or another.

    2. No vertigo.

    3. No tendency to fall consistently in one direction.

    4. No associated severe headache.

    5. No associated neurologic symptoms.

Patient Care Guidelines for Nurse Practitioners, 4th ed. by Axalla J. Hoole, C. Glenn Pickard, Jr., Ruth M. Ouimette, Jacob A. Lohr, and Robert A. Greenberg. Copyright © 1995 by J. B. Lippincott Company.

6. No symptoms of sinusitis or upper respiratory infection (URI).

7. No associated nausea or vomiting.

8. Feeling of faintness or sensation of loss of consciousness, but no actual loss of consciousness.

9. Attacks are neither precipitated by prior ingestion (1–1 1/2 hours before attack) of heavy carbohydrate meal nor relieved by ingestion of food.

10. No medications with side effect of dizziness.

B. **Signs**

1. Blood pressure between 100/70 and 150/100 mm Hg, with orthostatic drop of less than 10 mg Hg diastolic.

2. Normal neurologic examination.

3. No sinus tenderness or abnormality of tympanic membrane or oral mucosa.

4. No murmur of aortic stenosis.

IV. **Laboratory Studies**

Hematocrit or hemoglobin or both are normal.

V. **Differential Diagnosis**

A. Vasovagal syncope.

B. Vertiginous dizziness, as in labyrinthitis, Meniere's disease, and acoustic neuroma.

C. Sinusitis, otitis media, or other URI.

D. Postural hypotension, especially in patients being treated for hypertension.

E. Acute blood loss, as in gastrointestinal hemorrhage.

F. Unsteadiness associated with significant anemia (hematocrit reading less than 35%).

G. Dizziness associated with aortic stenosis.

H. Dizziness associated with other neurologic symptoms or signs, as in a stroke syndrome.

I. Hypoglycemic episodes.

VI. **Treatment**

A. Reassure patient as to the absence of serious disease.

B. Attempt to discover and alter psychosocial factors that often are associated.

VII. **Complications**

Prolonged disability.

VIII. **Consultation–Referral**

A. Severe, persistent (single attack lasting more than 24 hours), or recurring (more than 6 per week) attacks.

B. Patients >60 years old.

IX. Follow-Up

As needed.

▲ MIGRAINE HEADACHE: ADULT

I. Definition

A throbbing unilateral headache with familial tendency which in many cases is preceded by an aura and by other neurologic manifestations occurs with 3:1 predominance in females with onset usually between 10–30 years.

II. Etiology

Unknown. Pain is related to cerebral arterial spasm followed by dilation. It is during the dilation phase that pain occurs.

III. Clinical Features

A. Headache is usually unilateral, but not always on the same side.

B. Headaches are generally preceded by a visual aura, which may be followed by neurologic signs such as tingling and weakness in an extremity. There actually may be temporary paralysis.

C. Throbbing gradually increases in intensity to a peak in 1 hour and then may last for a few hours to several days. It may be associated with nausea and vomiting.

D. Photophobia may be present.

E. Eighty percent of patients have a family history of migraine.

F. Onset is usually in adolescence, and attacks tend to decrease in frequency with age. Migraine may, however, begin at a later age and actually accelerate in frequency during menopause.

G. Patients with migraine often have motion sickness as children.

IV. Laboratory Studies

None.

V. Differential Diagnosis

See Tension Headache: Adult, V, p. 270–271.

VI. Treatment

A. Patient can use either of the following at the first sign of headache:

    1. Ergotamine tartrate (Ergostat)—2 mg sublingually initially, followed by 2 mg every hour until headache is relieved, to a maximum of 6 mg per day or 10 mg per week.

    or

    2. A combination of 1 mg ergotamine tartrate and 100 mg caffeine (Cafergot)—2 tablets orally initially, followed by 1 tablet

every hour until headache is relieved, to a maximum of 6 tablets per day or 10 tablets per week. This may also be taken as a rectal suppository—(2 mg ergotamine tartrate and 100 mg caffeine), 1 suppository initially, followed by 1 suppository in an hour if needed (maximum, 2 per day)—if vomiting precludes oral administration.

3. Ergotamine may also be delivered sublingually, or by inhalation or suppository in those patients who can't take oral medicines.
4. Sumatriptan may be used after consultation.
5. Nifedipine.
6. Midrin.

Note: Ergotamine tartrate is contraindicated in moderate to severe hypertension, vascular diseases, renal disease, and pregnancy.

B. In established headache, an ergot preparation may be tried (see **A**), but generally the following measures are required:
1. Dark room.
2. Analgesic, such as codeine or meperidine HCl (Demerol). Both are controlled medicines requiring physician's orders.

C. One of the following may be used as preventive therapy under a physician's direction to decrease the frequency of attacks:
1. Bellergal (often effective when there seems to be a psychologic overlay to the problem).
2. Propranolol HCl (Inderal).
3. Methysergide maleate (Sansert).
4. Tricyclic antidepressants.

VII. Complications
Generally, there are no complications.

VIII. Consultation-Referral
A. Failure of treatment.
B. All new cases (first time to clinic or first time with headache).
C. Persistence of neurologic component.

IX. Follow-Up
Return visit if there is no improvement.

▲ TENSION HEADACHE: ADULT

I. Definition
A headache that is generally associated with periods of stress and is characterized by bandlike pressure across the forehead and occiput. May coexist with vascular headaches.

II. Etiology

The headache is generally associated with tension, but the cause may not be known. Pain may be associated with muscle spasm.

III. **Clinical Features**

A. **Symptoms**

1. Dull, aching pain often accompanied by occipital pain and tightness across the scalp.

2. Usually, middle-aged persons are affected, women more than men.

3. Headache is present for long periods.

4. Pain is not throbbing.

5. Usually not associated with nausea and vomiting.

6. Headaches may be associated with known periods of tension.

7. No aura or neurologic deficit is present.

B. **Signs**

1. Usually, there are no signs:

a. Blood pressure is normal.

b. Results of funduscopic examination are normal: pupils are reactive.

c. Results of the screening neurologic examination are normal.

d. No febrile disease is present.

e. The temporal arteries are nontender.

2. The scalp may be sore.

3. The muscles in the posterior neck may be tense and tender.

IV. **Laboratory Studies**

None.

V. **Differential Diagnosis**

Eliminate other major causes of headache.

A. **Sinus headache.** Pain is located over antrum, forehead, or around the eyes, most frequently in association with sinus congestion but sometimes in association with bacterial sinusitis. The overlying skin may be sensitive and the sinuses tender. Headache may begin at night and change sides with change in position.

B. **Migraine.** See Migraine Headache: Adult.

C. **Hypertension.** Hypertension may cause early morning headaches, but moderate hypertension does not usually cause severe headaches.

D. **Systemic febrile disease.**

E. **Acute glaucoma.** Pain is generally severe and is located around the orbits. It may be associated with nausea and vomiting. Pupils are fixed and semidilated with injected sclerae.

F. **Brain tumor.** Headache associated with brain tumor does not have a specific character but tends to be a more severe, deep-seated pain that may come and go and tends to worsen. It may occur at night and wake the patient; it may also occur in the early morning.

G. **Cluster headache (Horton's headache).** Cluster headache occurs at night, is generally localized to one orbit, and lasts approximately 1 hour. Intense pain associated with rhinorrhea, lacrimation, and flush is present. The pains tend to occur in clusters over a period of a few nights to weeks and then disappear.

H. **Temporal arteritis.** Usually a unilateral pain over the temple that may be initially described as soreness. Occurs in patients over fifty and is important because it may be associated with blindness.

VI. Treatment

A. **Reassurance**

B. **Analgesic.** Aspirin (325 mg per tablet), 2 tablets orally every 4–6 hours.

C. **A mild tranquilizer**, if stress is identifiable, may be added on physician's advice.

VII. Complications

Rare.

VIII. Consultation–Referral

A. **Tension headache** that does not improve after initial therapy has begun.

B. **All headaches not specifically diagnosed** as migraine, sinus, or tension headaches.

C. **Failure to resolve** after 2 weeks of treatment.

IX. Follow-Up

A. **Return visit** in 2 weeks, or sooner, if necessary.

B. Allow patient to initiate next visit.

▲ VASOVAGAL SYNCOPE (SIMPLE FAINT): ADULTS LESS THAN SIXTY YEARS OLD

I. Definition

A transient loss of consciousness and motor function due to a transient, reversible decrease in general cerebral blood flow.

II. Etiology

Vasovagal syncope is the result of a complex phenomenon involving, in part, vagal nerve stimulation with resultant bradycardia and venous pooling of blood in the extremities and viscera. It is often triggered by emotional factors, such as venipuncture or disturbing news. The cardiovascular phenomena are transient, lasting only a few minutes.

III. Clinical Features

A. Symptoms

1. Loss of consciousness preceded by a sensation of faintness often associated with slight nausea and mild diaphoresis.
2. No headache or localizing neurologic symptoms.
3. Prompt return of consciousness when placed in a supine position with no postictal state.
4. No history of organic heart disease, such as angina or arrhythmias.
5. No history of focal neurologic symptoms.

B. Signs

1. Weak, thready pulse.
2. Blood pressure during actual faint less than 70 mm Hg systolic.
3. Pallor.
4. Diaphoresis.
5. Sometimes, twitching of extremities, but no definite seizure activity.
6. No bladder or bowel incontinence.
7. No postictal confusion.
8. No demonstrable neurologic deficit in post faint evaluation.
9. No murmur of aortic stenosis.
10. Blood pressure rapidly returns to normal when patient is placed in a supine position.

IV. Laboratory Studies

A. Hematocrit may be obtained.
B. Obtain electrocardiogram if arrhythmias are present on clinical examination.

V. Differential Diagnosis

A. Grand mal or other seizure disorder.
B. Localized transient cerebral ischemia, as in stroke syndromes.
C. Syncope occurring with aortic stenosis.
D. Syncope occurring with tachycardia or bradycardia associated with organic heart disease.

VI. Treatment

A. Position patient so that the head is lower than the feet, or simply place the patient supine on the floor or ground.
B. Record blood pressure and pulse every 5 minutes.

VII. Complications

None.

VIII. Consultation–Referral

    A. Convulsion.

    B. Presence of any abnormal neurologic finding.

    C. Patient over 60 years of age.

    D. Orthostatic fall in blood pressure that persists after recovery from faint.

    E. Hematocrit reading below normal.

    F. Melena.

    G. Murmur of aortic stenosis.

    H. Arrhythmia.

    I. Failure of blood pressure and pulse to return to normal in 15 minutes.

IX. Follow-Up

As needed.

▲ ANXIETY: ADULT

I. Definition

State of apprehension, restlessness, nervousness, or fearfulness, which can be of long standing or relatively acute.

II. Etiology

    A. Life situations, usually associated with a family or personal crisis.

    B. Certain physical and mental illnesses, such as hyperthyroidism, pheochromocytoma, panic attacks.

III. Clinical Features

    A. Symptoms

        1. Anorexia, insomnia, increased sweating, thumping in the heart, irritability, weakness and fatigue, and headaches.

        2. Weight loss, nausea and vomiting, diarrhea, numbness and tingling of the extremities, shortness of breath, polyuria, and amenorrhea indicate complications other than, or in addition to, simple anxiety.

    B. Signs

        1. Trembling of fingers, increased sweating, drawn face and tight muscles, and tachycardia.

        2. Weight loss, slow speech, and flat affect indicate complications other than, or in addition to, simple anxiety.

IV. Laboratory Studies

None.

V. Differential Diagnosis

A. Hyperthyroidism.

B. Cancer.

C. Organic brain syndrome.

D. Unexplained weight loss due to other causes.

E. Hypertension.

F. Depression.

G. Alcoholism.

H. Drug abuse.

VI. Treatment

A. Supportive therapy using staff as much as possible or frequent *short* visits to health center, or both.

B. Buspirone.

C. Contraindications to drug therapy include:

1. First trimester of pregnancy, or if patient is near term.

2. Grief reactions (nighttime sedation is appropriate, but tranquilizers will only postpone normal grief and therefore should not be used).

3. Active liver disease.

4. Suspected drug abuse (if acute withdrawal is suspected, hospitalization is indicated).

VII. Complications

A. Drug abuse.

B. Buspirone

1. **Oversedation.** Patient should be warned that driving may be hazardous and should be urged to start drugs at time when he or she has no responsibility for driving, operating heavy machinery, and so on. If patient appears intoxicated, drug dose should be decreased.

2. **Potentiating effect.** Diazepam has a potentiating effect with other depressants, such as alcohol, tranquilizers, and narcotics; if patient is undergoing treatment with such drugs, use of depressants should be avoided and consultation sought.

3. **Confusion and agitation.** These complications may occur in the elderly with depressant drug treatment. Discontinue diazepam immediately if patient becomes confused or agitated.

VIII. Consultation–Referral

A. Evidence of underlying organic or other disease state, including manifestation of any of the symptoms or signs indicated as *not* consistent with simple anxiety (see **III.A** and **B**).

B. Mental health referral is indicated if:

1. There is evidence of depressant drug abuse (e.g., concurrent use of other depressants, such as Librium, barbiturates, or alcohol). Often such a patient demands drugs but gives an unclear or vague history that is judged to be unreliable.

2. There is evidence by history that the presenting symptoms are of long standing and have not been precipitated by a real life crisis.

3. At the end of 2 weeks of treatment symptoms persist, and the patient requires continued treatment with tranquilizers.

IX. Follow-Up

A. Return visit in 1 week if medication is prescribed.

B. Return visits as often as necessary, depending on severity of problem and need for continuing supportive therapy.

▲ DEMENTIA: ADULT

I. Definition

Loss of memory, judgment, and other cognitive functions due to a chronic progressive degenerative disease of the brain, leading to loss of occupational and social functioning.

II. Etiology

More than 60 causes. Alzheimer's disease is responsible for more than 55% of dementias; it is of unknown cause and is characterized by progressive worsening of memory and other cognitive functions in the absence of systemic or other brain diseases that could account for the deficits. Multi-infarct dementia tends to occur in a "stepwise" progression with associated neurologic deficits. Diagnostic tests in the workup of a patient with dementia are performed in the hope of finding a reversible cause. See V, Differential Diagnosis.

III. Clinical Features

A. Symptoms

1. Gradually increasing forgetfulness, especially for recent events (objects around the house, what's on the stove).

2. Decreased self-care.

3. The patient may or may not be aware of the change, or may deny any problem. The loss may have been gradual over years or relatively acute. Clear understanding of clinical course is essential to the etiologic and prognostic assessment. Often family or co-workers are the first to report a change in function.

B. Physical examination

1. A complete physical examination should be performed but

typically may reveal no abnormalities early in the course of potentially reversible dementia, such as cerebrovascular accidents, hypothyroidism, or anemia.

2. Careful mental status examination, such as the structured "minimental" state, must be supplemented by information from family and friends.

IV. Laboratory Studies

A. Complete blood count, creatinine, glucose, electrolytes, calcium, thyroid function tests, VDRI, vitamin B_{12}, and serum folate level and urine for culture and sensitivity.

B. Other studies, such as CT scans, should be performed only after physician consultation.

V. Differential Diagnosis

A. Potentially reversible dementias:

1. Metabolic disorders: hypothyroidism, hyperthyroidism, hypercalcemia, hyponatremia, Cushing's disease, Addison's disease.

2. Medication effect, including sedatives, cimetidine, anti-Parkinson drugs, and many others.

3. Vitamin B_{12} deficiency.

4. Psychiatric disorders. Depression may commonly cause a "pseudodementia."

5. A variety of neurologic diseases, including subdural hematoma, tertiary syphilis, and normal pressure hydrocephalus.

6. Infections such as pulmonary or urinary tract infections may unmask or worsen a dementia.

B. Nonreversible dementias:

1. Alzheimer's disease.

2. Multi-infarct dementia.

3. Dementia due to alcoholism.

Note: More than one type of dementia may coexist in a patient, and a deterioration in the functioning of a mildly demented patient should initiate consideration of a reversible cause. Any deterioration in general health may be reflected in worsening of cognitive function.

VI. Treatment

A. Treatment of the reversible dementias depends on the cause.

B. Most dementias are not curable, and treatment is supportive.

1. Personal autonomy, maximizing the patient's mental and physical capacities, should be maintained as long as is feasible.

2. Medication should be kept to a minimum.

3. Family support groups and newsletters can improve understanding.

4. Adult day care may increase socialization and provide the family with a respite.

5. A variety of home-care services may be available. The practitioner should become familiar with local agencies, including their expertise, costs and range of services.

VII. Complications

A. Safety at home may become compromised, with wandering, difficulty cooking or driving.

B. Inadequate nutrition.

C. Family stress.

D. Late in the course of the disease, decreased mobility, falls, and incontinence may occur.

VIII. Consultation–Referral

All new cases of dementia and acute deteriorations in mental status require physician consultation.

IX. Follow-Up

Patients and families may need follow-up every 1–3 months; however, provider availability for questions and crisis intervention is essential in the care of the demented patient.

12

DISORDERS OF THE ENDOCRINE SYSTEM

▲ DIABETES MELLITUS: ADULT

I. Definition

Diabetes mellitus is a chronic disorder that is characterized by hyperglycemia, associated with major abnormalities in carbohydrate, fat, and protein metabolism and is accompanied by a marked propensity to develop relatively specific forms of renal, ocular, neurologic, and premature cardiovascular diseases.

A. Types of diabetes mellitus. There are two clinical subtypes of diabetes mellitus:

1. **Type I.** Insulin dependent diabetes mellitus (IDDM)—ketosis prone. Insulin deficient due to islet cell loss. Occurs at any age, common in youth. Formerly called juvenile diabetes.

2. **Type II.** Non-insulin-dependent diabetes (NIDDM)—ketosis resistant. More frequent in adults but occurs at any age. Majority are overweight. May be seen in family aggregates as an autosomal dominant genetic trait. May require insulin for control of either chronic or acute hyperglycemia during stress. Patients

Patient Care Guidelines for Nurse Practitioners, 4th ed. by Axalla J. Hoole, C. Glenn Pickard, Jr., Ruth M. Ouimette, Jacob A. Lohr, and Robert A. Greenberg. Copyright © 1995 by J. B. Lippincott Company.

may have few or none of the classic symptoms of diabetes. Typically insulin resistance (decreased tissue sensitivity or responsiveness to exogenous and endogenous insulin) is present. Also known as adult or maturity onset diabetes.

B. **Other types of diabetes.** Diabetes secondary to:

1. Pancreatic disease.

2. Endocrinopathies (Cushing's syndrome).

3. Drug or chemical usage:

   a. Thiazide diuretics.

   b. Glucocorticoid stenosis.

   c. Psychoactive agents.

   d. Estrogen containing preparations.

   e. Catecholamines.

4. Associated with:

   a. Insulin receptor abnormalities.

   b. Genetic syndromes such as muscular dystrophies, Huntington's chorea.

C. **Gestational diabetes.** Patients with gestational diabetes mellitus have onset or discovery of glucose intolerance during pregnancy.

D. **Impaired glucose intolerance.** Previously called chemical, subclinical, borderline, or latent. Patients with impaired glucose tolerance have plasma glucose levels that are higher than normal but not diagnostic for diabetes mellitus. In this condition, fasting plasma glucose is less than 140 mg/dL. Following a 75 gm oral glucose dose the 2-hour plasma glucose level is between 140 and 200 mg/dL with an intervening plasma glucose value equal to or greater than 200 mg/dL.

II. Etiology

The cause of diabetes is unknown although in Type I, circulating antibodies to islet cells are almost always present. In Type II, patterns suggesting inheritance can often be demonstrated.

III. Clinical Features

A. **Symptoms**

1. **General.** Classical symptoms of Type I and II diabetes related to hyperglycemia with associated glycosuria. Many patients with Type II diabetes have few or no classic presenting symptoms.

2. Related to high blood glucose level:

   a. Polyuria.

   b. Polydipsia.

   c. Polyphagia.

   d. Weight loss.

  e. Blurred vision.

  f. Weakness or fatigue.

 3. Related to vascular complications:

  a. Microvascular.

   (1) Eyes. Decreased vision due to diabetic retinopathy, glaucoma, or early cataracts.

   (2) Nervous system. Numbness, burning of feet or hands, nonhealing foot ulcers, impotence.

   (3) Kidneys. Edema, hypertension, renal failure.

  b. Macrovascular.

   (1) Premature coronary artery disease. Myocardial infarction often silent, i.e., painless.

   (2) Cerebrovascular accidents.

   (3) Peripheral vascular insufficiency.

    (a) Cool extremities.

    (b) Claudication.

    (c) Nonhealing foot ulcer.

 B. Signs

 1. Microaneurysms, hemorrhages, and exudates in ocular fundus.

 2. Evidence of advanced atherosclerosis:

  a. Coronary artery disease.

  b. Vascular insufficiency in feet:

   (1) Poor or absent dorsal pedis, and posterior tibial pulses, and decreased capillary filling.

   (2) Loss of hair on toes and lower legs.

   (3) Bruits in abdomen or over femoral artery.

   (4) Ulcers between toes or on dorsum of foot.

   (5) Gangrene.

 3. Evidence of nervous system dysfunction:

  a. Absent or diminished vibration and proprioception in feet.

  b. Absent ankle jerks.

  c. Orthostatic hypotension without compensatory pulse increase.

IV. **Diagnostic Studies**

 A. Suggestive findings

 1. Elevated random blood glucose (serum or capillary). (This finding must be considered in relation to when the patient last ate. See criteria for glucose tolerance test.)

 2. Diagnostic criteria. Diagnosis of diabetes in nonpregnant adults should be restricted to those who have one of the following:

    a. Unequivocal elevation of random plasma glucose (>200 mg per dL) plus classic symptoms of diabetes; or

    b. Fasting plasma glucose of 140 mg per dL or greater on at least 2 occasions; or

    c. Fasting plasma glucose level less than 140 mg per dL plus sustained elevated plasma glucose levels during at least 2 oral glucose tolerance tests. Oral glucose testing is not necessary if the patient has fasting plasma glucose level of 140 mg per dL or greater.

  B. All abnormal glucose levels in an undiagnosed patient should lead to a physician consultation.

V. Differential Diagnosis

  A. Diabetes mellitus must be differentiated from other causes of hyperglycemia:

    1. Chronic pancreatitis (often due to alcoholism).

    2. Cushing's syndrome.

    3. Drug induced hyperglycemia from drugs such as oral contraceptives, corticosteroids, or thiazides.

    4. Gestational diabetes.

    5. Acromegaly.

    6. Pheochromocytoma.

VI. Treatment: Initial Evaluation

  A. Initial visit—Comprehensive medical history can uncover symptoms that will help establish the diagnosis in patients with previously unrecognized diabetes.

    1. Elements of the medical history of particular concern in patients with diabetes:

      a. Symptoms and previous laboratory test results related to diagnosis of diabetes.

      b. Dietary habits, nutritional status, and weight history.

      c. Details of previous treatment programs, including diabetes education.

      d. Current treatment of diabetes, including medications, diet, and results of glucose monitoring.

      e. Exercise history.

      f. Frequency, severity, and cause of acute complications such as ketoacidosis, and hypoglycemia.

      g. Prior and current infections, particularly skin, foot, dental, and genitourinary.

      h. Symptoms and treatment of chronic complications associated with diabetes: eye, heart, kidney, nerve, sexual function, peripheral vascular, and cerebral vascular.

    i. Other medications that may affect blood glucose concentration.

    j. Risk factor for atherosclerosis: smoking, hypertension, obesity, hyperlipidemia, and family history.

    k. Psychosocial and economic factors that might influence the management of diabetes.

    l. Family history of diabetes and other endocrine disorders.

    m. Gestational history: hyperglycemia, delivery of an infant weighing >9 lb., toxemia, stillbirth, polyhydramnios, or other complications of pregnancy.

2. Physical examination. Aspects requiring special attention:

    a. Height and weight management.

    b. Blood pressure measurement with orthostatic measurements.

    c. Ophthalmoscopic examination with dilation if possible.

    d. Thyroid palpation.

    e. Cardiac examination.

    f. Evaluation of pulses including auscultation for bruits.

    g. Foot examination.

    h. Skin examination including insulin injection sites.

    i. Neurological examination.

    j. Dental and periodontal examination.

3. Laboratory evaluation

    a. Fasting plasma glucose.

    b. Glycosylated hemoglobin (HgbA1 or HgbA1c).

    c. Fasting lipid profile: total cholesterol, high-density lipoprotein (HDL), low-density lipoprotein (LDL), and triglycerides.

    d. Serum creatinine.

    e. Urinalysis: ketones, glucose, protein, microscopic if indicated.

    f. Urine culture: if microscopic is abnormal or symptoms are present.

    g. Thyroid function tests (T4 or thyroid stimulating hormone).

    h. ECG.

VII. Treatment: Management

  A. **Implementation of the management plan** requires that the patient understand each aspect of it.

  B. **The treatment plan** should be individualized and contain the following components:

TABLE 12-1

LEVELS OF TREATMENT TYPE I DIABETES

MINIMAL

HgbA1c 11.0–13.0% and HgbA1 13.0–15.0%

Many SMGB values above 300 mg/dl

Almost constant glycosuria

Intermittent spontaneous ketonuria

AVERAGE

HgbA1c 8.0–9.0% and HgbA1 10.0–11.0%

Premeal SMBG 160–200 mg/dl

Intermittent glocosuria

Rare ketonuria

INTENSIVE

HgbA1c 6.0–7.0% and HgbA1 7.0–9.0%

Premeal SMBG 79–120 mg/dl; postmeal SMBG <180 mg/dl

Essentially no glycosuria or ketonuria

From *Physician's Guide to Insulin Dependent Diabetes.*

TABLE 12-2

LEVELS OF TREATMENT TYPE II DIABETES

TEST	NORMAL	AVERAGE	POOR
Plasma glucose*	115	140	>200 mg/dL
2-h postprandial glucose	140	200	>235 mg/dL
HgbA1c	6	8	>10%
Cholesterol*	200	<240	>240 mg/dL
Triglycerides*	150	200	>250 mg/dL

* = fasting.
From *Physician's Guide to Insulin Dependent Diabetes.*

1. Agreed to level of glycemic control (Tables 12-1 and 12-2).

2. Instruction regarding meal plan, medications, monitoring, prevention of acute complications (hypoglycemia, diabetic ketoacidosis or hyperosmolar hyperglycemic non-ketotic states), recommendations regarding life-style changes (exercise, smoking cessation).

3. All diabetic therapy is based on patient education. To a degree not found in any other disease, the patient manages his or her

own therapy. Good control and prevention of complications require a knowledgeable patient able to manipulate diet, exercise, and medication (insulin) based on home glucose monitoring results, as circumstances change.

C. **Diet.** Goals of the diet for the patient with diabetes, besides controlling blood sugar and normalizing blood cholesterol include:

1. Reaching and maintaining desirable or ideal body weight.

2. Selecting healthy foods, in predictable amounts, at predictable times.

Note: Reducing the number of calories per day by 500 kcal will result in a gradual weight loss of 1–2 lbs per week, and improve likelihood of patient adherence. A prudent heart diet is generally recommended for diabetes (50%–60% of calories from carbohydrates, 15%–20% of calories from protein, 30% of calories from fat). The exchange diet requires at least an eighth-grade education and a highly motivated patient. It is most appropriate for IDDM. Consider referral to a dietitian for patient instruction and follow-up.

TABLE 12-3

PRODUCTS FOR BLOOD GLUCOSE MONITORING

VISUALLY READ STRIPS			
PRODUCT	RANGE	HCT	COLOR
Chemstrips BG	20–800	35–55	Shades of blue
Glucostix	20–800	35–55	Shades of green and orange
Visidex	20–800	35–55	Shades of green and orange
Glucose V	20–800	35–55	Shades of blue

METER SYSTEMS			
Systems costing less than $60–70			
SYSTEM	WIPE	GLUCOSE RANGE	HCT RANGE
Tracer II	Yes	40–400	35–55
Glucometer 3	Yes	20–500	20–60
One Touch Basic	No	0–600	25–60
Accu-Chek Easy	No	20–500	30–55
Systems costing more than $60			
Accu-Chek III	Yes	20–500	35–55
One Touch II	No	0–600	25–60

D. Monitoring. All patients with diabetes should be encouraged to do regular glucose monitoring (Table 12-3).

1. Initially, patients should be asked to monitor 4 times a day (before each meal and the bedtime snack) and to keep a record of the results.

2. The patient should be instructed in the proper method of collecting and testing blood and/or urine.

3. As the condition stabilizes, the frequency of monitoring may be decreased.

Note: Urine testing does not correlate well with blood glucose in the individual with normal renal function. It may have a place in the individual who is treated with diet alone, or when blood glucose monitoring is not feasible because of cost or patient refusal to do self-monitored blood glucose.

Blood glucose monitoring is the preferred method for all patients on insulin, those with impaired renal function, a history of severe hypoglycemia, hypoglycemic coma, or seizures. A blood glucose meter is preferred to the colormetric strips.

E. Instruction on personal hygiene, especially foot care.

F. Exercise. A program of regular exercise offers many benefits to the patient with diabetes: it increases insulin sensitivity, helps to lower blood sugar, facilitates weight loss, and improves cardiovascular fitness.

1. Begin exercise at a low level—consult physician.

2. Consider referral to cardiac rehabilitation program if known to have coronary artery disease.

3. Modify exercise prescription if patient has retinopathy or peripheral neuropathy.

G. Drug therapy. Beginning therapy in an adult with Type II diabetes.

1. If blood glucose is between 200 and 300 mg per 100 mL and the patient has no symptoms and no ketosis, consider starting an oral agent as well as diet and exercise. If the patient is on diet alone, they should be monitored closely and if there is no improvement in blood glucose within one week, oral agent therapy should be started.

2. If the blood sugar is over 300 mg per 100 mL, consult the physician about starting oral agents or insulin. Tolbutamide, a first generation oral agent, was involved in a controversial trial that suggested a relationship to accelerated cardiovascular disease. Subsequent trials have not demonstrated the same result in Type II diabetics; second generation oral agents have not been similarly studied.

   a. Oral agents. Slowly (weekly) increase dose until blood sugars are within desired range or the maximum dose is reached.

(1) **First generation agents:**

(a) **Tolbutamide:** Start at 250 mg. given 2 or 3 times a day; maximum dose is 3000 mg a day; Duration of action is 6–12 hours.

(b) **Tolazamide:** Start at 250 mg/day, maximum dose is 1000 mg; duration of action is 12–24 hours.

(2) **Second generation agents:**

(a) **Glipizide (Glucotrol):** Start at 5 mg once a day. Maximum dose is 40 mg per day.

(b) **Glyburide (Micronase or Diabeta):** Start at 2.5 mg per day; maximum dose is 20 mg/day.

These second generation sulfonylureas have 12–24 hour duration of action, are hepatically metabolized with inactive or weakly active metabolites.

(3) Side effects of oral agents include: hypoglycemia, gastrointestinal disturbances, skin rashes including photosensitivity.

(4). Oral agents are contraindicated in patients with a history of coma or acidosis, ketosis, renal insufficiency, liver disease, or allergy to sulfonylurea compounds, or during pregnancy or lactation.

b. **Insulin.** Many patients with mild to moderate fasting hyperglycemia may be adequately controlled with one injection of intermediate insulin (NPH or Lente) before breakfast. An initial dose of 10–15 units of NPH or Lente may be used. However, most patients require 0.5–1.0 unit/kg/24 hours.

(1) Educational requirements (minimal): Insulin administration, home glucose monitoring, signs, symptoms and treatment of hypoglycemia.

Note: Hypoglycemia causes primarily central nervous system disturbances—confusion, abnormal behavior, and stupor; the symptoms of anxiety, sweating and tachycardia are caused by epinephrine.

(2) Patients starting insulin therapy should be in contact as often as daily until glucose control is achieved, the risk of hypoglycemia is low, and the patient is competent in the skills cited above.

c. Insulin dose adjustments can be made every 3–4 days, with the addition of a second injection or short acting insulin as needed based on home glucose data.

3. Maintenance

a. See patient regularly. Contact with the patient within a

week after a major change in the regimen.

b. Regular visits should be scheduled quarterly for insulin treated patients and for other patients at least twice a year.

c. Interim history and physical: assess frequency, causes, and severity of hypoglycemia and hyperglycemia; results of regular glucose monitoring; adjustments by the patient to the regimen; problems with adherence; symptoms suggestive of the development of complications; other medical illnesses and current medications.

d. Every regular visit: measure weight, blood pressure and blood sugar, and examination of the feet.

e. Laboratory studies. See Table 12-4.

4. Perform casual funduscopic, peripheral vascular and neurologic examination every year.

VIII. Complications

A. Hyperglycemia with glycosuria:

1. Diabetic ketoacidosis.

2. Hyperosmolar hyperglycemic non-ketotic states.

B. Hypoglycemia.

C. Recurrent difficult-to-treat infections.

D. Premature cardiovascular, cerebrovascular and peripheral vascular disease.

TABLE 12-4
SCHEDULE OF LABORATORY STUDIES

TEST	FREQUENCY
Glycosylated Hgb	
Patients on:	
Diet and oral agents	Q6 months
Insulin treated	Q3 months
Poor control	Q3 months
Lipid profiles	Yearly
Routine urinalysis	Yearly
Microalbumnuria Test*	Yearly
If proteinuria detected:	
BUN and creatinine	Yearly
ECG	Yearly

*IDDM after 5 years of disease
*NIDDM at diagnosis and yearly

    E. Diabetic retinopathy, premature cataracts, and glaucoma.

    F. Diabetic nephropathy and renal failure.

IX. Consultation–Referral

    A. All new diabetes.

    B. Blood glucose values greater than 400 mg per 100 mL.

    C. Moderate to large urine ketones.

    D. To ophthalmologist: ages 12 to 30 years after 5 years of IDDM; at time of diagnosis for patients over age 30 (NIDDM), or any patient with visual symptoms and/or abnormalities.

X. Follow-Up

See **VII.7.**

▲ GOUT AND HYPERURICEMIA: ADULT

I. Definition

Gout is an inflammatory arthritis that results from a variety of problems (usually an inborn error of metabolism) that lead to hyperuricemia which may be associated with monosodium nitrate deposits (tophi) or uric acid kidney stones, or both. Hyperuricemia, which may be asymptomatic, is defined as a serum level of monosodium urate greater than the generally accepted limits (7.5 mg/dL for males, and 6.6 mg/dL for females) using colorimetric methods.

II. Etiology of hyperuricemia

    A. Gout from an inborn error of metabolism leading to overproduction or underexcretion of uric acid. Only 10%–20% of cases with clinically apparent gout give a family history of gout.

    B. Drugs, such as thiazide diuretics.

    C. Myeloproliferative diseases.

    D. Chronic renal disease.

    E. Obesity.

    F. Starvation.

III. Clinical Features

Although acute arthritis and kidney stones may appear with a normal uric acid, attacks are rare with uric acid less than 7.0 mg per dL and occur more frequently with increasing serum levels.

    A. **Hyperuricemia.** The patient is asymptomatic until arthritis or symptoms of kidney stones appear.

    B. **Acute gouty arthritis** (first appearance or recurrent attacks):

        1. **Symptoms**

            a. Painful, swollen joints.

      b. No systemic symptoms other than those from a moderately elevated temperature.

  2. Signs

      a. Red, hot, tender joint, with inflammation extending into the surrounding tissue.

      b. Most often, involvement of only one joint, with a strong predilection for the joints of the feet, ankles, wrists, and hands. Classically, gout appears in the big toe (podagra). More than one joint may be affected in 10%–15% of patients. Temperature may be elevated.

C. Chronic gout

  1. Symptoms. Patient is asymptomatic between attacks of acute gout, 50% will have a recurrence within one year.

  2. Signs

      a. An elevated serum uric acid level (greater than 7.5 mg/dL) may be the only manifestation. With treatment, the uric acid level may fall to normal.

      b. Uric acid deposits (tophi) are found in only a small number of patients having an initial clinical attack of gout. Thereafter, with recurrence, the incidence of tophi increases. Tophi characteristically are found in and around joints, bursae, and subcutaneous tissue, especially around the olecranon bursa, the joints of the hand and foot, and the helix and anthelix of the ear.

      c. Uric acid kidney stones appear in about 20%–30% of gouty patients.

IV. Laboratory Studies

  A. Acute gout

    1. The serum uric acid may be greater than 7.0 mg per dL.

    2. Examination of joint fluid obtained by needle aspiration reveals urate crystals.

    3. White blood cell count usually is greater than $10,000/mm^3$.

    4. Erythrocyte sedimentation rate may be elevated.

  B. Chronic gout

    1. Serum uric acid level may be below normal, normal or elevated.

    2. Erythrocyte sedimentation rate is normal.

    3. White blood cell count is normal.

V. Differential Diagnosis

  A. Acute inflammatory monarthritis.

Note: Although a prescriptive diagnosis of gout may be made for patients with monarticular inflammatory arthritis with elevated uric acid, in almost all new cases of arthritis, the joint should be aspirated and the synovial fluid examined for bacteria and crystals.

1. Rheumatoid arthritis.
2. Pyogenic arthritis.
3. Pseudogout (chondrocalcinosis secondary to deposits of calcium pyrophosphate).
4. Reiter's disease.
5. Sarcoidosis.

B. Chronic recurrent arthritis (degenerative arthritis).

VI. Treatment

A. Description of drugs. Several drugs used in the treatment of gout have specific but different effects and must be used accordingly.

1. **Probenecid** (Benemid) blocks the reabsorption of uric acid by the proximal renal tubule. Probenecid, by causing increased excretion of uric acid, lowers the serum uric acid level. This drug is not of benefit in acute gout but is used in maintenance of normal uric acid levels.

2. **Allopurinol** (Zyloprim) blocks the production of uric acid and thus decreases the serum uric acid level. This drug is used in maintenance therapy and is contraindicated in acute gout.

3. **Colchicine** has been used for many years for acute attacks of gouty arthritis. Colchicine's specific effect in terminating an acute attack of gout has diagnostic significance. It is rarely used in maintenance therapy except in patients with chronic gout who have frequent acute attacks. In this situation colchicine may reduce the frequency and severity of attacks.

4. **Indomethacin** (Indocin) is a nonsteroidal antiinflammatory drug that frequently provides relief in acute gout. Other nonsteroidal anti-inflammatory drugs such as Motrin and Naprosyn have been used successfully.

B. Acute gout

1. Colchicine, 1.0–1.2 mg initially, then 0.5–0.6 mg every hour until symptoms are relieved or diarrhea, nausea, or vomiting begins. No more than 6 mg should be given for any one attack over a 72-hour period. Pain relief usually occurs within 6–12 hours and is complete within 48–72 hours. Unfortunately GI side effects occur in more than 50% of patients.

   or

2. Indomethacin, 50 mg 3 times a day for 2–3 days, tapering to 25 mg 4 times a day for a period of 1 week (may be continued 2–3 weeks). Side effects: gastrointestinal disturbances, headaches, rashes, and leukopenia have been reported. Other nonsteroidals may be substituted.

or

3. Rest and elevation of and cold applications to the affected joint are sometimes beneficial. Low-dose salicylates (1–2 gm per day) should be avoided.

4. Maintenance therapy with probenecid or allopurinol should not be given routinely following a first or even second attack of gout, because acute flares may be years apart. For patients with uric acid that is only mildly elevated (7.5–10 mg/dL), withhold allopurinol or probenecid until a pattern of increasing frequency is established.

C. **Chronic gout**

1. Known recurrent gout requires maintenance therapy with either:

   a. Probenecid, 250 mg twice a day for 1 week, then 500 mg twice a day thereafter.

   or

   b. Allopurinol, 100 mg a day for 1 week, then raise by 100 mg a day at weekly intervals until an average maintenance dose of 300 mg a day is reached.

   c. Which of these drugs to use depends upon the defect causing hyperuricemia. If a patient is excreting too much uric acid (as determined by a 24 hour urine uric acid collection), allopurinol is the drug of choice. Allopurinol is also preferred in patients with severe tophaceous gout, renal calculi, a history of renal calculi, or reduced renal function. In most other cases, however, probenecid is preferred because of the serious adverse reactions that may occur with allopurinol. For either drug, the goal of therapy is to lower the serum urate concentration to less than 7 mg/dL.

   d. The initial dose of either drug should be lower than maintenance dosage, because initiation of therapy may precipitate arthritis. To prevent acute attacks, colchicine, 0.5–0.6 mg 2–4 times a day, may be started several weeks before induction of therapy and continued for several weeks.

D. **Hyperuricemia.** Associated with no symptom of arthritis, tophi, or kidney stones.

1. Less than 10 mg/100 mL—no therapy.

2. Greater than 10 mg/100 mL on two successive occasions—physician consultation. Although there is a slight increased risk of renal stones or gouty arthritis, many physicians may elect not to treat those patients until symptoms occur.

VII. **Complications**

A. Recurrent acute attacks can lead to chronic joint disability.

    B. Untreated elevated serum uric acid level can result in:

       1. Acute gout.

       2. Renal stones with secondary infections or renal colic, or both.

       3. Tophaceous deposits in skin, joints, connective tissue.

VIII. Consultation–Referral

    A. New patient with acute gouty arthritis.

    B. Patient known to have gouty arthritis who has frequent attacks.

    C. Acute attack that persists beyond 72 hours.

    D. Serum uric acid greater than 10 mg/dL.

IX. Follow-Up

    A. Chronic gout. In asymptomatic chronic gout, uric acid levels need to be checked only yearly.

    B. Acute gout. The patient should be contacted or seen in 24 hours. A new patient should return in 4 weeks to discuss maintenance therapy.

▲ HYPOTHYROIDISM—
MAINTENANCE OF DIAGNOSED DISEASE: ADULT

I. Definition

Decreased function of the thyroid gland, causing reduced production of thyroid hormone and leading to progressive slowing of all bodily functions.

II. Etiology

Hypothyroidism is caused by thyroid failure due to a number of mechanisms:

    A. Treatment of hyperthyroidism (radioiodine, surgery, propylthiouracil.

    B. Following thyroiditis (primarily Hashimoto's thyroiditis).

    C. Idiopathic thyroid failure.

    D. Congenital defects in thyroid metabolism.

    E. Rarely, iodine insufficiency.

    F. Rarely, secondary hypothyroidism from pituitary or hypothalamic dysfunction.

III. Clinical Features

The adequately treated patient should be euthyroid, without signs of hypothyroidism or hyperthyroidism:

    A. Hypothyroidism (secondary to inadequate treatment).

       1. Symptoms

          a. Decreased energy, lethargy.

   b. Cold intolerance.

   c. Constipation.

   d. Menorrhagia.

   e. Sometimes, slight weight gain late in the disease.

   2. Signs

   a. Dry hair, which may fall out.

   b. Dry, rough skin.

   c. Hoarseness.

   d. Periorbital edema, dull expression.

   e. Slow Achilles tendon reflex (return phase).

   B. Hyperthyroidism

   1. Symptoms

   a. Nervousness.

   b. Heat intolerance.

   c. Weight loss.

   d. Increased appetite.

   e. Increased sweating.

   f. Emotional instability.

   2. Signs

   a. Sweating; moist skin.

   b. Tachycardia.

   c. Arrhythmia (primarily in the older age group).

   d. Fine tremor of fingers (cat's purr) and tongue.

   e. Lid lag.

IV. Laboratory Studies

   The TSH has replaced other thyroid tests. The TSH should be maintained in the normal range.

V. Differential Diagnosis

   If laboratory data do not reveal any evidence of thyroid dysfunction, one must find other causes of the symptoms and clinical findings.

VI. Treatment

   A. Continue replacement therapy, adjusting according to clinical response and laboratory findings.

   B. Usual doses of thyroid replacement:

   Sodium levothyroxine (Synthroid) 0.1–0.3 mg orally every day. Elderly patients may be managed on .075 mg of levothyroxine.

VII. Complications

   A. Hypothyroidism.

   B. Hyperthyroidism.

VIII. Consultation–Referral

Development of hyperthyroid signs and symptoms.

IX. Follow-Up

Laboratory tests of thyroid function approximately once a year, or when patient's condition changes.

▲ MULTINODULAR GOITER: ADULT

I. Definition

Enlargement of the thyroid, in which more than one nodule is identifiable; occurs in females 10–20 times more frequently than in males.

II. Etiology

Unknown. An inborn metabolic block may be responsible. In the United States today this disorder is very rarely secondary to iodine deficiency.

III. Clinical Features

A. Symptoms

1. Usually asymptomatic.

2. Symptoms of tracheal compression (stridor, difficult breathing) may develop if enlargement is great.

B. Signs

1. Visible enlargement of thyroid gland.

2. Palpable enlarged thyroid gland with more than one nodule.

3. Enlarged thyroid is nontender and nonpulsatile.

IV. Laboratory Studies

Usually, results of thyroid studies are normal, except in the rare case of hyperthyroid goiter. Obtain serum thyroxine (T_4) and serum triiodothyronine (T_3) uptake, and TSH.

V. Differential Diagnosis

A. Solitary thyroid nodule.

B. Hashimoto's thyroiditis.

VI. Treatment

A. If the patient is euthyroid, treatment is not indicated unless the gland is cosmetically disfiguring or causing obstruction. In these cases exogenous thyroid may be used for suppressing the pituitary production of thyroid-stimulating hormone (TSH), thus reducing the size of the thyroid gland. Consult physician for dose.

B. Significant compression may require surgery.

VII. Complications

A. Hyperthyroidism.

    B. Tracheal obstruction.

VIII. Consultation–Referral

    A. Obstructive symptoms.

    B. Hyperthyroidism.

    C. Solitary nodule.

    D. Goiter in males, especially young males.

    E. A tender thyroid gland.

    F. For initiation of exogenous thyroid.

IX. Follow-Up

    A. Every 6 months if gland is medically treated.

    B. Every year if untreated.

13

▼

DISORDERS OF THE HEMATOPOIETIC SYSTEM

▲

▲ IRON DEFICIENCY ANEMIA: PEDIATRIC

I. Definition

A. **Anemia** in general may be defined on the basis of a lowered hematocrit reading.

AGE	HEMATOCRIT (%)
3–6 months	<30
6 months—6 years	<33
6–14 years	<35
Over 14 years	
Female	<36
Male	<40

B. **Iron deficiency anemia** is a form of anemia resulting from an inadequate supply of iron for synthesis of hemoglobin.

Patient Care Guidelines for Nurse Practitioners, 4th ed. by Axalla J. Hoole, C. Glenn Pickard, Jr., Ruth M. Ouimette, Jacob A. Lohr, and Robert A. Greenberg. Copyright © 1995 by J. B. Lippincott Company.

II. Etiology

More than one of the following factors may be causative in an individual patient.

A. Inadequate supply of iron at birth due to:

   1. Prematurity.

   2. Fetal or perinatal blood loss without replacement.

B. Inadequate dietary iron.

C. Excessive demands for iron associated with growth:

   1. Prematurely born infant.

   2. Adolescent.

D. Blood loss without replacement:

   1. Blood loss may be obvious.

   2. The most common occult source of blood loss is the gastrointestinal tract.

III. Clinical Features

A. History. One or more of the following factors may be relevant:

   1. Premature birth without supplemental iron or iron-fortified milk during first year of life. Such an infant will often be anemic by age 9 months on an average diet.

   2. Iron-deficient diet. When milk not fortified with iron accounts for a large proportion of an infant's caloric intake, the overall diet will probably be poor in iron because of the low iron content of milk. Anemia from this cause is most common between 9 and 24 months of age. During the adolescent growth period, the incidence of iron deficiency anemia from an iron-deficient diet increases again, especially in females.

   3. Large intake of whole cow's milk during first two years of life. This may be associated with gastrointestinal blood loss as well as a diet poor in iron.

   4. Blood loss without replacement.

B. Symptoms

   1. Mild iron deficiency anemia (hematocrit reading 25%–33%):

      a. This condition is usually asymptomatic and discovered during routine health-maintenance screening.

      b. Results of some studies have suggested that decreased attention span may be associated with iron deficiency even before anemia develops.

   2. More severe iron deficiency anemia (hematocrit reading <25%)

      a. Pallor.

      b. Lethargy.

      c. Irritability.

      d. Anorexia.

      e. Occasionally, poor weight gain.

  C. Signs

      1. Mild iron deficiency anemia—normal physical examination.

      2. More severe iron deficiency anemia:

        a. Pallor.

        b. Occasional findings:

          (1) Poor weight gain.

          (2) Splenomegaly.

          (3) Systolic flow murmurs.

IV. Laboratory Studies

  A. Hematocrit. An abnormal value requires a repeat determination.

  B. Smear of the red blood cells for morphology. If anemia is more than mild, the red blood cells are hypochromic and microcytic, with some variety of size and shape.

V. Differential Diagnosis

  A. Anemia in general

      1. Acute or chronic hemorrhage.

      2. Excessive red blood cell destruction, as in hemolytic anemia such as sickle cell anemia and other hereditary anemia.

      3. Decreased or impaired production of red blood cells, as in iron deficiency anemia, chronic infection, renal failure, and leukemia.

  B. Iron deficiency anemia. One should try to establish why the patient is iron deficient (see **II** and **III.A**).

VI. Treatment

  A. Indications for treatment without consultation. Treatment for iron deficiency anemia may be started without consultation and before results of red blood cell smear are known if *all* the following circumstances apply:

      1. Hematocrit reading greater than 24% but less than normal.

      2. Patient more than 10 months of age.

      3. No history of a normal hematocrit or hemoglobin value in the past.

      4. No history of unexplained blood loss (e.g., red blood in stools or tarry stools).

      5. No history in siblings of anemia due to a cause other than iron deficiency.

      6. No abnormality on physical examination not explained by an unrelated diagnosis.

TABLE 13-1

ORAL DOSAGE OF FERROUS SULFATE (FER-IN-SOL) (15 MG ELEMENTAL IRON PER 0.6 ML) FOR *TREATMENT* OF IRON DEFICIENCY ANEMIA

DRUG FORM	BODY WEIGHT	DOSE	FREQUENCY
Ferrous sulfate drops (15 mg elemental iron per 0.6 mL)	8–10 kg (18–22 lb) 10–12 kg (22–26 lb)	0.6 mL* 0.9 mL*	3 times a day after meals for 2 mos
or			
Ferrous sulfate syrup (6 mg elemental iron per mL)	12–16 kg (26–35 lb) 16–22 kg (35-48 lb) 22–30 kg (48–66 lb)	5.0 mL 7.5 mL 10.0 mL	3 times a day after meals for 2 mos
or			
Ferrous sulfate tablets (60 mg elemental iron per tablet)	Over 30 kg (over 66 lb)	1 tablet	3 times a day after meals for 2 mos

*May be given in water, fruit juice, or vegetable juice.

B. **Therapeutic measures**
1. Discontinue whole cow's milk in infant under 18 months, substituting evaporated milk formula or commercial infant formula.
2. Decrease total milk intake to no more than 16 oz a day; increase other foods, especially those with high iron content, such as iron-fortified bran or whole cereals, dried fruit (raisins, prunes, peaches, apricots), beans (red kidney, pinto, lima, navy, soy), nuts, beef, and pork.
3. Start iron therapy, 6–7 mg/kg of body weight (3 mg/lb) of elemental iron per day in 3 divided doses for 2 months (see Table 13-1).

C. **Prevention**
1. Full-term infant:
   a. Breast milk.
   or
   b. Iron-fortified milk until age 18 months.
   or
   c. Medicinal iron supplement from 3–18 months of age (see Table 13-2 for dosage) unless baby consumes a solid diet with high iron content (see **VI.B.2**).
   d. Intake of iron-containing foods, e.g., iron-fortified cereal.
2. Premature infant
   a. Iron-fortified milk until age 18 months.

TABLE 13-2

ORAL PEDIATRIC DOSAGE OF FERROUS SULFATE DROPS (FER-IN-SOL) (15 MG ELEMENTAL IRON PER 0.6 ML) FOR *PREVENTION* OF IRON DEFICIENCY ANEMIA

BODY WEIGHT	DOSE*	FREQUENCY
4–7 kg (9–15 lb)	0.3 mL	Once a day
Over 7 kg (over 15 lb)	0.6 mL	Once a day until age 18 mos

*May be given in water, fruit juice or vegetable juice.

or

  b. Medicinal iron supplement from 2–18 months of age—ferrous sulfate drops (Fer-In-Sol) (containing 15 mg elemental iron per 0.6 mL) in a dosage of 0.6 mL once a day in water or fruit juice.

  or

  c. Breast milk and supplemental iron (see **VI.C.2.b**).

  d. Intake of iron-containing foods, e.g., iron-fortified infant cereal.

VII. Complications

  A. Progressive anemia, with increasing symptoms.

  B. Accidental ingestion of medicinal iron, especially capsules, resulting in fatal iron intoxication. Remind parents that, like all medications, it should be locked away from young children.

VIII. Consultation–Referral

  A. Hematocrit reading <25%.

  B. Patient less than 10 months of age.

  C. History of a normal hematocrit or hemoglobin in the past.

  D. History of unexplained blood loss (e.g., red blood in stools or tarry stools).

  E. History in siblings of anemia due to a cause other than iron deficiency.

  F. Abnormality on physical examination not explained by an unrelated diagnosis.

  G. Abnormal red blood cell morphology.

  H. Failure of hematocrit to return to normal in 1 month despite iron therapy.

IX. Follow-Up

  A. Clinic visit after 1 month of iron therapy:

   1. Determination of hematocrit reading (should be normal).

   2. Review of diet and further counseling as needed.

B. Clinic visit after 2 months of iron therapy.

1. Determination of hematocrit reading (should remain at or above 1-month level).

2. Review of diet and further counseling as needed.

C. Clinic visit 9 months after discontinuing iron therapy:

1. Determination of hematocrit reading (should remain normal).

2. Review of diet and further counseling as needed.

▲ IRON DEFICIENCY ANEMIA: MENSTRUATING FEMALE

I. Definition

Hematocrit reading <38% in menstruating females. The anemia is secondary to chronic iron loss and may be aggravated by intake of a diet that is low in iron as a result of food fadism or socioeconomic restrictions.

II. Etiology

See **I.**

III. Clinical Features

A. **Symptoms**

1. There may be none. Anemia may be discovered on routine blood examination.

2. Fatigue, weakness, headache, dizziness, and other nonspecific generalized complaints may be present, but these symptoms rarely appear with hemoglobin levels of greater than 10 gm/dL, unless related to another problem.

3. Heavy menstrual periods.

B. **Signs**

1. Often, there are none.

2. Pallor of skin and conjunctiva.

3. Fissure of lips.

4. Brittle nails.

IV. Laboratory Studies

A. **Studies required before treatment**

1. Complete blood count, which includes:

    a. Hematocrit.

    b. White blood cell count.

    c. White blood cell differential.

    d. Red cell indices.

    e. Red cell morphology.

2. Stool for occult blood.

    B. Optional studies:

        1. Serum iron and serum iron-binding capacity.

        2. Reticulocyte count

    C. Characteristic findings in iron deficiency anemia

        1. Hematocrit <38%.

        2. Normal white blood cell count.

        3. Normal white blood cell differential.

        4. Mean corpuscular volume <83 u^3; mean corpuscular hemoglobin <27 pg (microcytic, hypochromic RBCs).

        5. Red cells on peripheral smear are characteristically small (microcytic) and contain less hemoglobin (hypochromic).

        6. Low serum iron; high serum iron-binding capacity.

V. Differential Diagnosis

    A. Iron deficiency anemia secondary to menstruation must be differentiated from other causes of iron loss, which frequently are due to bleeding from the gastrointestinal tract. For this reason, results of stool test for occult blood must be negative.

    B. Anemia secondary to ineffective production:

        1. Bone marrow depression from drugs, infections, lead poisoning.

        2. Defective hemoglobin (e.g., sickle cell).

        3. Vitamin deficiency (B_{12}, folic acid).

        4. Chronic disease.

    C. Anemia from hemolysis.

VI. Treatment

Ferrous sulfate, 300 mg orally 3 times a day for 3 months.

VII. Complications

Rare.

VIII. Consultation–Referral

    A. Menstruating female with hematocrit reading <30%.

    B. Menstruating female with positive stool test for occult blood.

    C. Patients in whom serum iron or red blood cell indices, or both, do not fit iron deficiency anemia.

    D. All other cases of anemia.

    E. Failure to improve after 1 month of treatment.

IX. Follow-Up

Repeat hematocrit determination in 1 month.

14

OBSTETRICS AND GYNECOLOGY

▲ GUIDELINES FOR MANAGING THE OBSTETRIC PATIENT

I. Prenatal Care

All data should be recorded on the prenatal record (Figure 14-1).

A. The first visit

1. **Examination.** The first examination should be done by the family nurse practitioner (FNP), preferably shortly after the first missed period, unless the patient is having trouble, such as severe nausea, vomiting, pain, or bleeding.

   a. A complete history and physical examination should be performed.

      (1) History should include questions for genetic screening:

         (a) Eastern European Jewish origin—Tay-Sachs disease.

         (b) African-American ancestry—sickle cell disease.

         (c) Italian or Greek ancestry—thalassemia.

Patient Care Guidelines for Nurse Practitioners, 4th ed. by Axalla J. Hoole, C. Glenn Pickard, Jr., Ruth M. Ouimette, Jacob A. Lohr, and Robert A. Greenberg. Copyright © 1995 by J. B. Lippincott Company.

FIGURE 14.1

ACOG ANTEPARTUM RECORD

DATE _____

NAME _____

LAST   FIRST   MIDDLE

ID# _____ HOSPITAL OF DELIVERY _____ FINAL EDD _____

NEWBORN'S PHYSICIAN _____ REFERRED BY _____

BIRTH DATE	AGE	RACE	MARITAL STATUS	ADDRESS	
Mo Day Yr			S M W D Sep	Zip	Phone (H)	(O)

OCCUPATION   EDUCATION   Insurance Carrier/Medicaid#
☐ Homemaker   (Last Grade Completed)
☐ Outside Work _____

Type of Work _____

☐ Student

EMERGENCY CONTACT _____ RELATIONSHIP _____ PHONE _____

Total Preg	Full Term	Premature	Abortions Induced	Abortions Spontaneous	Ectopics	Multiple Births	Living

MENSTRUAL HISTORY

LMP ☐ Definite ☐ Approximate (month known)   MENSES MONTHLY ☐ Yes ☐ No   FREQUENCY: Q ___ days   MENARCHE ___ (age onset)

☐ Unknown ☐ Normal Amount/Duration   PRIOR MENSES ___ Date   On BCP's at Concept ☐ Yes ☐ No   hCG+ __/__/__

304

PAST PREGNANCIES (LAST SIX)

Date Mo/Yr	GA Weeks	Length of Labor	Birth Weight	Type Delivery	Anes	Place of Delivery	Perinatal Mortality Yes/No	Treatment Preterm Labor Yes/No	Comments/ Complications

PAST MEDICAL HISTORY

	O Neg + Pos	Detail Positive Remarks Include Date & Treatment		O Neg + Pos	Detail Positive Remarks Include Date & Treatment
1. Diabetes			15. Alcohol		
2. Hypertension			16. Rh Sensitized		
3. Heart Disease			17. Tuberculosis		
4. Rheumatic Fever			18. Asthma		
5. Mitral Valve Prolapse			19. Allergies (Drugs)		
6. Kidney Disease/UTI			20. Gyn Surgery		
7. Neurologic/Epilepsy			21. Operations/Hospitalizations (Year & Reason)		
8. Psychiatric			22. Anesthetic Complications		
9. Hepatitis/Liver Disease			23. History of Abnormal Pap		
10. Varicosities/Phlebitis			24. Uterine Anomaly		
11. Thyroid Dysfunction			25. Infertility		
12. Major Accidents			26. In Utero DES Exposure		
13. History of Blood Transfus.			27. Street Drugs		
	Amt/Day Prepreg	Amt/Day Preg	#Yrs Use	28. Other	
14. Tobacco					

COMMENTS: _____

(cont'd)

ACOG ANTEPARTUM RECORD (CONT'D.)

GENETICS SCREENING

INCLUDES PATIENT, BABY'S FATHER, OR ANYONE IN EITHER FAMILY WITH:

	YES	NO			YES	NO
1. Patient's Age ≥ 35 years				10. Huntington Chorea		
2. Thallassemia (Italian, Greek, Mediterranean, or Oriental Background) MCV < 80				11. Mental Retardation If Yes, Was Person Tested for Fragile X?		
3. Neural Tube Defect (Meningomyelcele, Open Spine, or Anencephaly)				12. Other Inherited Genetic or Chromosomal Disorder		
4. Down Syndrome				13. Patient or Baby's Father Had a Child with Birth Defects Not Listed Above		
5. Tay-Sachs (eg, Jewish Background)				14. ≥3 First Trimester Spontaneous Abortions or a Stillbirth		
6. Sickle Cell Disease or Trait				15. Medications or Street Drugs Since Last Menstrual Period		
7. Hemophilia				If Yes, Agent(s)		
8. Muscular Dystrophy				16. other significant family history (see comments)		
9. Cystic Fibrosis						

COMMENTS: _____

INFECTION HISTORY

	YES	NO			YES	NO
1. High Risk AIDS				4. Patient or Partner Have History of Genital Herpes		
2. High Risk Hepatitis B				5. Rash or Illness Since Last Menstrual Period		
3. Live with Someone with TB or Exposed to TB				6. History of STD. GC. Chlamydia. HPV. Syphilis		
				7. Other (See Comments)		

COMMENTS: _____

_____ INTERVIEWER'S SIGNATURE _____

INITIAL PHYSICAL EXAMINATION

Date _____ / _____ / _____   Height _____   BP _____

Prepregnancy Weight _____

1. Heent	☐ Normal	☐ Abnormal		
2. Fundi	☐ Normal	☐ Abnormal		
3. Teeth	☐ Normal	☐ Abnormal		
4. Thyroid	☐ Normal	☐ Abnormal		
5. Breasts	☐ Normal	☐ Abnormal		
6. Lungs	☐ Normal	☐ Abnormal		
7. Heart	☐ Normal	☐ Abnormal		
8. Abdomen	☐ Normal	☐ Abnormal		
9. Extremities	☐ Normal	☐ Abnormal		
10. Skin	☐ Normal	☐ Abnormal		
11. Lymph Nodes	☐ Normal	☐ Abnormal		

12. Vulva	☐ Normal	☐ Condyloma	☐ Lesions
13. Vagina	☐ Normal	☐ Inflammation	☐ Discharge
14. Cervix	☐ Normal	☐ Inflammation	☐ Lesions
15. Uterus	☐ Normal	☐ Abnormal	☐ Fibroids
16. Adnexa	☐ Normal	☐ Mass	
17. Rectum	☐ Normal	☐ Abnormal	
18. Diagonal Conjugate	☐ Reached	☐ No	_____ CM
19. Spines	☐ Average	☐ Prominent	☐ Blunt
20. Sacrum	☐ Concave	☐ Straight	☐ Anterior
21. Arch	☐ Normal	☐ Wide	☐ Narrow
22. Gynecoid Pelvic Type	☐ Yes	☐ No	

COMMENTS (Number and explain abnormls): _____

_____

_____

EXAM BY _____

(cont'd)

ACOG ANTEPARTUM RECORD (CONT'D.)

INITIAL LABS	DATE	RESULT	REVIEWED	COMMENTS/ADDITIONAL LAB
Blood Type	/ /	A B AB O		
Rh Type	/ /			
Antibody Screen	/ /			
HCT/HGB	/ /	____ % ____ g/dl		
Pap Smear	/ /	Normal / Abnormal / ____		
Rubella	/ /			
VDRL	/ /			
GC	/ /			
Urine Culture/Screen	/ /			
HBsAg	/ /			

8–18 WEEK LABS (WHEN INDICATED)	DATE	RESULT		
Ultrasound	/ /			
MSAFP	/ /	____ MOM		
AMNIO/CVS	/ /			
Karyotype	/ /	46. xx or 46. xy / Other ____		
Alpha-Fetoprotein	/ /	Normal ____ Abnormal ____		

24–28 WEEK LABS
(WHEN INDICATED)

	DATE	RESULT	REVIEWED	COMMENTS/ADDITIONAL LAB
HCT/HGB	/ /	_____ % _____ g/dl		
Diabetes Screen	/ /	1 Hr. _____		
GTT (If Screen Abnormal)	/ /	FBS _____ 1 Hr. _____ _____ 2 Hr. _____ 3 Hr.		
Rh Antibody Screen	/ /			
Rhig Given (28 weeks)	/ /	Signature _____		

32–36 WEEK LABS
(WHEN INDICATED)

	DATE	RESULT	REVIEWED	
Ultrasound	/ /			
VDRL	/ /			
GC	/ /			
HCT/HGB	/ /	_____ % _____ g/dl		

OPTIONAL LABS
(HIGH RISK GROUPS)

	DATE	RESULT	REVIEWED	
HIV	/ /			
HGB Electrophoresis	/ /	AA AS SS AC SC AF TA₂		
Chlamydia	/ /			
Other	/ /			

(cont'd)

ACOG ANTEPARTUM RECORD (CONT'D.)

PLANS/EDUCATION   (Counseled ☐)

☐ Anesthesia Plans _____

☐ Toxoplasmosis Precautions (Cats/Raw Meat) _____

☐ Childbirth Classes _____

☐ Physical Activity _____

☐ Premature Labor Signs _____

☐ Nutrition Counseling _____

☐ Breast or Bottle Feeding _____

☐ Newborn Car Seat _____

☐ Postpartum Birth Control _____

☐ Environmental/Work Hazards _____

☐ Tubal Sterilization _____

☐ VBAC Counseling _____

☐ Circumcision _____

☐ Travel _____

REQUESTS _____

_____

_____

TUBAL STERILIZATION	**DATE**	**INITIALS**
Consent signed	___/___/___	___

AA128   1   / 2

NAME _____

LAST _____ FIRST _____ MIDDLE _____

DRUG ALLERGY: _____

ANESTHESIA CONSULT PLANNED   ☐ YES   ☐ NO

PROBLEMS/PLANS

1. _____
2. _____
3. _____
4. _____

MEDICATION LIST:

	Start date	Stop date
1.		
2.		
3.		
4.		

EDD CONFIRMATION

Initial EDD:

LMP ___/___/___ = ___/___/___ = EDD ___/___/___

Initial Exam ___/___/___ = _____ wks = EDD ___/___/___

Ultrasound ___/___/___ = _____ wks = EDD ___/___/___

Initial EDD ___/___/___ initialed by _____

18–20-WEEK EDD UPDATE:

Quickening ___/___/___ + 22 wks = ___/___/___

Fundal HT at umbil. ___/___/___ + 20 wks = ___/___/___

FHT w/fetoscope ___/___/___ + 20 wks = ___/___/___

Ultrasound ___/___/___ = ___ wks = ___/___/___

Final EDD ___/___/___ initialed by _____

(cont'd)

▶ 311 ◀

ACOG ANTEPARTUM RECORD (CONT'D.)

32–34-WEEK EDD–UTERINE SIZE CONCORDANCE (±4 OR MORE CM SUGGESTS THE NEED FOR ULTRASOUND EVALUATION)

VISIT DATE (YEAR _____)													
Weeks gest. (best est.)													
Fundal height (cm)													
FHR present F = fetoscope D= doptone													
Fetal movement (+ = present; 0 = absent)													
Prematurity: Signs/symptoms* (+ = present; 0 = absent)													
Cervix exam (DIL./EFF./STA.)													
Blood pressure initial													
repeat													
Edema (+ = present; 0 = absent)													
Weight (prepreg: _____)													
Cumulative weight gain													
Urine (glucose albumin/ketones)													
Next appointment													
Provider (initials)													
Test reminders CVS/AMNIO/MSAFP	8–18 weeks GLUCOSE SCREEN/Rhig						24–28 weels						

COMMENTS: _____

*For example: vaginal bleeding, discharge, cramps, contractions, pelvic pressure.

Copyright © 1989 Revised November 1991. The American College of Obstetricians and Gynecologists, 409 12th Street SW, Washington DC 20024-2188

    (d) Family history of spina bifida, hydrocephalus, anencephaly.

    (e) History of muscular dystrophy.

    (f) History of Down syndrome—how old will the patient be when the baby is born?

    (g) Bleeding problems or mental retardation in the family.

  b. The pelvic examination should include obtaining a Papanicolaou (Pap) smear and culture of the cervix for *Neisseria gonorrhoeae*, Chlamydia, and Group B streptococcus.

  c. The initial laboratory work for the pregnant patient should include the following studies:

    (1) Serological test for syphilis.

    (2) Blood type and Rh factor.

    (3) Antibody screening for Rh antibody.

    (4) Rubella titer.

    (5) Hematocrit.

    (6) Urinalysis and urine culture.

    (7) Tuberculin skin test.

    (8) Pap smear.

    (9) Sickle cell preparation in African-American patients.

    (10) Cervical culture for *N. gonorrhoeae*, Chlamydia, and Group B streptococcus in high-risk populations.

    (11) Hepatitis BsAg, BsAb

    (12) (HIV screening may be offered.)

2. Medications

  a. A routine prenatal vitamin with folic acid (0.8–1.0 mg) should be started at this time.

  b. Ferrous sulfate, 325 mg orally twice a day, should also be started if the hematocrit reading is below 36%.

3. Patient instruction

  a. The FNP should instruct the patient about diet and personal hygiene.

  b. The patient should be told to report to the FNP any of these conditions:

    (1) Persistent vomiting.

    (2) Continuous or severe headaches.

    (3) Persistent or recurring abdominal pain or cramping.

    (4) Vaginal bleeding.

    (5) Dimness or blurring of vision.

(6) Chills or fever.

(7) Loss of fluid from vagina (not vaginal discharge, but a gush of watery-type fluid or a continuous loss of this fluid).

(8) Swelling of hands, feet, or face that becomes persistent.

(9) Urinary symptoms, such as dysuria or hematuria.

B. **The second visit**

1. The second visit is made 4 weeks later.

2. Examination is done together by the obstetrician and the FNP.

3. The obstetrician should confirm the diagnosis of pregnancy, measure the pelvis, and confirm the estimated date of confinement.

C. **Subsequent visits**

1. **Scheduling.** Unless some special instructions are given by the obstetrician, the subsequent prenatal examinations should be done by the FNP at these intervals:

a. Every 4 weeks until 28 weeks of gestation.

b. Every 2 weeks from 28 to 36 weeks of gestation.

c. Every week from 36 weeks until delivery.

2. **Routine studies**

a. Every routine prenatal examination should include:

(1) Questioning the patient about any present problems.

(2) Blood pressure.

(3) Urinalysis for protein, glucose, and albumin.

(4) Measurement of the uterine fundus.

(5) Auscultation of the fetal heart with fetoscope or doptone, or both.

(6) Determination of the position of the fetus, if possible.

(7) Physical examination for edema.

(8) Weighing the patient.

b. Hematocrit determination should be repeated at 28 and 36 weeks in each patient, and at the following visit if the patient's previous reading was below 36%.

c. Glucose screen for gestational diabetes should be done at 28–30 weeks or initial visit if history is positive for diabetes: 50 cc of glucola orally followed by a blood glucose in one hour. A plasma glucose value of >160 mg/dL requires a glucose tolerance test.

d. Serum alpha fetal protein (AFP) should be offered at 16 weeks gestation.

3. **Examination.** If possible, prenatal examinations should be done by the FNP on the same day the obstetrician is to be at

the clinic, but before he or she arrives, so that any problem case may be held over for review by the obstetrician.

4. **Assessment of Rh-negative patients.** At the initial prenatal screening examination, blood is drawn for blood type and Rh factor determination. All Rh-negative patients are to be handled as follows:

   a. Antibody titer is measured when the patient is discovered to be Rh negative.

   b. Rh antibody titer determination is repeated in Rh-negative patients at 26–28 weeks of gestation and RhoGAM given.

   c. Patients found to have a *positive* Rh antibody titer, initially should be referred to the obstetrician. Titer will be positive after RhoGAM is given.

   d. Patients who are Rh *negative* are treated as if they were *Rh positive* (That is, there is no need for antibody titer determination or use of RhoGAM.)

   e. If the newborn is Rh positive, human RhoD immune globulin (RhoGAM) is given immediately after delivery to all unsensitized Rh-negative women to protect them against being sensitized in future pregnancies.

5. **Management of miscellaneous complaints of pregnancy**

   a. **Constipation**

      (1) Advise patients that this common complaint of pregnancy may be minimized by maintaining adequate fluid intake and by promoting the softening of stools through dietary intake of fruits, juices (especially prune juice), and high-fiber foods (e.g., bran).

      (2) Persistent cases may be treated with any of these stool softeners and laxatives:

         (a) Dioctyl sodium sulfosuccinate (100 mg), 1 capsule twice a day as needed.

         (b) Psyllium hydrophilic mucilloid (Metamucil), 1 teaspoon by mouth 2 or 3 times a day as needed.

         (c) Milk of Magnesia, 30 cc (2 tablespoons) at bedtime as needed.

      (3) Constipation persisting for more than 10 days should be evaluated by the obstetrician.

   b. **Headaches**

      (1) Nonspecific occasional headaches may be treated with acetaminophen (325 mg tablets), 1 or 2 tablets every 4 hours as needed.

      (2) Persistent, recurrent, or migraine-like headaches should be evaluated by physician.

c. **Heartburn**

(1) This complaint is seen throughout pregnancy but may be especially prominent in the last trimester. It is due to esophageal reflux through the relaxed esophagogastric sphincter.

(2) Calcium carbonate (a mild antacid) is also a good source of calcium.

(3) Liquid antacids, 30 mL taken 30–60 minutes after meals and at bedtime as needed. May be more effective than tablets since they coat the esophagus and stomach more effectively.

(4) Elevation of the head with pillows may reduce night-time symptoms.

d. **Upper respiratory infections**

(1) The same diagnostic and etiologic considerations as for the nonpregnant patient (see Upper Respiratory Tract Infection: Common Cold, pp. 155–158) will apply.

(2) Antibiotics should be withheld until the results of the throat culture are known.

(3) Although the use of antihistamines and decongestants is not contraindicated in pregnancy, it is prudent to restrict their use to patients in whom local agents have failed to provide relief of symptoms.

(4) Nasal sprays and nose drops are more desirable as initial therapies, since their limited absorption is less likely to expose the fetus to higher doses of medications. The following agents are acceptable for use up to 10 days; oxymetazoline HCl (Afrin) *or* xylometazoline HCl (Otrivin), nasal spray or drops every 8–10 hours as needed.

e. **Anemia**

(1) Patients with hematocrits below 33% should have:

(a) Repeat hematocrit. If still below 33%, proceed with studies in **(b)**.

(b) Complete blood count, sickle cell preparation (in African-American patients), serum iron, reticulocyte count, and red cell indices. If these studies show iron deficiency, begin iron therapy (325 mg ferrous sulfate 3 times a day). If serum iron is normal, refer to obstetrician *and* order bilirubin (direct and indirect), urine culture, and Coombs' test.

(c) Test stool guaiac in all anemic patients.

D. **Consultation–Referral**

1. The FNP should consult with or refer the patient to the obstetrician if any of the following are noticed:
   a. No fetal heart tones are heard by 22 weeks.
   b. The patient feels no movement by 22 weeks or none for 1 week at any time after this.
   c. Blood pressure is above 140/90 mm Hg on two checks after bed rest.
   d. Patient has albuminuria or persistent edema.
   e. Patient has glycosuria.
   f. Patient has proteinuria.
   g. There is a lack of regular fetal growth.
   h. Late in pregnancy the FNP questions the position of the fetus (e.g., breech or transverse lie).
   i. At any time the FNP is in doubt about the patient's status.
   j. Hematocrit reading is below 33%.
   k. Symptoms of pyelonephritis.
   l. Significant condylotomy or herpes develop.
   m. Uterus size is 2 weeks greater or smaller than expected from estimated weeks of gestation.

2. *All* prenatal patients should again be reviewed with and examined by the obstetrician at 36 weeks.

E. **General instruction relative to labor and delivery.** At some time, preferably between 28 and 32 weeks, but certainly before 36 weeks, the FNP should discuss with each patient when to go to the hospital.

1. **Contractions**
   a. Primigravidas should usually wait until contractions are regular, at least 6–8 minutes apart, lasting more than 30 seconds, and increasing in intensity.
   b. Multigravida probably should wait until the contractions are regular and 10–15 minutes apart.
   c. Instructions to patients, especially multigravidas, should be individualized according to the distance they must travel or history of previous rapid labor.

2. **Rupture of the membranes.** Patients should go directly to the hospital when they think their membranes may have ruptured.

3. **Any active bleeding** (even without associated labor contractions). The patient should be instructed to go to the hospital. Discussion here should include differentiation of a small bloody mucus type of discharge from active bleeding. Explain to the patient that a bloody mucous discharge associated with contractions is a good sign that the contractions are true

instead of false. A bloody mucous discharge by itself *without any contractions* may occur in the latter part of the pregnancy without indicating the immediate onset of labor.

4. **Onset of active labor**

a. The patient should be instructed not to eat if she believes labor has started. She may drink clear fluids.

b. She should be directed to report to the obstetrician at the hospital, who will then perform a vaginal examination to determine whether active labor has started. In most cases this cannot be determined on the telephone by either the FNP or the physician. The decision whether the patient will be admitted in active labor or sent home if it is false labor will be made at the time of the examination.

5. The patient should understand the various types of anesthetics available and should discuss this subject with the FNP or obstetrician. Preference for breast- or bottle-feeding should also be discussed at this time. If there are any special questions about the foregoing, they may be discussed with the obstetrician when he or she sees the patient at 36 weeks.

II. Postpartum Period

A. **Family planning.** The FNP should discuss with the patient during pregnancy the type of birth control desired post partum:

1. **Oral contraceptives** may be started upon leaving the hospital. If they are not started then, the patient should telephone the FNP within the first 2 weeks after returning home to obtain the pills. If the patient is breast-feeding, OCPs may decrease milk production but are safe to take. However, a patient may want to delay taking OCPs for four weeks or more postpartum when breast feeding.

2. **Intrauterine contraceptive device.** Two IUDs are currently available, the Progestasert (a progesterone containing IUD) which is effective for 1 year and the Para Gard (a copper wound IUD which is effective for 8 years). Appropriate counseling should be done and the patient instructed to arrange for insertion at the postpartum visit or during her menses.

3. **Norplant and Depo-Provera.** Norplant is a continuous release progestin which is delivered by 6 subcutaneously placed Silastic rods and is effective for 5 years. Depo-Provera is a progestin which is given by injection every 3 months. Appropriate counseling is important for satisfaction with these methods.

4. **Postpartum tubal sterilization.** Candidates for sterilization should be informed about the procedure and then evaluated by the obstetrician before delivery. Consent papers should be signed more than 30 days before delivery and attached to the hospital record.

5. **Diaphragm/cervical cap.** Patient should return to the clinic at 6 weeks postpartum for fitting and instructions.

B. **Postpartum examinations**

1. All patients should be seen 4–6 weeks postpartum for a **general physical examination, including breast and pelvic examination, plus laboratory work, including hematocrit determination and urinalysis.** These examinations should be done by the obstetrician in association *with the FNP.*

2. **A Pap smear** should be done at this time if there is any question about the previous smear, or if for some reason a smear was not obtained during pregnancy.

▲ NAUSEA AND VOMITING DURING PREGNANCY

I. Definition

Nausea or vomiting, or both, occurring during the course of pregnancy, usually during the first trimester.

II. Etiology

Unknown. Nausea and vomiting probably are related to the hormonal changes occurring with pregnancy, with psychologic factors playing a secondary but important role.

III. Clinical Features

A. **Symptoms**

1. Nausea and vomiting, typically occurring early in the morning and then disappearing later in the day.

2. No abdominal pain or disturbance in bowel function.

B. **Signs**

1. No signs of dehydration.

2. Soft abdomen, with no tenderness. Normal bowel sounds.

IV. Laboratory Studies

None.

V. Differential Diagnosis

A. Hyperemesis gravidarum.

B. Viral gastroenteritis.

C. Multiple gestations.

D. Molar pregnancy (placenta tumor).

VI. Treatment

Advise patient on the following measures:

A. Frequent small feedings.

B. Avoid spicy and greasy foods.

C. Clear fluids.

Note: Pyridoxine (VIT B_6) 10 mg daily may be effective.

VII. Complications

Dehydration, ketosis.

VIII. Consultation–Referral

A. Nausea or vomiting occurring later than the twentieth week of pregnancy.

B. Dehydration, ketosis.

C. Persistence of nausea and vomiting that is annoying to patient even in the absence of dehydration.

IX. Follow-Up

A. Maintain daily contact for severe nausea and vomiting.

B. Maintain weekly or less frequent contact if problem is mild.

▲ CANDIDAL VAGINITIS: ADULT

I. Definition

An inflammatory process involving the vagina caused by a common skin fungus.

II. Etiology

Candida albicans. Infection often occurs in association with uncontrolled diabetes mellitus, pregnancy, antibiotic usage, and use of birth control pills.

III. Clinical Features

A. **Symptoms**

  1. Vaginal discharge.

  2. Commonly, intense vulval itching or burning, or both.

  3. No vaginal bleeding.

B. **Signs**

  1. Intense vulval inflammation is commonly found.

  2. Copious cheesy vaginal discharge.

  3. A cheesy discharge is often present in labial folds.

  4. Satellite lesions apart from the main area of inflammation may be found.

IV. Laboratory Studies

A. Potassium hydroxide preparation is positive for *Candida*.

B. Wet preparation is negative for *Trichomonas*.

C. Urine should be tested for glycosuria.

D. If there is a family history of diabetes or any symptoms suggestive of diabetes are present, or both, a blood glucose specimen is drawn 2 hours after eating.

V. Differential Diagnosis

  A. Other causes of vaginitis.

  B. Carcinoma of the vagina or cervix, or both.

VI. Treatment

  A. If candidal vaginitis occurs in a patient with diabetes mellitus, the diabetes must be controlled before it is possible to control or cure the vaginitis.

  B. Patient can use miconazole nitrate 2% (Monistat), *or* clotrimazole 1% (Gyne-Lotrimin, Mycelex-G) vaginal cream, or terconazole 0.4% (Terazol) cream. Use 1 applicator full intraregionally at bedtime for 7 days; or Monistat 3 Dual Pack—3 vaginal suppositories (insert 1 suppository intravaginally at night for three nights) and cream for use as needed; or butoconazole 2% (Femstat)—1 applicator full intravaginally at bedtime for 3 days.

  C. Cool compresses may be applied to irritated vulval lesions twice a day. Instruct patient to dry the skin thoroughly before using a compress.

VII. Complications

  None.

VIII. Consultation–Referral

  A. Refractory cases not responding to treatment in 2 weeks.

  B. Patient with coexisting uncontrolled or newly diagnosed diabetes.

IX. Follow-Up

  As needed.

◢ ABNORMAL PAPANICOLAOU SMEAR FINDINGS IN AN ASYMPTOMATIC PATIENT: ADULT

I. Definition

  A report on a cytologic examination of a cervical scraping taken from an *asymptomatic* patient that is read as abnormal, with abnormalities classified as follows:*

  A. Atypical Cells of Uncertain Significance (ASCUS).

  B. Low Grade Squamous Intraepithelial Lesion (LGSIL).

  C. High Grade Squamous Intraepithelial Lesion (HGSIL).

  D. Carcinoma.

II. Etiology

---

*Bethesda Classification.

A. Many factors may lead to abnormal findings on Papanicolaou or Pap smears, but **inflammation secondary to infections** is probably the most common cause.

B. The possibility of a **malignancy** must always be considered.

III. Clinical Features

Pap smears are most commonly done as a screening procedure, and usually no complaints are present.

IV. Purpose

Early detection of cervical carcinoma (rarely, endometrial carcinoma).

V. Frequency

See Table 1-3, p. 54, for frequency of routine Papanicolaou smears for detection of cervical cancer. A Papanicolaou smear should also be done if any of the following are present:

A. **Symptoms** or signs suggesting gynecologic disease: obtain Pap smears when pelvic examination is performed.

B. Sexual activity prior to age 18: obtain Pap smears on first visit.

C. History of abnormal Pap smears: perform as indicated by physician.

D. After hysterectomy:
1. If performed for benign disease such as fibroid uterus, Pap smear should be done every 3 years.
2. If hysterectomy was performed for dysplasia or carcinoma, Pap smear should be done as indicated by physician.

VI. Equipment

A. Dacron or saline-soaked cotton swab. The endocervical brush is not recommended during pregnancy.

B. Ayer's spatula (wood or plastic).

C. Glass side, labeled.

D. Fixation spray.

VII. Technique

A. Use Dacron or saline-soaked cotton swab to obtain endocervical specimen from endocervical canal. Spread evenly on slide.

B. Use spatula to obtain a 360-degree exocervical scraping, being sure to include the squamocolumnar junction. Spread evenly on slide.

C. One or two slides may be used, but both endocervical and exocervical specimens must be obtained.

D. Spray the slide rapidly in order to avoid drying artifact.

VIII. Interpretation

Follow-up is predicated on the appearance of the smear.

A. If no atypical cells are present, follow-up on a routine basis.

B. ASCUS—Repeat in 6 months: refer to physician if second ASCUS.

C. If there is LGSIL:

   1. Treat any infection, if present, and repeat Pap smear in 2–3 months (LGSIL reverts in many patients).

   2. If second smear shows LGSIL refer to gynecologist for coloscopy.

D. If there is HGSIL or carcinoma, refer to gynecologist for colposcopy.

⚠ TRICHOMONAL VAGINITIS: ADULT

I. Definition
An inflammatory process involving the vagina caused by a common flagellate parasite.

II. Etiology
Trichomonas vaginalis.

III. Clinical Features
A. Symptoms

   1. Vaginal discharge.

   2. Vulval itching.

   3. No vaginal bleeding.

B. Signs

   1. Minimal vulval inflammation.

   2. Frothy, bubbly vaginal discharge.

   3. Small petechial lesions on cervix and vagina.

IV. Laboratory Studies
A. Wet preparation is positive for *Trichomonas*.

B. Potassium hydroxide preparation is negative for *Candida*.

V. Differential Diagnosis
Other causes of vaginitis.

VI. Treatment
A. **Nonpregnant patient.** Metronidazole (Flagyl), 250 mg tablets—2 gm dose (8 tablets) orally at one time or 1 tablet 3 times a day for 7 days for both patient and sexual partner. Avoid alcohol for 24 hours, because a disulfiram type of reaction may occur.

B. **Pregnant patient**

   1. **Before 16 weeks of gestation,** use Trimo-San vaginal cream twice daily for 7 days for control of symptoms.

   2. **After 16 weeks of gestation,** use metronidazole gel—1 applicator twice a day for 5 days.

VII. Complications
None.

VIII. Consultation-Referral.

Refractory cases not responding to treatment in 2 weeks.

IX. Follow-Up

As needed.

▲ NONSPECIFIC OR BACTERIAL VAGINITIS: ADULT

I. Definition

An inflammation of the vagina caused by one or more bacteria.

II. Etiology

Various bacteria, especially *Gardnerella vaginalis.*

III. Clinical Features

  A. Symptoms

    1. Minimal vulval pruritus.

    2. Vaginal discharge.

  B. **Signs.** Yellowish white vaginal discharge.

IV. Laboratory Studies

  A. Potassium hydroxide preparation is negative for *Candida.*

  B. Hanging-drop preparation is negative for *Trichomonas* and positive for CLUE cells.

  C. Sniff test positive (fishy odor on addition of potassium hydroxide to vaginal discharge).

  D. Culture of *Neisseria gonorrhoeae* is negative.

V. Differential Diagnosis

Other causes of vaginitis, principally *Candida* and *Trichomonas.*

VI. Treatment

  A. Local measures:

    1. Povidone-iodine (Betadine) douche once, followed by triple sulfa (Sultrin) vaginal cream *or* 10% sulfisoxazole (Koro-Sulf) vaginal cream *or* Trimo-San twice a day for 7 days.

    2. Vinegar douche once (if not pregnant) followed by triple sulfa (Sultrin) or Trimo-San vaginal jelly twice a day for 7 days.

    3. Triple sulfa (Sultrin) *or* 10% sulfisoxazole (Koro-Sulf) vaginal cream twice a day for 7 days.

    4. Trimo-San vaginal jelly twice a day for 7 days.

  B. Metronidazole (Flagyl), 250 mg tablets—500 mg twice a day for 7 days for resistant cases; also treat partner simultaneously.

  C. If patient cannot tolerate metronidazole, use ampicillin, 500 mg 4 times a day for 10 days; treat partner with identical dosage.

  D. MetroGel, 1 applicator vaginally twice a day for 5 days.

VII. Complications

None.

VIII. Consultation–Referral

Refractory cases not responding to treatment in 2 weeks.

IX. Follow-Up

As needed.

▲ PRIMARY DYSMENORRHEA

I. Definition

Painful menstruation occurring in the absence of any demonstrable abnormality of the pelvic organs.

II. Etiology

Unknown. Psychologic factors, endocrine layers involving imbalance of estrogen and progesterone, and factors relating to prostaglandins have all been implicated.

III. Clinical Features

A. **Symptoms.** Cramping lower abdominal pain occurring just prior to or coincident with the onset of menstruation. May be associated with systemic symptoms, including headache, nausea, and diarrhea.

B. **Signs.** Physical examination (including abdominal and pelvic examination) reveals no structural abnormalities. In a symptomatic patient, there may be demonstrable uterine tenderness on examination.

IV. Laboratory Studies

None indicated.

V. Differential Diagnosis

A. Secondary causes of dysmenorrhea

1. Endometriosis.

2. Pelvic inflammatory disease.

3. Adenomyosis.

B. Other causes of abdominal pain that may coincidentally occur with menstruation, such as urinary tract infections and appendicitis.

VI. Treatment

A. Counseling and reassurance as to the probable causes of dysmenorrhea and the absence of abnormalities of the pelvic organs.

B. Ibuprofen, 400–800 mg orally 3–4 times a day for 5 days, beginning 2 or 3 days before expected onset of menses.

C. Indomethacin, 25 mg orally 3 times a day for 5 days, beginning 2–3 days before expected onset of menses.

  D. Mefenamic acid (Ponstel), 500 mg initially followed by 250 mg every 6 hours with food.

  E. Naproxen (Anaprox) 550 mg initially then 275 mg every 6–8 hours with food for 5 days beginning 2–3 days before expected onset of menses.

VII. Complications

Gastritis, diarrhea, tinnitus, platelet dysfunction.

VIII. Consultation–Referral

Refractory cases not responding to therapy.

IX. Follow-Up

As needed.

▲ BARTHOLIN'S DUCT ABSCESS AND CYST

I. Definition

Soft swelling within the labia minora at the juncture of its mid and lower thirds. This abnormality, which is almost invariably the result of pyrogenic infection, may present as a cystic nontender mass, but often it presents as an abscess with a tender mass, with surrounding erythema and induration.

II. Etiology

Usually the result of pyogenic infection. May be caused by *Neisseria gonorrhoeae, Escherichia coli,* other GI/vaginal pathogens.

III. Clinical Features

  A. Symptoms

    1. Pain.

    2. Dyspareunia.

    3. Tenderness.

  B. Signs

    1. One or both labia are swollen.

    2. Introitus is distorted.

    3. Fluctuant swelling.

    4. Low grade fever.

IV. Laboratory Studies

  A. Culture of cervix for *N. gonorrhoeae,* Chlamydia.

  B. Culture abscess material.

V. Differential Diagnosis

  A. Inclusion cysts.

  B. Large sebaceous cysts.

C. Hidradenoma.

D. Congenital anomalies.

E. Primary cancer or secondary malignancy metastic to vulvovaginal area.

VI. Treatment

A. Antibiotics—ampicillin or cephalexin, 500 mg 4 times a day for 7 days.

B. Bed rest, local or moist heat.

C. Codeine 30 mg with acetaminophen 325 mg (Empracet #3, Tylenol #3, Phenaphen #3), 1–2 tablets every 3–4 hours as needed (controlled substance—physician consultation required).

D. Fluctuant abscess should be incised and drained by the nurse practitioner.

E. When lesion is quiescent, physician should decide if the duct should be incised and marsupialized, or the diseased duct and gland should be removed.

VII. Complications

Cellulitis of surrounding tissues.

VIII. Consultation–Referral

None required.

IX. Follow-Up

A. Telephone contact in 24 hours to ensure response to therapy.

B. Examination by physician in 1–2 weeks.

▲ FAMILY PLANNING: METHODS OF BIRTH CONTROL

Changing mores now allow people to inquire about contraception at a time when scientific developments and technologic advances provide reasonable means of birth control. Indeed, birth control pills, if taken correctly, offer 98%–99% protection against pregnancy. Other methods are almost as effective and many women who are not willing or able to take birth control pills may benefit from one of these methods.

For any broad group of people, one method is predictably most appropriate—for example, birth control pills for the young woman who wants certain protection. An individual woman, however, may need several methods during her reproductive life. Characteristically, a young couple starts out with birth control pills until they decide to have their first child. If the effects of the pills become intolerable on resumption after delivery, an IUD or Nor plant may be excellent alternatives.

Once a family is complete, tubal sterilization or vasectomy may be preferred. Other effective methods include condoms and diaphragms. Less effective methods are sponges and spermicidal suppositories. Least effective is withdrawal.

In the literature the success of the various methods of contraception is expressed as both *method* effectiveness and *use* effectiveness. Method effectiveness is the idealized effectiveness if the method is used properly; use effectiveness is the actual effectiveness found in practice. It is important to understand method (theoretical) and use (actual) effectiveness.

Comparison of relative effectiveness is shown in Table 14-1. Discussion of the various methods of birth control follows:

I. Coitus Interruptus

Not recommended as an effective method of contraception.

II. Rhythm Method

Defined as avoiding intercourse 4 days before and after ovulation. This method may be used successfully by some mature couples; however, it is very unreliable and difficult to teach. Improvement in reliability can be achieved by recording basal body temperatures and following cervical mucous.

III. Condom

Fairly reliable method when used properly. Problems with condom use:

A. Condom may break.

B. Condom may slide upward during intercourse or be left behind upon removal of penis.

C. Condom must be applied before intromission.

D. Condom must be held in place for removal of penis.

TABLE 14-1

EFFECTIVENESS OF METHODS OF BIRTH CONTROL

METHOD	METHOD EFFECTIVENESS (%)	USE EFFECTIVENESS (%)
Diaphragm/cap	97–98.5	80–90
Condom	97–98.5	85–95
Birth control pill	99.6–99.9	97–99
IUD	97.0–99.0	97–98
Withdrawal	85	50–60
Sponge	85	60–70
Norplant	99+	98–99
Depo-Provera	99+	98–99
Sterilization	99+	99+

Benefits: Reduce risk of disease transmission.

IV. **Diaphragm With Spermicide**

A. **Indications.** This method may be especially appropriate for breast-feeding mothers, premenopausal women, and for women who need only occasional contraception. It may be the method of choice in women who are fearful about the systemic side effects of hormonal methods or IUDs. The effectiveness of a diaphragm is due to the spermicidal agent (*any* spermicidal cream or jelly) used with it, to the regularity of its use, and proper fitting and insertion.

B. **Types.** The arching diaphragm is most frequently used, although patients who are accustomed to using a flat, non-arching diaphragm may choose to continue using that type. Do not use if patient has latex allergy.

C. **Fitting a diaphragm.** Diaphragms are measured according to their external diameter, ranging from 55 mm to 95 mm. Expertise in measuring and fitting individuals for diaphragms can be attained easily and quickly by any practitioner. Because of the risk of dislodgment at the time of orgasm, the diaphragm should be as large as can be inserted and worn without discomfort. Most patients are adept at learning how to insert and remove a diaphragm and can easily master this skill in a few minutes. Fitting of postpartum patients should be delayed until 6 weeks after delivery to allow for complete vaginal involution.

D. **Spermicidal cream or jelly.** Any spermicidal jelly or cream intended for use with a diaphragm may be used, according to personal patient preference.

E. Must be left in place 6 hours after intercourse. If there is more than one episode of intercourse, insert additional spermicide into the vagina without removing the diaphragm.

F. Do not use petroleum products with latex products.

V. **Birth Control Pills**

A. **Physiology.** Birth control pills suppress pituitary gonadotropins—follicle-stimulating hormone (FSH) and luteinizing hormone (LH)—which in turn suppress ovulation.

Neither estrogen nor progestin effectively suppresses ovulation alone, and thus combination pills of the two hormones are required for this effect. Progestin also affects the endometrium and prevents implantation, changing the composition and consistency of cervical mucus so that sperm penetration of the mucus is decreased. Progestins alone (the "minipill") can be used for birth control but are not as effective as combinations of estrogen and progestin. The more recent triphasic combinations of estrogen and progestin appear to result in fewer unfavorable changes in serum lipids than do the standard combination pills. The new triphasic combination pills reduce the total amount of progestin dose by varying the daily dose to more closely mimic the natural hormonal flow during each cycle.

B. **Side effects.** In general, side effects are dose related and, in some cases, age related. Most problems are much less frequently seen with low-dose birth control pills.

   1. Most side effects are nonspecific complaints such as bloating, nausea, edema, and cyclical weight gain and are less severe and less frequently seen with low-dose pills.

   2. Thromboembolic side effects such as thrombophlebitis, CVAs, and myocardial infarction are primarily related to estrogen and are dose related. Progestin affects cholesterol, but clinical significance of this finding is not clear. Thromboembolic side effects greatly increase in pill takers who are over 35, smoke cigarettes, or are obese.

   3. Headaches. Occur in a small number of patients. In patients with migraine the effect is unpredictable.

   4. Hypertension. Occurs in a small percentage of patients. Blood pressure will usually return to normal when birth control pills are stopped.

   5. Acne may occur or be worsened in progestin-dominant BCPs.

   6. Incidence of breast and endometrial cancer is not increased.

   7. Incidence of cancer of cervix may be slightly increased. This is believed not to be related to BCP usage.

C. **Side effects from low estrogen dose**

   1. Decreased menstrual flow.

   2. Amenorrhea.

   3. Breakthrough bleeding for a few months after initiation of low-dose pills.

   4. Sporadic breakthrough bleeding.

D. **Contraindications**

   1. History of deep venothrombophlebitis.

   2. History of embolus.

   3. Undiagnosed abnormal uterine bleeding.

   4. Impaired liver function.

   5. Cerebral vascular accidents/stroke.

   6. Estrogen dependent cancer, breast cancer.

   7. Pregnancy.

E. **Relative contraindications**

   1. Diabetes mellitus.

2. Thyroid dysfunction.

3. Leiomyomata (fibroids).

4. Cigarette smoking and over 35 years of age.

5. Undiagnosed amenorrhea.

6. Seizure disorders.

7. Undiagnosed breast masses.

8. Severe depression.

9. Migraine headaches.

F. **Types of birth control pills**

1. **Combination**

   a. Estrogen component is either mestranol or ethinyl estradiol; these have approximately equal hormonal activity for a given weight. Because many side effects are dose related it is important to start on the lowest dose possible, usually 30–35 mg of estrogen.

   b. Progestin component—several, which have varying degrees of progestin androgenic properties. Theoretically, one might base the selection of a pill on physical characteristics of the patient. (Norethindrone acetate, the least androgenic, to levonorgestrel, the most androgenic.)

2. Biphasic or triphasic combination pills vary the progestin dose. These are effective but have not been shown to be a significant improvement over the standard combination pill.

3. Progestin only.

4. Morning-after pill.

G. **Patient evaluation**

1. History. Specifically, obtain information about side effects and contraindications.

2. Physical examination. Complete physical with special attention to:

   a. Blood pressure.

   b. Breast examination.

   c. Pelvic examination.

3. **Laboratory studies**

   a. Papanicolaou (Pap) smear.

   b. Blood sugar (suggested).

   c. Cholesterol (suggested).

H. **Selection of pill**

1. Birth control pills offer maximum protection against pregnancy when used correctly, and are therefore an appropriate

choice for anyone who does not want to get pregnant.

2. Patients should be started on the low-dose pills. Only combinations containing a low-dose estrogen (usually 30–35 mg) are recommended.

I. **Follow-Up**

1. Check weight and blood pressure and assess side effects after three cycles in first-time user.

2. After initial follow-up visit, annually.

3. Breast examination and Pap smear annually.

4. Return visit as necessary for problems.

J. **Consultation-referral.** Any persistent side effect (see **V.B**).

VI. Intrauterine Devices

A. **General aspects.** The intrauterine device (IUD) has proved to be 95–97% effective as a contraceptive method and is especially suited to women over age 30, who may be at increased risk from oral contraceptive use. Nulliparous patients are somewhat less suitable candidates, because they are more prone to dysmenorrhea and because of the risk that salpingitis (known to be more common in IUD users) may impair future fertility. Relative contraindications include documented previous or present pelvic inflammatory disease, pregnancy, uterine fibroids, abnormal uterine bleeding, and dysmenorrhea. After approval by the consulting gynecologist, IUDs may be inserted by a nurse practitioner who has the proper training and experience. IUDs should be inserted during the menstrual period, if possible. If not, ascertain that the woman is not pregnant. IUDs currently available include ParaGard and Progestasert.

B. **Types of IUDs**

1. The ParaGard IUD is a copper containing IUD which is effective for 8 years. Before insertion, there is an extensive informed consent booklet must be read, explained, and signed before insertion. Insertion is best accomplished during menses.

2. **Progesterone IUD (Progestasert)** releases a minute amount of progesterone into the endometrial cavity. Its significantly greater cost and limited duration of effectiveness (1 year) have largely restricted its use to patients with dysmenorrhea or menometrorrhagia, or both, in whom no other form of contraception is acceptable.

C. **Side effects and complications**

1. **Cramps, intermenstrual bleeding, menorrhagia.** These complaints occur more frequently among IUD users but are not indications for removal unless the patient finds them to be unacceptable in duration and degree.

2. **Pelvic infection.** Salpingitis and pelvic abscess, often unilat-

eral, are seen with slightly increased frequency in IUD users; they are indications for removal of the device.

3. **Uterine perforation.** Difficult insertion of an IUD may lead to perforation of the device through the uterine wall. Although bleeding or unusual pain, or both, may result, often the only symptom of a perforation may be disappearance of the IUD string from its usual cervical position. Suggestion of uterine perforation requires physician consultation.

4. **Spontaneous expulsion.** Most common in the first two or three cycles, but can happen at any time; may be accompanied by severe cramping and bleeding but may go undetected.

D. **Removal of IUDs**

1. **Indications for removal**

   a. **Partial expulsion**

      (1) The IUD is found in the vaginal vault, or the tip of the device is visualized on external or speculum examination or is palpated during bimanual examination.

      (2) This possibility must be considered when either the patient or her sexual partner complains of pain with intercourse or of feeling the device during intercourse; when the patient complains of pelvic pain or excessive bleeding; or when the patient suddenly believes the string to be longer. The cervix must be palpated very carefully, with the possibility of embedded IUD in mind.

   b. **Infection.** If the patient exhibits symptoms of uterine or pelvic infection, such as elevated white blood cell count (greater than 10,000), pelvic tenderness, fever, and abnormal vaginal discharge.

   c. **Pregnancy.**

   d. **Patient request.**

   e. The ParaGard is not effective after 8 years and should be removed at that time.

2. **Procedure for removal**

   a. May be removed at any time in the menstrual cycle. Instruct patient that she is no longer protected against pregnancy until a new method of contraception is initiated.

   b. Obtain patient history.

   c. Obtain pregnancy test when indicated by patient history.

   d. Perform bimanual examination to determine uterine size and position.

   e. Insert speculum to visualize cervix; observe for IUD string.

   f. Warn patient that menstrual-like cramping may occur with removal.

  g. Grasp string with uterine dressing forceps and exert smooth, gentle traction on the IUD. *Do not use jerky motion.* IUD removal should be accomplished quite easily.

  h. Allow patient to rest briefly after removal of device.

E. **Laboratory studies**

  1. Complete blood count and endocervical culture if patient exhibits symptoms of endometritis or pelvic inflammatory disease.

  2. Pregnancy test, if pregnancy is a possibility.

F. **Treatment**

  1. Remove IUD. See **VI.D.2** for procedure.

  2. Advise patient on possible complications.

VII. Post-Coital Birth Control

(Morning After Pill)

In some situations, postcoital birth control has become a frequently used form of birth control, particularly when unprotected intercourse occurs in circumstances in which a pregnancy would be extremely undesirable. Diethylstilbestrol (DES) in large doses was the first compound used for this purpose, and large doses of conjugated equine estrogens (Premarin) have also been used. Currently the treatment of choice is Ovral (0.5 mg Norgestrel and 0.05 mg ethinyl estradiol). Two tablets stat and repeated in 12 hours, within 72 hours after intercourse. Ovral causes fewer gastrointestinal side effects than DES or large doses of premarin and is as effective as a birth prevention measure.

A. Consult with physician.

B. Therapy must be initiated.

C. Patients should be warned that:

  1. It is necessary to take all medication, despite the high incidence of nausea (with Premarin), to achieve complete effectiveness.

  2. The medication is highly effective but not absolutely guaranteed to prevent pregnancy.

  3. If pregnancy occurs, therapeutic abortion should be strongly considered because of possible adverse effects of the drug on the fetus.

  4. Patient receiving such treatment should return in 4 weeks.

   a. Ascertain that pregnancy has been prevented.

   b. Provide contraceptive counseling.

VIII. Norplant

A. A birth control system consisting of 6 Silastic capsules that contain levonorgestrel. The capsules are inserted in the subcuticular tissue, usually in the inner aspect of the upper arm (the nondominant arm is usually chosen). Bruising is very common at the site of insertion. It is inserted using local anesthesia in the office. This method is cost effective after 2 years and is an effective means of birth control for 5 years.

B. **Side effects**
1. The most common side effect is irregular vaginal bleeding during the first 9–12 months. This can be controlled by using supplemental estrogens.
2. Depression, especially in those so predisposed.
3. Possible increase in migraine pattern or generalized headaches.
4. Possible hair loss.
5. Weight gain of approximately 1 lb per year.
6. Breast tenderness.
7. Increase in acne.

C. **Contraindications**
1. Hormonally related thrombosis or thromboembolic events.
2. Undiagnosed uterine bleeding.
3. Known or suspected uterine bleeding.
4. Acute liver disease or dysfunction.
5. Known breast carcinoma

D. **Effectiveness.** 98%–99%

Note: Thorough counseling is necessary for this birth control method to be accepted by the patient. The most common reason for removal is irregular/unpredictable vaginal bleeding. Placing a patient on progestin-only birth control pills for two cycles may determine if the patient will experience bothersome side effects. There have been reports of increased failure rates in those patients on rifampin or anticonvulsants.

IX. **Depo-Provera**

A. An injectable means of birth control that has been used for decades overseas. This progesterone is medroxyprogesterone acetate suspension. The injection is given in the deltoid or gluteus muscle. Fertility usually returns within 6–9 months of the last injection. The standard dosage is 150 mg every 3 months. If it has been more than 14 weeks since the previous injection, it is mandatory that the patient have a negative pregnancy before another injection is given.

B. **Side effects**
1. The most common side effect is irregular vaginal bleeding during the first 6–9 months. This can be controlled by using supplemental estrogens.
2. Amenorrhea is common after 1–2 years.

3. Depression, especially in those so predisposed.

4. Possible increase in migraine pattern or generalized headaches.

5. Weight gain of approximately 3–5 lbs per year.

6. Breast tenderness.

7. Increase in acne.

8. Possible decreased libido.

9. Insignificant change in cholesterol profile.

C. **Contraindications**

1. Hormonally related thrombosis or thromboembolic events.

2. Undiagnosed uterine bleeding.

3. Known or suspected uterine bleeding.

4. Acute liver disease or dysfunction.

5. Known breast carcinoma.

D. **Effectiveness.** 98%–99%

Note: Thorough counseling is necessary for this birth control method to be accepted by the patient. Placing a patient on progestin-only birth control pills for two cycles may determine if the patient will experience bothersome side effects. Backup contraceptive methods should be used if the injection is not given in the first 5 days of onset of menses or it has been more than 14 weeks since the last injection. In patients who are morbidly obese, dosages should be increased to 200–250 mg every 3 months.

X. Therapeutic Abortions

In the United States, legal abortions are available through the second trimester. Although recent changes in federal regulations have made third-party reimbursement by Medicaid problematic and dependent on state decisions, termination of pregnancy can still be obtained through a number of sources, with tremendous regional variations. Health care providers should acquaint themselves with the local capabilities and alternatives. For some health care practitioners, abortion may present a crisis of values—an understandable point of view, but one which should not conflict with a balanced presentation to patients.

Discussion of the various methods of abortion follows:

A. **Before eight weeks of gestation.** Aspiration of uterine contents with a flexible catheter is the preferred procedure. Because this removal may be done before pregnancy tests are positive, it is euphemistically called menstrual extraction. An advantage is that aspiration may be done on an outpatient basis.

B. **Eight to twelve weeks gestation.** Dilation and curettage of uterine contents now has been largely replaced by curettage and vacuum procedures.

C. **Second trimester.** Several methods may be used:

1. Intra-amniotic prostaglandin injection.

2. Intra-amniotic injection of saline and urea.

3. Dilation and evacuation, in selected circumstances.

4. Rarely, direct removal of contents by vaginal or abdominal hysterotomy.

XI. Permanent Contraception

A. **Vasectomy** (male)

1. This procedure is 99%+ effective.

2. Reanastomosis is usually successful regarding potency of the vas, but not as successful regarding viable sperm. The longer the time between the initial procedure and anastomosis, the worse the prognosis.

3. Psychosexual problems are occasionally reported. Adequate counseling is necessary.

4. Of males who have a vasectomy, 50%–60% will develop antibodies to sperm that can cause sterility.

B. **Tubal ligation** (female)

1. Laparoscopic techniques permit outpatient surgery with early return to work (1–3 days).

2. This procedure is 99+% effective.

3. Reversals are possible but the risk of ectopic pregnancy is significantly increased.

4. Psychosexual problems have been reported. Adequate and thorough counseling is necessary.

▲ MENOPAUSE

I. Definition

Strictly speaking, menopause is the physiologic cessation of menstruation due to the normal aging of the ovary. In many women, this event occurs with few, if any, associated symptoms. In others, many associated symptoms lead them to seek medical care.

II. Etiology

A complex and poorly understood interaction of factors involving hormonal changes (decreased estrogen, increased gonadotropin levels) vasomotor phenomena, neurotransmitters and psychological factors.

III. Clinical Features

A. **Symptoms**

1. Vasomotor phenomena are manifested as episodes of flushing/hot flashes and sweating.

    2. Irritability, fatigue, insomnia, headaches, palpitation, dizziness, frequent mood swings.

    3. Dyspareunia, vaginal irritation, and pruritus.

B. Signs

    1. Atrophy and inflammation of the vaginal mucosa.

    2. Elevated FSH/LH.

IV. Laboratory Studies

A. Cervical Papanicolaou smear to rule out malignancy.

B. Potassium hydroxide and saline vaginal preparations to rule out other causes of vaginitis.

C. Estrogen index of vaginal mucosa shows decreased maturation manifested by lack of superficial cells (large, flat mucosal cells found in inactive mucosa). Wet smear shows atrophic basal cells.

V. Differential Diagnosis

A. Pregnancy and other causes of missed menstrual periods; other irregularities or abnormalities of menstruation; or both.

B. Anxiety and other physiologic states occurring in the absence of menopause.

C. Alternative explanations for any of the nonspecific symptoms of menopause, such as irritability, headaches, fatigue, stress, and tension.

VI. Treatment

Note: Hormonal replacement therapy (HRT) is a sensitive subject for many patients. It is apparent that replacement would be beneficial for most women. The major benefits are: 1) a significant reduction in the incidence of osteoporosis and prevention of the morbidity/mortality associated with major bone fractures that will occur in these elderly patients; 2) a significant reduction in the effects of cardiovascular disease and myocardial infarcts/ischemia (50% reduction); 3) prevention of vaginal atrophy, vaginal dryness, dyspareunia, and continual support for the pelvic tissues and bladder; 4) relief of menopausal and vasomotor symptoms. Compliance in a woman convinced against her will is poor, so careful counseling is essential.

A. Initial therapy

    1. Conjugated estrogen, 0.625 mg or equivalent by mouth each day. Estraderm patch (0.05 mg) may also be used initially with a Sunday/Wednesday change cycle.

    and

    2. Medroxyprogesterone acetate, 10 mg by mouth the first 10–12 days of each month. This medication counteracts the unopposed estrogen effect on the endometrium and facilitates the occurrence of withdrawal bleeding.

or

3. Alternatively, medroxyprogesterone acetate (2.5 mg) by mouth can be given every day. This will generally produce an amenorrheic state after 6–8 months and may be more acceptable to the patient.

   Note: Progesterone must be given if the patient still has her uterus.

B. **Long-term maintenance therapy** (consultation with physician required). If long-term maintenance estrogen replacement is deemed necessary by the consulting physician, then the following guidelines should be applied:

   1. The dosage of conjugated estrogen may be reduced to the dose that will control symptoms. Reduction in dosage should be attempted after the first 4 weeks of therapy; however, 0.625 mg is the optimal dose for preventing osteoporosis.

   2. Progestin should be added each month to facilitate withdrawal bleeding (see **VI.A.2,3.**)

   3. Blood pressure must be followed closely to identify the small percentage of patients who develop hypertension on estrogen replacement therapy.

Note: Hormonal replacement therapy (HRT) may stimulate breast tissue (mastodynia) and initially produce irregular vaginal bleeding. A few patients may experience headaches, depression, and/or nausea.

C. **Atrophic vaginitis.** Atrophic vaginitis, in the absence of other menopausal symptoms, may respond to conjugated estrogen vaginal cream (Premarin)—1 gm (1/4 applicator-ful) twice a day for 4 weeks. Any intercurrent vaginal infection must be treated specifically; see Candidal Vaginitis: Adult, **VI**, pp 320–321. Certain patients may require long-term therapy with a conjugated estrogen vaginal cream used 2 or 3 times a week, but the health-care provider should note that estrogen vaginal creams are absorbed and exert a systemic effect. Oral estrogen therapy may prove more convenient and equally effective.

VII. Contraindications and Complications

A. **Contraindications**

   1. Thrombophlebitis, hormone related.
   2. Pulmonary embolus.
   3. Stroke.
   4. Allergy to estrogen preparations.
   5. Known or suspected pregnancy.
   6. Undiagnosed genital bleeding.

7. Known or suspected estrogen-dependent neoplasm of the breast or reproductive tract.

All patients with a history of any of these conditions must be referred to the physician before estrogen replacement therapy is considered.

B. Complications

1. Possible carcinoma of the endometrium if estrogen is given unopposed by progestin.

2. Breast pain.

3. Hypertension.

4. Thrombophlebitis and thromboembolia phenomena.

VIII. Consultation–Referral

A. All patients after first 1–2 months of therapy.

B. Any patient with a history of a contraindication.

C. Any patient who develops genital bleeding while on therapy.

D. Any patient who develops complications of therapy.

IX. Follow-Up

A. Blood pressure check every 6 months for first year of replacement therapy.

B. Pap smears obtained annually while on estrogens.

C. Frequent follow-up is needed to counsel patient and deal with psychologic and other aspects of menopausal syndrome.

▲ PREGNANCY: DIAGNOSIS AND REFERRAL

I. Definition

Although pregnancy is properly not regarded as a "disease," the process of making a diagnosis of pregnancy, which includes a pelvic examination for estimating length of gestation on the basis of uterine size, does constitute medical practice and should be covered by a protocol. This requirement is particularly applicable when the patient desires to terminate the pregnancy.

II. Clinical Features

(Usually apparent 2 weeks after first missed period.)

A. Symptoms

1. Missed menstrual period occurring in a patient whose periods are usually regular.

2. Breast engorgement.

3. Nausea or vomiting, or both, particularly in the early morning on arising.

    4. Tiredness or easy fatigability.

B. Signs

    1. Cervical softening (Goodell's sign).

    2. Cervical and vaginal cyanosis (Chadwick's sign).

    3. Softening of the uterine isthmus (Hegar's sign).

    4. Enlargement of the uterus consistent with duration of pregnancy:

        a. 8 weeks—approximately two times normal size.

        b. 12 weeks—palpable on abdominal examination above symphysis pubis.

        c. 20 weeks—palpable at level of umbilicus.

        d. 36 weeks—palpable at xiphoid process.

III. Laboratory Studies.

Test for human chorionic gonadotropin should be positive by the first missed period. The more sensitive assays are positive within a few days of conception.

IV. Differential Diagnosis

    A. Ectopic pregnancy.

    B. Menopause.

    C. Other causes of amenorrhea.

    D. Uterine fibromyomata.

V. Treatment

    A. Enrollment in prenatal care program

    or

    B. Referral for therapeutic abortion after careful counseling of patient and when consistent with local laws, customs, and religious beliefs.

    C. Referral if etiology is not intrauterine pregnancy.

VI. Complications

    A. See Guidelines for Managing the Obstetric Patient, **I.C.5,** p. 315, for complications of pregnancy.

    B. Psychologic and social complications of therapeutic abortion are frequent and often severe. Appropriate arrangements for ongoing counseling and care should be ensured.

VII. Consultation–Referral

    A. See Guidelines for Managing the Obstetric Patient, **I.D.,** p. 316, for consultation requirements in pregnancy.

    B. Therapeutic abortion. In the great majority of cases, nurse practitioners refer patients who desire a therapeutic abortion to a physician who, in some instances, may practice in a different community. The nurse practitioner should explore the alternatives and arrangements for referral of patients in advance of the need for such services. Because of the psychologic and social impact of the termination of an unwanted pregnancy, every effort should be expended to ensure proper transfer of information and continuity of care, including psychologic and social support services.

VIII. Follow-Up

A. Scheduled prenatal visits; See Guidelines for Managing the Obstetric Patient, **I.C.1.**, p. 314.

or

B. Careful follow-up for patients who elect therapeutic abortion.

15
▼

|

PARASITIC INFESTATIONS

▲

▲ ASCARIASIS: PEDIATRIC AND ADULT

I. Definition

Ascariasis is an infestation of the intestine by a species of roundworm *(Ascaris lumbricoides)* capable of infesting a human host.

II. Etiology and Life Cycle

Infestation begins when ascaris eggs are ingested. Children may ingest eggs by playing in or eating soil that is contaminated with eggs. Some people ingest eggs by eating unwashed, raw vegetables that were grown in contaminated soil. The soil becomes contaminated when sanitary facilities are not adequate, when infected persons (usually children) defecate directly on the ground near living quarters, or when human excrement is used for fertilizing gardens. After ingestion, the eggs hatch into larvae that migrate from the small intestine to the liver and lungs through the venous circulation. The larvae enter the alveoli of the lungs and then migrate to the trachea, where they can be coughed up or swallowed. Swallowed larvae enter the small intestine, where they mature. The adult female worms produce numerous eggs,

Patient Care Guidelines for Nurse Practitioners, 4th ed. by Axalla J. Hoole, C. Glenn Pickard, Jr., Ruth M. Ouimette, Jacob A. Lohr, and Robert A. Greenberg. Copyright © 1995 by J. B. Lippincott Company.

which are passed in the stool. Individual adult worms may be passed in the stool and are easily identified on visual inspection.

III. Clinical Features

A. **Symptoms**

1. Many patients are asymptomatic (likely due to infestation with only a small number of worms).

2. Cough and fever may be present during the lung migration phase of the life cycle.

3. Small children with large numbers of worms may have anorexia, digestive disturbances, irritability and weight loss.

4. Children with pica (a tendency to ingest dirt) are more likely to become infested. Pica is sometimes associated with iron deficiency anemia. Therefore, the presence of pica should prompt an evaluation for possible anemia and for ascariasis.

B. **Signs**

1. Adult worms may be seen in the stool.

2. Failure to gain weight may be noticed in a small child when large numbers of worms are present.

3. Acute pneumonitis (particularly if associated with eosinophilia) should suggest the possibility of ascariasis.

4. Ascariasis does not cause blood loss or diarrhea.

IV. Laboratory Studies

A. None are needed if adult worms are seen.

B. Microscopic examination (by an experienced observer) of the stool of an infested person will reveal ascaris eggs.

V. Differential Diagnosis

A. Pulmonary symptoms during lung migration by larvae can be confused with bacterial or viral pneumonia or asthma.

B. Other causes of failure to gain weight or of vague digestive symptoms should be ruled out.

C. Because many patients are asymptomatic, case finding can be a problem. Many cases present when an adult worm is noticed in the stool or when patients have a stool examination for eggs because of eosinophilia on peripheral blood smear.

VI. Treatment

A. Correction of poor sanitation (particularly the practice of indiscriminate defecation near houses), improvement in personal hygiene (handwashing), and care in food preparation (washing of raw foods prior to eating) are important.

B. Elimination of pica by treating iron deficiency anemia and counseling parents on proper nutrition for children.

C. Either of two drugs may be used to treat infected persons:

1. Pyrantel pamoate (Antiminth) suspension given as a single oral dose of 1 mL (50 mg) per 5 kg (10 lb) of body weight (maximum dose is 20 mL).

or

2. Mebendazole (Vermox), 100 mg per tablet—1 tablet twice a day for 3 days (tablets may be chewed, swallowed, or crushed and mixed with food).

Warning: Mebendazole should not be used in children under 2 years of age or in pregnant females.

VII. Complications

Rarely, intestinal obstruction results from a tangled worm mass.

VIII. Consultation–Referral

Generally, not needed in routine cases.

IX. Follow-Up

High risk families with proved infection should be followed with periodic stool examinations because of the possibility of reinfection.

▲ PEDICULOSIS: PEDIATRIC AND ADULT

I. Definition

Infestation of the skin or hair by one or both of the two species of lice capable of infesting the human host.

II. Etiology

A. *Pediculus humanis* infests the head or body.

B. *Phthirus pubis,* the "crab" louse, infests the genital region.

C. Both species of lice are transmitted either by close personal contact or through shared clothing, bedclothes, etc.

III. Clinical Features

A. **Symptoms.** Intense itching.

B. **Signs**

1. Head (pediculosis capitis):

   a. The nits (ova) are seen as small (1–2 mm) oval objects attached to individual hair shafts.

   b. The lice themselves are difficult to find.

   c. Secondary changes in the scalp, including impetiginous changes and furuncles, may develop.

2. Body (pediculosis corporis):

   a. The lice feed on the skin, but may live in clothing or bedding.

    b. Skin lesions are characterized by changes secondary to scratching such as excoriative or secondary impetigo.

  3. Genital or pubic region (Phthirus pubis):

    a. As seen in head lice, nits may be seen on hair shafts.

    b. The lice are often difficult to find.

    c. Small black dots, which are probably excreta, may be seen.

IV. Laboratory Studies

Suspected nits should be examined under the microscope at 10X to confirm that the morphology is typical and that there is attachment of the hair shaft. Casual inspection may misdiagnose hair root casts (which can appear as white objects on hair shafts) as nits.

V. Differential Diagnosis

A. The presence of nits or mature lice is pathognomonic.

B. The secondary lesions or excoriations and impetigo can be of multiple origins. Their location on the scalp, pubic areas, or the skin folds may be helpful in diagnosing pediculosis.

VI. Treatment

A. Hygiene. Contaminated clothing, bed linens, towels, hats, and other personal articles should be dry cleaned, washed in hot water, or dried at high heat to destroy nits and lice.

B. Pediculosis capitis (head lice)

  1. Permethrin Liquid 1%.

    a. Apply to hair and scalp until hair is thoroughly wet.

    b. After 10 minutes rinse off with warm water.

    c. Remove any remaining nits with a fine-tooth comb.

    d. repeat application in 7–10 days if nits are still present.

  2. Gamma benzene hexachloride 1%, shampoo

    a. Apply a sufficient quantity of gamma benzene hexachloride shampoo to thoroughly wet hair and adjacent hairy skin.

    b. Add small quantities of water to produce a lather and continue to shampoo for 4 minutes.

    c. Rinse thoroughly and towel briskly.

    d. Remove any remaining nits with a fine-tooth comb or tweezers.

    e. Repeat application in 7–10 days if nits are still present.

    Warning: Gamma benzene hexachloride should not be used in pregnant females or in children under 3 years of age.

C. Pediculosis corporis (body lice)

  1. Bathing plus management of clothing and bed linens as mentioned above are the necessary measures.

2. Gamma benzene hexachloride 1% lotion or shampoo should be used for occasional nits on body hair.

D. **Phthirus pubis (pubic lice, "crabs").** Use gamma benzene hexachloride 1%, cream or lotion, as follows:

1. Apply liberally to hair and skin of pubic area.

2. Remove with a thorough washing after 4 minutes and then rinse with warm water.

3. Repeat application in 7–10 days if nits are still present.

4. Treat sexual contacts simultaneously.

E. Family and close contacts should be carefully examined but treated *only* if they are infested.

F. Oral antihistamines, such as diphenhydramine HCl (Benadryl), may be helpful to relieve itching (see Table 3-1, p. 95, for dosage).

VII. Complications

Secondary infection with impetigo, furuncles, or regional lymphadenitis, or a combination of these.

VIII. Consultation–Referral

Questions about diagnosis.

IX. Follow-Up

As needed.

▲ PINWORMS: PEDIATRIC AND ADULT

I. Definition

An infestation of pinworms *(Enterobius vermicularis)* in the human intestinal tract. It is the most common parasitic infestation in the United States.

II. Etiology and Life Cycle

Infestation is initiated by the oral ingestion of pinworm eggs. Eggs from the perianal skin of infected persons (especially small children) are easily spread by hands, toys, rugs, and other objects to the hands of other persons. If hands are not washed, eggs are then transmitted from contaminated hands to the mouth. Once swallowed, the eggs hatch into larvae that mature into adult worms over the next 15–28 days as they pass through the intestinal tract. Mature female worms migrate from the anus and deposit thousands of eggs on the perineum. Pinworms can attach to the mucosa of the colon and rectum, thereby causing local irritation. The life cycle does not, however, include migration into the blood or into other tissues.

III. Clinical Features

A. **Symptoms**

1. Patients may be asymptomatic.
2. The primary symptoms are anal pruritus and sometimes secondary skin excoriation and infection.
3. Young females may wake up crying at night with genital irritation as worms migrate into the vulval area. Such migration can also cause vulvovaginitis and dysuria.

B. **Signs**

1. Adult pinworms are sometimes seen on the perineum. The worms are approximately 1 cm in length and resemble white threads.
2. Perineal excoriation is sometimes present.
3. Heavy infestations (large numbers of worms in the colon and rectum) may cause perineal pain and bleeding on defecation.

IV. **Diagnostic Studies**

A. Observation of worms by a responsible person is sufficient for diagnosis.

B. Examination for pinworm eggs will also establish the diagnosis.

1. Press a piece of clear tape (Scotch tape) directly over the anus and surrounding skin, preferably early in the morning.
2. Remove tape and place on glass slide with sticky side down.
3. Examine microscopically (10X) for characteristic eggs.
4. Do not send stool for egg examination, since eggs are primarily deposited on perianal skin.

C. Pinworms do not usually cause eosinophilia.

V. **Differential Diagnosis**

A. Other causes of anal pruritus and excoriation (e.g., poor hygiene, localized skin infection, and anal fissure).

B. Other causes of local irritation of the female genitalia (e.g., poor hygiene, chemical irritants like bubble baths, other causes of vaginitis).

C. Other causes of dysuria (especially urinary tract infection).

VI. **Treatment**

A. **General measures**

1. Stress personal hygiene, particularly handwashing before eating and after using the toilet.
2. Pajamas and bed linens of symptomatic family members should be washed in regular laundry detergent after treatment.

B. **Specific therapy** (treat all family members at the same time)

1. Pyrantel pamoate (Antiminth) suspension given as a single oral

dose of 1 mL (50 mg) per 5 kg (10 lb) of body weight (maximum single dose is 20 mL). The dose should be repeated in 2 weeks.

or

2. Mebendazole (Vermox), 100 mg per tablet—1 tablet given as a single dose (tablets may be chewed, swallowed, or crushed and mixed with food). The dose should be repeated in 2 weeks.

Warning: Mebendazole should not be used in children under 2 years of age or in pregnant females.

VII. Complications

A. Patients may present with minor complications from localized irritation and migration (vulvovaginitis, secondary skin infection at sites of excoriation, dysuria).

B. Rarely, pinworms can cause acute appendicitis by obstructing the lumen of the appendix.

VIII. Consultation–Referral

None in uncomplicated cases.

IX. Follow-Up

Return visit only for recurrence.

16

MISCELLANEOUS INFECTIONS

▲ Measles: Pediatric and Adult

I. Definition

A highly contagious, febrile, exanthematous, viral disease associated with a high rate of serious complications.

II. Etiology

Measles virus.

III. Clinical Features

A. Symptoms

 1. The incubation period is 8–12 days.

 2. The catarrhal, or prodromal period before the rash lasts 3–5 days.

  a. The patient is usually very ill, with fever up to 104 °F (40 °C).

  b. Coryza, cough, and conjunctivitis are prominent.

  c. Marked malaise and anorexia are present.

  d. Vomiting or diarrhea may occur.

Patient Care Guidelines for Nurse Practitioners, 4th ed. by Axalla J. Hoole, C. Glenn Pickard, Jr., Ruth M. Ouimette, Jacob A. Lohr, and Robert A. Greenberg. Copyright © 1995 by J. B. Lippincott Company.

3. The rash usually begins on the head and neck and spreads caudally, reaching the feet on the second or third day:

   a. The fever and symptoms of the prodromal period continue after the appearance of the rash, and symptoms are most severe as the rash reaches its peak.

   b. By the second or third day of rash, the fever usually falls and symptoms begin to decrease.

   c. Fever persisting after day 4 of rash suggests the presence of complications.

B. **Signs**

1. Fever is present throughout the prodromal period, increasing stepwise until the height of the rash and rapidly declining on day 2 or 3 of the rash.

2. Marked nasal discharge, conjunctivitis, and pharyngeal infection begin prodromally and continue into the rash period.

3. Koplik's spots are pathognomonic and appear on the buccal mucosa 2 days before the rash appears.

4. The maculopapular rash begins about the face and hairline and descends, gradually becoming confluent and eventually desquamating.

IV. Laboratory Studies

A. Paired serum samples (from the acute and convalescent periods) should be drawn and sent to state laboratories for confirmation of diagnosis.

B. Other laboratory tests should be done on the basis of the presence of complications, after consultation.

V. Differential Diagnosis

A. Rubella.

B. Roseola.

C. Rocky Mountain spotted fever.

D. Scarlet fever.

E. Enteroviral exanthems.

F. Drug rashes.

VI. Treatment

A. Prevention*

1. Live measles vaccine should be given alone or as part of combined measles–mumps–rubella vaccine as soon as possible after the age of 15 months.

---

*See Chapter 1, III.D, for immunization contraindications.

2. Adults and adolescents born after 1954, who have not had measles and who are unimmunized or who received only the killed measles vaccine, should be immunized with live measles vaccine unless there are contraindications to vaccine administration.

3. Individuals who received vaccine as infants should be reimmunized during adolescence.

B. **Therapy**

1. No specific therapy.

2. Isolation of patient beginning with the onset of the catarrhal stage through the third day of the rash.

3. Immediate notification of appropriate public health authorities so that control measures may be instituted. Be certain to confirm suspected cases by obtaining serum specimens for serologic studies.

4. Investigation of immune status of family and immediate contacts, and appropriate steps to limit spread of measles.

5. Antipyretic therapy: see Chapter 5, Upper Respiratory Tract Infection (Common Cold): Pediatric and Adult, **VI.C**, p. 156–157.

6. Antibiotic therapy only as indicated for specific complications.

7. Adequate fluid and nutritional intake.

8. Darkened room (this may be more comfortable, but is not necessary for conjunctivitis).

VII. **Complications**

A. **Pneumonia**

1. Pneumonia may occur at any time during the course of measles.

2. It should be treated as bacterial pneumonia, because it usually represents superimposed bacterial disease.

B. **Otitis media**

1. A very common complication.

2. It should be treated according to the guidelines in Chapter 5, Acute Purulent Otitis Media: Pediatric and Adult, **VI**, pp. 136–137.

C. **Encephalitis**

1. A very serious complication, occurring in 0.1% of cases.

2. Onset is most commonly between 2 and 6 days after the onset of the rash.

D. **Tuberculosis**

1. Tuberculin sensitivity is depressed during and immediately after measles.

2. Inactive tuberculosis may be activated, and children with positive tuberculin tests should be on antituberculosis therapy.

VIII. Consultation-Referral

A. Consultation is indicated for all cases of suspected measles because an immediate decision needs to be made on methods to prevent the spread of the infection.

B. Patients with clinically diagnosed measles who develop signs of encephalitis should be referred immediately.

C. Consultation is indicated for patients who develop pneumonia.

D. Public health authorities should be notified immediately when suspected cases of measles are seen, and decisions should be made on steps required to limit the spread of the virus.

IX. Follow-Up

All patients should be seen 3 or 4 days after the onset of the rash.

▲ INFECTIOUS MONONUCLEOSIS: PEDIATRIC AND ADULT

I. Definition

A disease primarily of children and young adults characterized mainly by fever, sore throat, enlarged lymph nodes, malaise, and lassitude.

II. Etiology

Epstein–Barr virus (EBV).

III. Clinical Features

A. Symptoms

1. Sore throat.
2. Malaise and lassitude.
3. Usually, *no* nasal congestion, earache, cough, or other symptoms commonly present in respiratory infections.

B. Signs

1. Fever (often 101 °F–103 °F).
2. Inflammation of the pharynx (often exudative).
3. Bilateral, usually nontender, enlargement of the lymph nodes. The cervical lymph nodes are almost always involved; the axillary and inguinal nodes, frequently.
4. Often splenomegaly.
5. Sometimes, erythematous maculopapular rash.
6. Periorbital edema.
7. Sometimes, jaundice.

IV. Laboratory Studies

A. Throat culture is done to rule out streptococcal pharyngitis.

B. White blood cell and differential count usually show lymphocytosis, with 10%–20% atypical lymphocytes by the seventh day of illness.

C. Heterophil antibody determination, or slide agglutination test (Monospot), is usually positive.

V. Differential Diagnosis

A. Streptococcal pharyngitis.

B. Hepatitis of other origin in patients who develop jaundice.

C. Viral exanthems and other causes of skin rash.

D. Other causes of cervical lymphadenopathy and splenomegaly that have negative heterophil, such as cytomegalovirus or Toxoplasma infection.

VI. Treatment

A. Acetaminophen for fever; see Table 5-5, p. 156, for dosage.

B. Increased fluid intake.

C. Rest, according to degree of illness. Forced bed rest in mildly ill patient is *not* necessary.

D. Do not give a penicillin (especially ampicillin or amoxicillin) for coexisting problems in patients with infectious mononucleosis, because a rash often develops.

VII. Complications

A. Hepatitis.

B. Ruptured spleen.

C. Hemolytic anemia.

D. Aseptic meningitis.

E. Polyneuritis.

F. Thrombocytopenia.

G. Agranulocytosis.

H. Orchitis.

I. Myocarditis.

VIII. Consultation–Referral

A. Splenomegaly.

B. Tender spleen.

C. Jaundice.

D. Marked tonsillar enlargement, with difficulty in swallowing.

E. Evidence of cardiac, hematologic, or nervous system involvement.

F. Illness persisting for more than 2 weeks.

IX. Follow-Up

Weekly until patient has recovered.

▲ MUMPS: PEDIATRIC AND ADULT

I. Definition

Mumps is a clinical syndrome characterized by acute salivary gland enlargement, particularly of the parotid gland.

II. Etiology

A. Mumps is usually caused by mumps virus, a member of the myxovirus family.

B. Other myxoviruses, particularly the parainfluenza viruses, can cause clinical mumps and may account for second cases of mumps and for mumps in immunized children.

III. Clinical Features

A. Symptoms

1. Incubation period lasts 14–21 days, with an average of 18 days.

2. Fever may precede development of parotid swelling by 1–2 days.

3. Constitutional symptoms include headache, lethargy, anorexia, myalgia, and vomiting.

4. Parotitis produces pain anterior to the ear, which is increased by eating, local pressure, and jaw movement and is accompanied by visible swelling.

5. Symptoms related to complications (see **VII**) may *precede*, accompany, or follow parotitis.

B. **Signs**

1. Fever may be present.

2. Upper respiratory symptoms may accompany illness.

3. Parotid swelling is characteristic.

a. The swelling is diffuse and difficult to demarcate.

b. Twenty-five percent of cases have unilateral involvement.

c. Swelling obliterates the angle of the mandible and is usually maximal near the earlobe.

d. Stensen's duct may be inflamed.

e. There is marked variation in the amount of parotid swelling seen with mumps.

f. Other salivary glands may be involved.

4. Complications, particularly meningoencephalitis and orchitis (see **VII.A and C**), are common and should be looked for.

IV. Laboratory Studies

None.

V. Differential Diagnosis

A. Parotitis may be confused with the following:

1. Anterior, cervical, or preauricular lymphadenitis.
2. Idiopathic recurrent parotitis.
3. Parotid duct stone with secondary infection.
4. Mikulicz's syndrome—painless bilateral enlargement of the salivary and lacrimal glands, usually with dryness of the mouth and absence of tears.

B. Meningoencephalitis may occur with or without parotid swelling and must be distinguished from other causes of meningitis.

VI. Treatment

A. **Prevention**

1. Live mumps virus vaccine* should be given as combined measles-mumps-rubella vaccine after 15 months of age. The combined vaccine should be given again either before entering school or before adolescence. Mumps vaccine is particularly recommended for persons approaching puberty and for adult males with no history of natural mumps infection or immunization.
2. Exposed pubertal males with no history of natural mumps or immunization should be given live mumps vaccine.
3. The value of mumps immune globulin is not established, and it is not recommended.

B. **Therapy**

1. No specific treatment.
2. Acetaminophen for fever or pain; see Table 5-5, p. 156, for dosage.
3. Supportive care as required for specific complications.
4. Isolation (mumps is contagious from as much as 7 days before to 9 days after parotid swelling is evident).

VII. Complications

A. **Meningoencephalitis**

1. This is a very common and usually benign complication.
2. It usually follows parotitis by 3–10 days but may precede or occur in absence of parotitis.
3. Hospitalization for symptomatic care may be necessary in severe cases.

---

*See Chapter 1, III.D, for immunization contraindications.

B. **Nerve deafness** is usually unilateral; occurring after mumps.

C. **Orchitis**

1. Orchitis is usually unilateral, occurring in postpubertal males.

2. There is marked variation in the severity of symptoms. Gonadal enlargement and pain, fever, headache, nausea, vomiting, and abdominal pain all may occur.

3. Impotence does not result, and sterility is extremely rare.

D. **Pancreatitis** is uncommon but can be severe.

VIII. Consultation–Referral

All patients with evidence of complications should be discussed with physician.

IX. Follow-Up

A. Patients with complications should be checked in 24 hours, at least by telephone. Continue close follow-up until there is improvement.

B. Follow-up is not required in uncomplicated cases.

▲ ROSEOLA INFANTUM (EXANTHEMA SUBITUM): PEDIATRIC

I. Definition

Roseola infantum is an acute, benign febrile illness limited almost exclusively to children from 6 months to 3 years of age and characterized by cessation of fever as a rash appears.

II. Etiology

Human herpesvirus 6 (HHV6).

III. Clinical Features

A. **Symptoms**

1. High fever of sudden onset lasts 1–6 days, usually 3–4 days. Fever may be sustained or intermittent.

2. There is a marked contrast between the high fever and the paucity of symptoms.

3. Symptoms, usually minimal, may include malaise, vomiting, and coryza.

4. Fever and the other minimal symptoms clear with the onset of the rash.

5. By age 4, most individuals are seropositive, suggesting most infections are asymptomatic or atypical.

6. Incubation period is estimated to be 5–15 days.

B. **Signs**

1. Fever occurs prior to onset of rash.

2. Minimal coryza, slight injection of the pharynx, and cervical and occipital adenopathy are the only clinical findings prior to the rash.

3. Rash occurs with lysis of fever:

   a. Faint maculopapular rash first occurs on the trunk and neck, with minimal involvement of the upper face and the extremities.

   b. The rash usually clears in 24–48 hours.

IV. **Laboratory Studies**

If a rash is not present and fever is the only abnormal finding, perform urinalysis and urine culture to rule out urinary tract infection.

V. **Differential Diagnosis**

A. Urinary tract infection before onset of rash.

B. Rubella.

C. Other acute febrile illnesses, including asymptomatic bacteremia.

VI. **Treatment**

A. **Prevention.** None.

B. **Therapy**

1. No specific treatment.

2. Antipyretic therapy with acetaminophen; see Table 5-5, p. 156, for dosage.

VII. **Complications**

Febrile seizures.

VIII. **Consultation-Referral**

A. Seizures.

B. Fever.

1. Lasting more than 4 days.

2. Continuing after rash develops.

3. Associated with more than the minimal symptoms (see **III.A**).

IX. **Follow-Up**

Maintain daily contact with family until diagnosis is confirmed.

▲ RUBELLA: PEDIATRIC AND ADULT

I. **Definition**

Postnatally acquired rubella is a usually mild disease associated with a 3-day rash and lymph node enlargement. Congenital infections are associated with a high incidence of congenital malformations.

II. Etiology

Rubella virus.

III. Clinical Features

A. **Symptoms**

1. Incubation period lasts 14–21 days.
2. Transmission is by droplet spread or direct contact with infected persons or by exposure to material freshly contaminated by nasopharyngeal secretions, feces, or urine.
3. Prodromal symptoms either are absent or consist of minimal lethargy, anorexia, and upper respiratory tract symptoms.
4. Transient polyarthralgia is common in adolescents and adults.

B. **Signs**

1. The maculopapular rash begins about the face and neck, with rapid spread to the trunk and extremities. It usually disappears by the third day, with slight desquamation occasionally occurring.
2. Generalized lymphadenopathy is usually most pronounced in the suboccipital, postauricular, and cervical nodes.
3. Fever is usually of low grade or absent during the period of the rash.
4. Polyarthritis may occur in adolescents and adults.

IV. Laboratory Studies

A. Paired serum samples, separated by a 2-week interval, should be submitted to the state laboratory for confirmation of the diagnosis if the patient has been in contact with pregnant women. Several sensitive immunologic essays are available and a fourfold titer rise confirms the diagnosis.

B. Pregnant women whose immunity to rubella is unknown and who have contact with a suspected case of rubella should have a rubella titer drawn immediately. The presence of antibody indicates immunity, and the individual can be reassured that she is immune. Blood specimens should be obtained at 3 and 6 weeks post-exposure from nonimmune pregnant individuals. The presence of antibody in a previously nonimmune individual documents infection, and the pregnant woman should be referred to a physician for a decision regarding possible termination of pregnancy.

V. Differential Diagnosis

A. Measles.
B. Scarlet fever.
C. Roseola.
D. Infectious mononucleosis.
E. Enteroviral exanthems.
F. Drug rashes.

VI. Treatment

A. Prevention

1. Rubella vaccine should be given at 15 months of age, either combined with measles or as combined measles–mumps–rubella vaccine.

2. Repeat immunization of all adolescents is recommended using MMR.

3. Emphasis should be placed on ensuring that all females in the child-bearing age or approaching puberty are immune. Post-pubertal, nonimmune females should receive rubella vaccine and avoid pregnancy by use of a medically acceptable method of contraception for 3 months following immunization.

4. The use of immune globulin is *not* recommended but may be considered for nonimmune females who have been exposed to rubella and who will not consider therapeutic abortion.

5. Officials of colleges and institutions where young adults congregate should require immunization for entry. Unless there are contraindications, unimmunized young adults, both male and female, should receive the vaccine.

6. Pregnant nonimmune individuals should be identified and immunized in the immediate post-partum period.

B. Therapy

1. No specific treatment is available.

2. Antipyretic therapy may be used, but is rarely necessary; see Table 5-5, p. 156, for dosage.

3. Contacts should be evaluated to determine if pregnant women are at risk.

4. Patient should be isolated while rash is present.

5. Cases must be reported immediately to the appropriate public health authorities.

VII. Complications

A. Severe damage to the fetus if the infection occurs in a pregnant woman.

B. Polyarthralgia and polyarthritis can occur in adults following both natural disease and immunization.

C. Encephalitis is rare.

VIII. Consultation–Referral

A. Consultation for all patients with complications.

B. Consultation for exposure of nonimmune pregnant women.

IX. Follow-Up

A. Follow-up is needed only when there is a need to obtain convalescent serum to confirm the diagnosis for public health reasons.

B. Follow-up is needed to obtain convalescent serum samples from patient and exposed nonimmune pregnant women to confirm the diagnosis of rubella so that appropriate steps may be taken to terminate pregnancy, if desired.

▲ VARICELLA (CHICKENPOX): PEDIATRIC AND ADULT

I. Definition

An acute, usually benign, highly contagious disease of childhood associated with a pruritic, vesicular rash.

II. Etiology

Varicella–zoster virus causes both chickenpox and herpes zoster.

III. Clinical Features

A. **Symptoms**

1. The incubation period ranges from 11–20 days, with an average of 14–16 days.

2. A prodrome is usually absent in children; adolescents may have 1 or 2 days of prodromal fever, malaise, and anorexia.

3. Rash is characterized as follows:

   a. Lesions appear in crops, with rapid evolution (in 6–8 hours) of individual lesions from macule to papule to vesicle to crusting. Lesions in all stages are present at the same time in any given area.

   b. Lesions begin on the trunk and spread peripherally, with least involvement of the extremities.

   c. Oral mucous membranes frequently are involved with vesicles that ulcerate.

   d. Rash is usually very pruritic.

   e. New lesions usually occur for 3–5 days.

4. Onset of fever is usually at the time of the rash, and its severity is proportional to the degree of skin involvement of the rash.

5. Headache, malaise, and anorexia are usually related to the height of the fever.

B. **Signs.** Major physical findings are related to the rash (see **III.A.3**).

IV. Laboratory Studies

None.

V. Differential Diagnosis

A. Diagnosis is usually not a problem.

B. Chickenpox may be confused with the following:

1. Herpesvirus hominis infections.

2. Drug eruptions.

3. Impetigo.

4. Secondary syphilis.

5. Erythema multiforme.

6. Hand-foot-and-mouth disease (Coxsackie virus).

VI. Treatment

A. Prevention

1. No vaccine is available.

2. If exposed to varicella, children and nonimmune adults receiving steroid or immunosuppressive therapy, patients with AIDS, immunologic disorders or malignant disease, and newborns should be referred immediately for consideration of varicella–zoster immune globulin (VZIG).

3. Normal, nonimmune adults, particularly pregnant women, in close contact with an infected individual should be referred immediately for consideration for varicella immune globulin (VZIG).

B. Therapy

1. Symptomatic care for skin:

   a. Fingernails should be kept short to minimize excoriation and scarring by scratching.

   b. Drying lotion (calamine) may be applied to lesions to decrease pruritus.

   c. Soap and water washing does not spread virus and does reduce secondary infection.

   d. Antipruritic—diphenhydramine HCL (Benadryl) or hydroxyzine HCl (Atarax, Vistaril)—may be helpful to control itching in some cases; see Tables 3-1 and 3-2 (pp. 95–96) for dosage.

2. Antipyretic-acetaminophen (Tylenol); see Table 5-5, p. 156, for dosage.

Note: Aspirin should *not* be used if varicella (chickenpox) is suspected because use of salicylates is associated with the development of Reye's syndrome in patients with influenza or chickenpox.

3. Isolation. The disease is contagious from as early as 1–2 days before the rash appears until the lesions have crusted.

VII. Complications

A. Secondary bacterial infections (streptococcal or staphylococcal, or both).

B. Pneumonia. Primary viral pneumonia is extremely rare as a complication in children but relatively common in adults.

C. **Encephalitis** is a rare complication that has a better prognosis than most postinfection encephalitides.

D. **Severe disseminated disease** may occur in newborns, patients receiving steroid or immunosuppressive therapy, or patients with AIDS, immunologic deficiency or malignant disease.

E. **Bleeding disorders** occur very rarely.

F. **Reye's syndrome.**

VIII. Consultation–Referral

A. Refer all patients with suspected chickenpox and with conditions predisposing to severe disseminated disease (see **VII.D**) immediately for consideration of antiviral therapy, usually acyclovir.

B. Refer all nonimmune contacts with conditions predisposing to severe chickenpox (see **VI.A.2** and **3**) immediately for consideration of varicella-zoster immune globulin (VZIG).

C. Development of pneumonia, bleeding problems, or central nervous system symptoms.

D. Severe secondary bacterial infections.

IX. Follow-Up

A. In routine cases, no follow-up is required.

B. Patient should return in 48 hours if there is concern about secondary bacterial infection.

▲ THE ASYMPTOMATIC HIV-INFECTED ADULT

I. Definition

Asymptomatic adult patients who have known positive risk factors (see Etiology below) and who test positive for the HIV antibody. All other patients with positive HIV antibody test (symptomatic patients or those with no risk factors) should be referred.

II. Etiology

Infection with the HIV virus.

A. **Risk factors for infection include**

1. IV drug abuse.

2. Homosexuality.

3. Heterosexual activity with multiple partners.

4. Partners at risk, or infected partners.

5. Transfusion of blood or blood products before 1985, or occupational exposure to blood or blood products.

B. Transmission is only through exchange of body fluids (blood, sperm, vaginal fluids), usually in sexual contact, sharing of needles, or through transfusion of blood products.

III. Clinical Features

In order to define the patient as asymptomatic, one must conduct a directed review of symptoms and perform a directed physical exam.

A. **Symptoms**

1. **General or constitutional**—fatigue, fever for several days, night sweats, chills, anorexia, lymph node enlargement, weight loss.

2. **Skin**—genital herpes, shingles, tinea, bruises, folliculitis, seborrhea, moles, dark colored bumps.

3. **HEENT**—sore throat, coated tongue, oral thrush, aphthous ulcer, oral hairy leukoplakia, blurred vision.

4. **Respiratory**—cough, shortness of breath.

5. **GI**—odynophagia, dysphagia, bloating, flatulence, belching, diarrhea, ulcerative lesions, hemorrhoids, recurrent or severe Candida infection, guaiac positive stool, lower abdominal pain.

6. **Neurological**—headaches, memory loss, numbness and/or tingling sensations in extremities, weakness.

7. **Psychiatric**—depression, anxiety.

B. **Signs**

1. Vital signs including height (once), weight, temperature, blood pressure, each visit.

2. Skin—detailed exam with patient fully disrobed.

3. Eyes—funduscopic exam.

4. Ears—external ear (common site of Kaposi's sarcoma).

5. Nose, oral cavity, throat—careful detailed exam. (Note warts, ulcers, white plagues, violaceous macules or papules). Check lateral margin of tongue for hairy leukoplakia.

6. Lungs—auscultate (wheezes, rales, rhonchi).

7. Heart—murmurs (particularly in IV drug abusers), cardiac enlargement.

8. Abdomen—palpate for enlarged liver or spleen, penile discharge.

9. Genital—ulcerative lesions, vesicles, crusted lesions, genital warts. Pelvic exam, PAP smear every 6 months.

10. Rectal—rectal tone, discharge, tenderness.

11. Neurological—mental status, cranial nerves, reflexes, gait, motor strength, fine motor skills.

IV. Laboratory Studies

A. CD_4 count.

B. PPD and control.

C. Chest X-ray.

  D. VDRL, G-6 PD, Hepatitis B core antibody, CBC with differential and platelets, liver function tests, Hepatitis B surface antibody, Hepatitis B surface antigen.

  E. Toxoplasmosis antibodies.

V. Differential Diagnosis

  A. Extensive.

VI. Treatment (Prevention of Complications)

  A. Vaccines

   1. Pneumovax—single dose.

   2. Influenza—yearly.

   3. Hepatitis B if seronegative.

   4. Measles if only one vaccination after age 1 and if born after 1956. Check measles serology first.

VII. Complications

  A. Anemia.

  B. Neutropenia.

VIII. Consultation–Referral

Consult physician after initial evaluation and whenever patient becomes symptomatic or CD_4 count drops to 500 or less, consistently.

IX. Follow-Up

  A. PRN for any symptoms.

  B. Every 3–6 months for ROS and PE.

  C. CD_4 count every 6 months.

▲ Index

To avoid unnecessary repetition of the major outline headings in the text, these topics have not been indexed under the specific diseases and disorders. Rather, only inclusive page numbers for a disease or disorder are given, followed by subentries for lengthy discussions on these pages.

Sodium Sulamyd. *See* Sodium sulfacetamide
Sodium sulfacetamide (Sodium Sulamyd), for conjunctivitis, 130
Solu-Medrol, for bronchospasm, 58
Sore throat, 146–150
Spectinomycin, for gonococcal infection, 237
Spermicide, 329
Sprain, minor, 255–257
  ankle, 254–255
Stasis ulcer, of lower extremity, 201–202
Staticin. *See* Erythromycin
Sterilization, 318, 327–328, 337
Stimulation guidelines
  birth to six months, 39
  six to twelve months, 39–40
  one to three years, 40–43
  three to five years, 29, 43–45
  at eight years, 31–32
Stool softener, 207
Strain
  lumbosacral, 258–260
  minor, 255–257
Streptococcal pharyngitis, 146–150
Stress, adult health screening, 47
Stye, 130–131
Sudafed. *See* Pseudoephedrine
Sulfisoxazole (Gantrisin)
  for adult female cystitis, 228–229
  for pediatric urinary tract infection, 233–234
Sulfisoxazole (Koro-Sulf) cream, for nonspecific vaginitis, 324
Sultrin cream. *See* Triple sulfa cream
Sutures, for small open wounds, 88–89
Syncope, vasovagal, 271–273
Synthroid. *See* Sodium levothyroxine

Tactile stimulation
  birth to six months, 39

  six to twelve months, 40
Tagamet. *See* Cimetidine
Temporal arteritis, 271
Tension headache, 269–271
Terazol. *See* Terconazole
Terbutaline, for bronchial asthma, 171
Terconazole (Terazol), for candidal vaginitis, 321
Tetanus-diphtheria toxoid, 35, 37, 54
Tetanus prophylaxis
  for animal bite, 59–60
  for burns, 66
  for open wounds, 89
  for snake bite, 63
Tetracycline
  for acne, 92
  for acute lower respiratory tract infection, 165
  for adult female cystitis, 228
  for gonococcal infection, 237
  for nonspecific urethritis, 239
Theophylline
  for bronchial asthma, 170–172
  for chronic obstructive pulmonary disease, 179
Therapeutic abortion, 336–337, 341
Thrush, 150–151
Thyroid function testing, 49
Tinactin. *See* Tolnaftate
Tinea corporis, 118–120
Tinea pedis, 120–121
Tinea versicolor, 121–122
Tobramycin, for hordeolum, 131
Tolazamide, for diabetes mellitus, 286
Tolbutamide, for diabetes mellitus, 286
Tolnaftate (Tinactin), for tinea corporis, 119
Tourniquet
  for anaphylaxis, 57
  for snake bites, 63
Tracheobronchitis, acute, 161–163
Transdermal nicotine patch, 53
Trental, for occlusive arterial disease of extremities, 200–201
Tretinoin. *See* Retin A
Triamcinolone, for bronchial asthma, 170